How the Brain Got Language

Oxford Studies in the Evolution of Language

General Editors

Kathleen R. Gibson, *University of Texas at Houston,*
and James R. Hurford, *University of Edinburgh*

PUBLISHED

1
The Origins of Vowel Systems
Bart de Boer

2
The Transition to Language
Edited by Allison Wray

3
Language Evolution
Edited by Morten H. Christiansen
and Simon Kirby

4
Language Origins
Perspectives on Evolution
Edited by Maggie Tallerman

5
The Talking Ape
How Language Evolved
Robbins Burling

6
*Self-Organization in the Evolution
of Speech*
Pierre-Yves Oudeyer
Translated by James R. Hurford

7
Why We Talk
*The Evolutionary Origins of
Human Communication*
Jean-Louis Dessalles
Translated by James Grieve

8
The Origins of Meaning
Language in the Light of Evolution 1
James R. Hurford

9
The Genesis of Grammar
Bernd Heine and Tania Kuteva

10
The Origin of Speech
Peter F. MacNeilage

11
The Prehistory of Language
Edited by Rudolf Botha and
Chris Knight

12
The Cradle of Language
Edited by Rudolf Botha and
Chris Knight

13
*Language Complexity as an
Evolving Variable*
Edited by Geoffrey Sampson,
David Gil, and Peter Trudgill

14
The Evolution of Morphology
Andrew Carstairs McCarthy

15
The Origins of Grammar
Language in the Light of Evolution 2
James R. Hurford

16
*How the Brain Got Language:
The Mirror System
Hypothesis*
Michael A. Arbib

How the Brain Got Language

The Mirror System Hypothesis

Michael A. Arbib
Computer Science, Neuroscience, and the USC Brain Project
University of Southern California

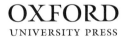
OXFORD
UNIVERSITY PRESS

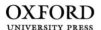

Oxford University Press, Inc., publishes works that further
Oxford University's objective of excellence
in research, scholarship, and education.

Oxford   New York
Auckland   Cape Town   Dar es Salaam   Hong Kong   Karachi
Kuala Lumpur   Madrid   Melbourne   Mexico City   Nairobi
New Delhi   Shanghai   Taipei   Toronto

With offices in
Argentina   Austria   Brazil   Chile   Czech Republic   France   Greece
Guatemala   Hungary   Italy   Japan   Poland   Portugal   Singapore
South Korea   Switzerland   Thailand   Turkey   Ukraine   Vietnam

Copyright © 2012 by Oxford University Press, Inc.

Published by Oxford University Press, Inc.
198 Madison Avenue, New York, New York 10016
www.oup.com

Oxford is a registered trademark of Oxford University Press

Library of Congress Cataloging-in-Publication Data
Arbib, Michael A.
   How the brain got language : the mirror system hypothesis / Michael A. Arbib.
      p. cm.
   Includes bibliographical references and index.
   I SBN 978-0-19-989668-4 (hbk . : acid-free paper)
   1. Brain–Evolution.   2. Brain–Anatomy.   3. Language and languages–Origin.
   4. Mirror neurons.   5. Evolutionary psychology.   6. Neurolinguistics.
   7. Macaques–Anatomy.   8. Anatomy, Comparative.   I. Title.
   QP399.A73 2012
   612.8'2—dc23
                              2011047813

9 8 7 6 5 4 3 2 1
Printed in the United States of America
on acid-free paper

To the Memory of
Marc Jeannerod
True Friend, Admired Colleague

Preface

Let's cut to the chase.

- Humans have language; other creatures do not.
- This is the result of both biological and cultural evolution.
- Humans have language because their brains are different from those of other creatures.

But, of course, each of these claims needs unpacking.

Don't bees have language? Haven't apes been taught sign language? Not really. Bees have a dance that lets them tell other bees the location of a source of pollen they have found. And a bonobo (a species of ape also called a pygmy chimpanzee) has learned to understand spoken English at roughly the level of a 2-year-old child. But when it comes to the ability to put a large number of symbols together in new and complex combinations (like this sentence) and have others understand what is meant (hopefully also true of this sentence), nonhumans are out of the running. Human language is not just speech but includes the gestures that accompany speech, and the sign languages of the deaf as well. It both builds upon and differs immensely from the communication systems of our primate cousins. So one aim of this book is to discuss how monkeys and apes communicate using vocalizations, hand gestures, and facial expressions, whether in the wild or raised by humans. This will let us develop the notion of protolanguages, forms of communication used by our distant ancestors that were richer and more open than those now used by non-human primates but lacked the astounding subtlety and flexibility of human languages as we know them today.

What about evolution? Some people deny it, claiming that each species was created in its present form and will ever remain so. Yet the key idea behind Darwin's theory of evolution is simply that organisms vary, and that some of the resulting variants reproduce more successfully than others. Let bacteria loose in a hospital, and random variation will mean that some are more resistant to antibiotics than others—and it is hardly surprising that those bacteria with the greater resistance to antibiotics reproduce more successfully while other strains tend to die out, so that over time the population changes completely from its original form. It was Darwin's genius to understand that random variation when coupled with selection for success at reproduction yields creatures that had never appeared before, so that variation and selection over many many generations can yield species that are completely new. Evolution does not just "stir the pot," increasing the population size for some species and decreasing that of others. Some species go extinct, while new species arise.

What I have talked about so far is *biological* evolution, as the accumulated changes in the genes passed down from parents to children eventually yield gene patterns sufficiently different from those of the ancestors that a new species emerges. But I want also to talk about *cultural* evolution. When I talk of culture, I do *not* want to say that there is such a thing as a monolithic French culture in the sense that all aspects of "French-ness" are determined by a small causal nexus. Rather, I want to say that a culture has many aspects—the food, the attitude to education, the interpretation of history, the language, the architecture, the taboos and ideas of politeness, and on and on—that reflect the history of a people. Some of these strongly influence each other, while yet others seem rather independent. For example, a tradition of excellence in cheese seems to me unrelated to the language or architecture of France but might well relate to patterns of gastronomy considered more generally, and these in turn might interact with traditions of wine making, and thus in turn with agriculture.

When I speak about *cultural evolution*, I will be talking about the processes that shape facets of a human culture in ways that are relatively independent of human biology. Thus, we might ask how hunter-gatherers became farmers or how scattered tribes gathered into cities, or how Latin gave rise to the whole range of Romance languages from Brazilian Portuguese to Romanian. The key point here is that we cannot hope to understand how the brain changed so that humans "got" language unless we understand that much of this "getting" involves historical change—cultural evolution—and not just the evolution of the biological substrate.

This brings us to brains and brain evolution. If we say a human brain is different from a frog brain or a rat brain or a monkey brain, what does this really mean? Are humans smarter than frogs just because their brains are bigger? Well, whales have much bigger brains than humans, and frogs have much better eye-tongue coordination. Different brains can be good at different things and size is only one difference among many. So another task of the book is to offer some sense of "how brains work" and the way in which a brain has many different subsystems that compete and cooperate to allow a creature to conduct a variety of tasks. Here my major focus will be on a comparison of human brains with those of macaque monkeys. I will look not only at what is different about them but also at what is held in common to try to anchor some ideas about what the brain of our last common ancestor looked like, more than 25 million years ago. This will provide the basis for my later attempts to chart the changes that must have occurred during human evolution to make us uniquely equipped for language.

Only the human brain is *language ready*, in the sense that a normal human child will learn a language—an open-ended vocabulary integrated with a syntax that supports the hierarchical combination of words into larger structures which freely express novel meanings as needed—while infants of other species cannot. Indeed, humans not only can learn an existing language but can take an active role in the shaping of new languages, as dramatically demonstrated in the study of emerging sign languages. Syntax refers to the set of "rules" that tell us how words can be put together to make the sentences of a particular language, while semantics refers to the meanings of these words and sentences. But are the rules of syntax innately wired into the human brain? I will argue that the specifics of our capability for language—like our ability to drive cars or surf the Web—rest only indirectly on the genes, and express the outcome of cultural developments that exploited prior biological evolution.

This perspective makes it clear that no discussion of the brain will be complete without some sense of its social role in allowing creatures of the same family or grouping to interact with one another and its adaptive role in allowing a child to learn the fruits of the cultural evolution of its community. A new dimension in our understanding of how the brain serves social interaction came with the discovery of mirror neurons in the area for hand control in the brains of macaque monkeys. These are neurons that fire both when the monkey is generating a specific set of grasps and when it observes similar grasps performed by others. This led us to ask whether the human brain, too, contains a mirror system for grasping—a region that would show up as especially active in brain imaging both when a person performed grasps and when she observed them. We found such one such area is Broca's area, a part of the human brain that had traditionally been associated with the production of speech. This book presents the *Mirror System Hypothesis*, namely that the brain mechanisms that support language evolved on top of the basic mechanisms of the mirror system. But grasping is very different from speech. To understand how one could provide the basis for the other, we will trace the path whereby the mirror system's involvement in both grasping and observing grasping evolved across millions of years to provide the basis for *language parity*. This is what makes the shared meaning of language possible, with an utterance meaning roughly the same for both speaker and hearer.

Language is far more than speech; we use face, voice, and hands when we talk, and the deaf have sign languages that let them communicate with full human subtlety without use of the voice. Crucially, the Mirror System Hypothesis shows how language readiness evolved as a multimodal system, explaining how protolanguage evolved with gestural communication or protosign providing the scaffolding for protospeech by transforming the semantic openness of pantomime into a system of shared conventionalized symbols. Protosign and protospeech then evolved together in an expanding spiral to yield the neural circuitry and social structures that enabled modern language to emerge.

Part I of the book sets the stage. It introduces schema theory as a way of talking about the brain processes underlying praxis, our practical interaction with the world, providing perspectives on manual skill, the use of language, and socially constructed knowledge. We next take a deeper look at linguistics, stressing that human languages include sign languages as well as spoken ones. We take an admiring look at generative linguistics while rejecting its claims for autonomy of syntax or an innate Universal Grammar, and we suggest that construction grammar may provide a more suitable framework for studying the evolution, historical change, and acquisition of language. To enrich our understanding of how different the communication systems of other primates are from human language, we assess vocalization and gesture in ape and monkey, stressing that vocalization patterns seem to be innately specified, whereas some manual gestures seem to be "culturally" specified. An introduction to neural circuitry serving visual perception and manual action as well as the auditory system and vocalization in the brains of macaque monkeys and humans then sets the stage for the detailed introduction to mirror neurons in the macaque brain and mirror systems in the human brain that closes Part I.

Part II then develops the Mirror System Hypothesis. Chapter 6, Signposts: The Argument of the Book Revealed, both summarizes the background set forth in Part I and outlines the arguments of each chapter of Part II. Thus, some readers may prefer to start with Chapter 6 before (or instead of) reading Part I. Part II is informed by the general view—consistent with the greater openness of manual gesture as compared to vocalization in nonhuman primates—that protosign (i.e., communication based on conventionalized manual gestures) provided the essential scaffolding for the development of protolanguage. Noting that the ability to recognize a known action is not the same as learning to imitate a novel behavior, we go beyond the mirror system to assess the forms of imitation used by monkeys, chimps, and humans, claiming that only the form available to humans, so-called complex imitation, whose brain mechanisms evolved to support the transfer of manual skills, is powerful enough to support the succeeding stages. In particular we will see that an apparent weakness of humans as compared to chimpanzees, over-imitation, is instead a powerful engine for cultural evolution. Biological evolution supports, in turn, the emergence of brain mechanisms for pantomime and then protosign. Once protosign has opened up the relatively free invention of protosign symbols, the way is open for evolution of the neural control of the speech apparatus. When all these brain mechanisms are in place, complex imitation applied in the communicative domain provides the mechanisms whereby languages can emerge from protolanguages by cultural evolution. The final chapters chart how the brain mechanisms that made the original emergence of languages possible perhaps 100,000 years ago are still operative: in the way children acquire language, in the way in which new sign languages have emerged in recent decades, and in the historical processes of language change on a time scale from decades to centuries. Languages keep changing.

Acknowledgements   I would like to express my thanks to Marc Jeannerod for setting me on the path to an understanding of how the brain controls hand movements, to Giacomo Rizzolatti for our collaboration on mirror neurons and language, to Mary Hesse for getting me to think about neuroscience from a social perspective, and to Jane Hill for modeling the linkage of individual and social schemas in language acquisition. Beyond that, I thank the hundreds of friends and colleagues and students and strangers with whom I have discussed aspects of the facts, models, and hypotheses presented in this book, and in particular those whose coauthorship of books and papers formed so integral a part of my intellectual development.

Michael A. Arbib
La Jolla, California

July 4, 2011

Contents

Expanded Contents

PART I

SETTING THE STAGE

1

Underneath the Lampposts

Lampposts and the Specialization of Science

There is an old story about a gentleman walking home one dark night when he sees a drunk searching under the light from a lamppost. He asks the drunk what he is doing, and the drunk replies, "I'm looking for my keys." The gentleman joins in the search but finds no trace of the keys. "Are you sure you lost them here?" "No, I lost them up the street, but it's too dark to look for them there...."

The point of the story for us is that science has become very specialized. A physicist may have no expertise in biology. But worse than that, the physicist who is an expert in string theory may know nothing about biophysics, and the biologist expert in DNA may have no more than a general knowledge of animal behavior. A scientist (often serious, sometimes convivial, rarely drunk) makes his living by determining that a problem needs to be solved and then looking for a solution (keys, if you will) using the specialized theoretical and experimental techniques she or he has mastered (the light shed by the lamppost). The problem, of course, is that the keys may only be found under another lamppost or, indeed, only if a new lamppost is first constructed. Who would have guessed that a key to understanding the formation of biological species might be found under the lamppost of X-ray crystallography—but it was this technology that illuminated the structure of DNA as a double helix, thus opening the floodgates of molecular biology.

In this case, Watson and Crick found the key—they solved the problem of the structure of DNA—but in doing so they contributed to the development of the new field of molecular biology. If we continue speaking metaphorically, and think of an open field in the countryside, we can imagine a whole area where new lampposts can be constructed and new keys can be found. But I want to expand the metaphor in a somewhat different way. We've been thinking about a key or a neatly joined set of keys. But now let's imagine, instead, that a wind has scattered the pieces of a jigsaw puzzle far and wide. We may have to search under many lampposts and still not find enough pieces to put the whole puzzle together. We may be pleased to get enough pieces to put together a small scene—a person standing by a windmill, say—with a few pieces missing. The ultraspecialist might then try to figure out what was on just one missing piece from this scene, while generalists might begin to analyze what other fragmentary scenes may be needed to fill out the whole picture.

And so we move from one drunk, one lamppost, one set of keys, and one helpful but misled gentleman to a new metaphor for science as an interdisciplinary enterprise with many men and women searching a dark landscape, each looking for pieces of the puzzle, with very varied techniques (searchlights, lampposts, spotlights) at their disposal, sometimes finding a piece of the puzzle they are working on, and sometimes finding a puzzle piece that clearly does not belong to that puzzle but is so interesting that they decide to work on that new puzzle instead. In any case, the puzzlers may move from one lamppost to another or talk to puzzlers under other lampposts to coordinate their searches. And some will instead work on building new light sources (developing new technologies) to help others find pieces of the puzzle where none have been seen before.

Enough for now. The point I want to make is this: The problem of language evolution is not a box to be opened with a single key but a puzzle of many pieces. To put that puzzle together, we need the illumination from many different lampposts. At present, a few areas of the puzzle have been crudely assembled, and interesting patterns have begun to emerge. My task in this book is to show a few of these patterns and suggest what must be done to fill in missing pieces and extend the pattern. I devote the rest of this chapter to the first "lampposts" that illuminated my own efforts to probe the mysteries of language evolution.

My First Lamppost: Schema Theory for Basic Neuroethology

As an undergraduate at Sydney University, I soon decided that I was going to be a pure mathematician—someone who delighted in theorems for their formal structure and elegance, rather than for their applicability in physics or other areas of the real world. But although my love for pure mathematics continued, I got waylaid. I spent three undergraduate summers working with computers (with perhaps one-millionth of the capacity of the laptop I use today), and there I was introduced to Norbert Wiener's (1948) seminal book, *Cybernetics: or Control and Communication in Animal and Machine*. From this book, and the reading of other books and papers that it triggered, I learned that mathematics had many fascinating applications very different from the applied mathematics of forces and accelerations on which I had taken lectures. I learned that mathematical techniques developed to study control systems could also be used to model feedback systems in the neural networks of the spinal cord that control movement in vertebrates. I studied Turing machines and Gödel's incompleteness theorem and the formal models of neural networks developed by Warren McCulloch and Walter Pitts. I studied the mathematical theory of communication developed by Claude Shannon. These defined the new field of automata theory, and I went on to read a set of key papers called *Automata Studies*, edited by Shannon and John McCarthy, which included a paper on neural networks by Marvin Minsky. And Bill Levick and Peter Bishop of the Sydney University Physiology Department allowed me to sit in on their experiments on the neurophysiology of the cat visual cortex. It was Bill Levick who introduced me to the then just published paper, "What the Frog's Eye Tells the Frog's Brain," which McCulloch and Pitts had coauthored with the neurophysiologist Jerry Lettvin and the Chilean neuroanatomist Humberto Maturana (Lettvin, Maturana, McCulloch, & Pitts, 1959). From this paper I learned that McCulloch and Pitts had moved since writing their earlier papers and that they were now—along with Wiener, Shannon, McCarthy, and Minsky—at the Massachusetts Institute of Technology (MIT) in Cambridge, Massachusetts. And so it was to MIT that I went for my Ph.D. There I wrote a thesis on probability theory, but my career was set with the title of the lectures I gave during the winter term at the University of New South Wales in Sydney during the summer vacation midway through my time at MIT: *Brains, Machines, and Mathematics* (Arbib, 1964).

This experience, plus the work I did with my first doctoral students at Stanford, defined my first lamppost, which I call "Computational Neuroethology and Schema Theory."

Let me unpack what this means. Ethology is the study of animal behavior, while neuroethology is the study of the brain mechanisms that make that behavior possible. Computational neuroethology, then, says that we not only look at the brain mechanisms underlying behavior, but we seek to represent them mathematically so we can study the sort of computations the brain carries out. And, even though the brain is a highly parallel, adaptive computer quite unlike today's electronic computers, we can use these electronic computers to simulate our mathematical models and test whether they really can explain the behaviors that interest us. In this book, I will avoid all mathematical formalism and all details of computer simulations, but much of what I write will be based on my experience with computational modeling. The idea of "simulation," though, may be familiar to anyone who watched the harrowing movie *Apollo XIII*. A crucial element of the spaceship's successful return to Earth was that the engineers at Houston could make a mathematical model of how firing the rockets in different ways would affect the spaceship's trajectory, taking into account the gravitational pull of Earth and Moon. The dilemma was that the less one fired the rockets, the better one conserved fuel, but the less one fired the rockets, the longer the flight back to Earth would take. The challenge, successfully met, was to find a plan that got the crew all the way back to Earth but did so before the oxygen ran out. Simulation can thus be used to explain the observed behavior of a system and to calculate a control strategy for getting the system to behave in a desired way—or, when we model animal behavior, to understand how the animal's brain and body work together to increase the probability that the animal will behave in a successful way.

"What the Frog's Eye Tells the Frog's Brain" had shown that the ganglion cells of the frog—the output cells of the retina, whose axons course back to the tectum, the key visual area in the frog's midbrain—are of four kinds, and that each provides the tectum with a different map of the world. What was exciting was that one of these maps would have peaks of activity that signaled the location of small moving objects (a map of "prey"), whereas another had peaks to indicate the location of large moving objects (could these be predator detectors?). But the frog has a lot more brain than its retina and tectum; it also has to have machinery to use the information on those maps to plot a course of action. If several flies and enemies are present, the animal has to "decide" whether to escape or to snap at one of the flies, and whichever it "chooses," it must then pass the correct instructions down to its brainstem and spinal cord to get its muscles to move it away from the predators or toward the "selected" prey. We want to know what the frog's eye tells the *frog*. Note, then, that we are rejecting the camera metaphor of the retina relaying a photograph to the brain and instead trying to understand how the visual system starts transforming patterns as soon as they hit the retina's rods and cones in a way that will help the animal's brain find appropriate courses of action. My slogan for this is *action-oriented perception*—the idea that the animal (and human) actively seeks out information it needs from the environment. We do not act as passive stimulus-response machines, reacting to every stimulus that impinges upon us; rather, what we perceive is heavily influenced by our current goals or motivation.

Before going further, let me comment on the quotes around "decide," "chooses," and "selected" in the previous paragraph. Often, when we use these terms, we may think of ourselves consciously reviewing courses of action—take selecting from the menu at a restaurant for a trivial case—and evaluating their merits before consciously deciding how to proceed. But all this involves subtle patterns of activity in our brain, and this subtle neural activity can commit us to a course of action without any awareness on our part that a decision is being made. We touch a hot stove. Should we keep our hand in contact with the stove or withdraw it? Our hand has been withdrawn even before we first become aware of the burning pain. More subtly, we may grasp a glass, the grasp may begin to slip ever so little, and we tighten our grasp to stop the slipping; in many cases we never become aware of our "decision" to grasp the glass more firmly. In what follows, I will stop using quotes and use expressions like "the animal decides" or "the brain decides" without implying that the decision is conscious—and without ruling it out either. Yes, we are conscious of much of our language use—of what we say and what we hear, and even more of what we read and what we write. But I know, to my own cost, there are many cases in which I should have thought more carefully about what I was about to say, and we may often be aware of the general nature of what we want to say yet have no awareness of which words we will choose until we actually say them. And when we are fluent in a language, we rarely stop to consider how to pronounce a word, or what aspects of grammar to employ in constructing a sentence.

Trying to think through how a neural network could make choices was motivated for my student Rich Didday (1970) and myself by experiments by the neuroethologist David Ingle (1968). He was able to get frogs to snap at wiggling pencil tips—presumably, these activated the frog's retinal "prey detectors" in much the same way a fly would do. If he wiggled two pencils rather than one, the frog would normally snap at just one of them. But, intriguingly, if the two stimuli were close together, the frog would snap in between them "at the average fly." Thus, the challenge for Rich and me was to design a neural network that could take as its input a map of activity and serve as a "maximum selector," providing as output a map with just one peak of activity corresponding to the location of the maximal input value (the "juiciest fly"). The issue was to avoid a serial computation—search one at a time through the locations on the input array and find the largest value—but instead to let the neurons of the network excite and inhibit each other in such a way that only the strongest input would win through to the output. We succeeded, and the result is what is now called a *Winner-Take-All network*. Where a conscious search might take several seconds, the Winner-Take-All network can make its decision in a fraction of a second.

The next example explaining some aspect of behavior introduces the idea of "schemas" by considering approach and avoidance in the frog. While this may appear a digression from our survey of lampposts to illuminate the search for pieces of the puzzle of language evolution, the details will provide the reader with a basic understanding of the interaction between *perceptual schemas* (defined as processes that recognize specific objects or situations or events in the world) and *motor schemas* (akin to control systems that specify some course of action).

A frog surrounded by dead flies will starve to death, but we have seen that the frog will snap with equal "enthusiasm" at a moving fly or a pencil tip wiggled in a fly-like way. On the other hand, a larger moving object can trigger an

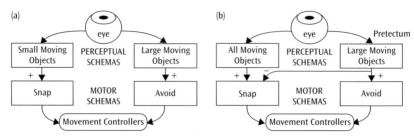

FIGURE 1-1.   (*a*) A "naive" model that incorporates the perceptual and motor schemas for frog approach behavior (snap at small moving objects) as completely separated from those for avoidance. For example, if the Small Moving Objects perceptual schema is activated, it triggers the Snap motor schema, which formulates the neural commands that get the movement controllers to move the frog to snap at its prey. (*b*) A schema program for approach and avoidance that takes into account data on the effect of lesioning the pretectum. In particular, the "approach schema" is not localized in the tectum alone since it depends on pretectal inhibition for its integrity. Instead, the nonlesioned animal will snap at a moving object, which activates the All Moving Objects perceptual schema but does not activate the Large Moving Objects perceptual schema. Then the excitation (+) from the former, in the absence of the inhibition (−) from the latter, will trigger the Snap motor schema. Activity of the Large Moving Objects perceptual schema will trigger the Avoid motor schema to issue the neural commands, which get the movement controllers to move the frog to avoid the predator while inhibiting the Snap. (Adapted from Arbib, 1990.)

escape reaction. A first schema-level model of this (Fig. 1-1a) has signals from the eye routed to two perceptual schemas, one for recognizing small moving objects (food-like stimuli) and one for recognizing large moving objects (enemy-like stimuli). If the small-moving-object perceptual schema is activated, it will in turn trigger the motor schema that gets the animal to approach and snap at what is apparently its prey. If the large-moving-object schema is activated, it will trigger the motor schema for avoidance, causing the animal to escape an apparent enemy.

To turn this schema model into a biological model, we need to relate the four schemas to anatomy. Each eye of the frog projects to regions on the opposite side of the brain, including the tectum (which we have already met) and the pretectum (just in front of the tectum). If we hypothesize that the small-moving-object schema is in the tectum, while the large-moving-object schema is in the pretectum, the model (Fig. 1-1a) predicts that animals with a pretectal lesion (i.e., frogs in which the pretectum has been surgically removed) would approach small moving objects since the small-moving-object schema would remain in the tectum. Moreover, according to this model, the lesioned frog would not respond at all to large moving objects since the large-moving-object schema would have been removed with the pretectum. However, the neuroethologist Peter Ewert in Kassell, Germany, studied toads with the pretectum removed and found that they responded to both large and small moving objects with approach behavior! This observation leads to the new schema-level model shown in Figure 1-1b (inspired by Ewert & von Seelen, 1974):

We replace the perceptual schema for small moving objects of Figure 1-1a by a perceptual schema for all moving objects and leave the right-hand column the way it was. We also add an inhibitory pathway from the large-moving-object perceptual schema (in the pretectum) to the snap schema. This inhibition ensures that the model yields the normal animal's response to small moving objects with approach but not avoidance. The transition here is from schemas as purely functional units to neural schemas as functional units constrained by neural data. The resultant model of Figure 1-1b explains our small database on the behavior of both normal frogs and toads and those with a lesion of the pretectum.

We have thus shown how models expressed at the level of a network of interacting schemas can really be testable biological models.[1] Further details are not important here. What is important is that we now have the following concepts at our disposal:

- **Action-oriented perception:** We are interested in the overall behavior of the animal. In particular, we look at perception in terms of the role it serves in providing the animal with the information it needs to carry out a course of action.
- **Schemas and neural networks:** We can model the brain either at the level of neural networks or at the higher level of interacting functional units called schemas. In each case, we can either rest content with the model as a functional model that yields the patterns of behavior of the animal or human as seen "from the outside" or probe further and restructure our models in the light of lesion studies or brain imaging or single-cell recording to help us understand how this behavior is mediated by the inner workings of the brain.
- **Cooperative computation (competition and cooperation) and the action-perception cycle:** The classic computational style of an electronic computer is serial, with masses of data stored passively and with a single central processing unit carrying out one instruction at a time on just one or two pieces of data at a time, to either combine them in some way and store the result, or test them as a basis for determining which instruction to carry out next.[2] By contrast, in the brain—whether described at the level of a neural network or a schema network—activity is distributed across the whole network, with excitation and inhibition between neurons, or patterns of competition and cooperation between schemas eventually yielding a pattern of activity (like the output pattern of our winner-take-all network) that commits the organism to one course of action rather than another. Moreover, as the animal acts, its sensory input changes, and the

action-perception cycle (see Figure 2-7) and the dynamics of competition and cooperation continue as the animal makes sense of, and interacts with, the dynamic world around it.

We shall have little to say about frogs in what follows, but these three key ideas will play important roles in our attempt to understand the brains of humans (who do have language) and those of monkeys (which do not) and thus chart the evolutionary paths that created the human, language-ready brain from that of their common ancestor.

My Second Lamppost: Schema Theory for Vision and Dexterity

We saw that much of my early searching under the "Computational Neuroethology" lamppost was inspired by the study of "What the Frog's Eye Tells the Frog's Brain." My second lamppost differs from the first in that it provides ways for schema theory to illuminate aspects of action and perception that are far more complex than those seen in the frog. The construction of this lamppost began when David Ingle—he of the frog and the "average fly"— invited me to a conference at Brandeis University in 1979. One of the speakers there was the French neuropsychologist Marc Jeannerod who reported on his study with Jean Biguer of what happens when reaching to grasp an object (Jeannerod & Biguer, 1982). They had charted the way in which the hand, as it moves to grasp a ball, is preshaped so that as it approaches the ball, it is of the right shape and orientation to enclose the ball prior to gripping it firmly. Moreover, to a first approximation,[3] the movement can be broken into a fast initial movement and a slow approach movement, with the transition from the fast to the slow phase of transport coming just before closing of the fingers from the preshape so that touch may take over in controlling the final grasp. I was intrigued by this and tried to formalize it in terms of the ideas about perceptual and motor schemas that I had developed to talk about frogs. The result is shown in Figure 1-2. When it was published in a chapter (Arbib, 1981) of *The Handbook of Neurophysiology* it created the (at that time erroneous) impression that I was an expert on the visual control of hand movements, and I got invited to talk at conferences on the topic. To avoid embarrassment, and with the help of PhD students Thea Iberall and Damian Lyons, I eventually became the expert I had appeared to be.

The top half of Figure 1-2 shows three perceptual schemas: Successful location of the object activates schemas for recognizing the size and orientation of the object. The outputs of these perceptual schemas are available for the control

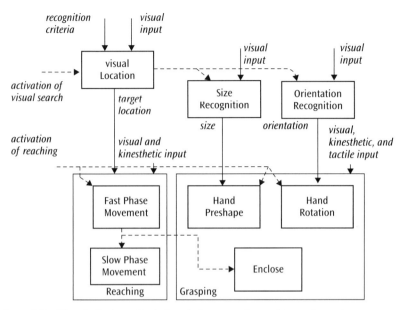

FIGURE 1-2.   Hypothetical coordinated control program for reaching and grasping. Perceptual schemas in separate visual pathways analyze the visual input to set parameters for the motor schemas required for control of arm (Reaching) and hand (Grasping = Preshape/Rotation + Enclose). Different perceptual schemas (top half of figure) provide input for the motor schemas (bottom half of figure) for the control of "reaching" (arm transport ≈ reaching) and "grasping" (controlling the hand to conform to the object). Note the timing relations posited here between subschemas within the "Reaching" motor schema and those within the motor schema for "Grasping." Dashed lines indicate activation signals; solid lines show transfer of data. Reaching was hypothesized to involve a ballistic phase followed by a feedback phase, with the transition between the two also activating the Enclose motor schema. (Adapted from Arbib, 1981.)

of arm and hand movement by concurrent activation of two motor schemas (shown in the bottom half of the figure), one controlling the arm to transport the hand toward the object and the other preshaping the hand, with finger separation and orientation guided by the output of the appropriate perceptual schemas. Once the hand is preshaped, it is only the completion of the fast phase of hand transport that "wakes up" the final stage of the grasping schema to shape the fingers under control of tactile feedback. (This model anticipates the much later discovery, reported in Chapter 5, of perceptual schemas for grasping located in an area [AIP] of parietal cortex and motor schemas for grasping situated in an area [F5] of premotor cortex.)[4]

The schemas are akin to the blocks in a conventional block diagram for a control system, but they have the special property that they can be activated and deactivated. Thus, where control theory usually examines the properties of a fixed control system, schema theory allows the control system to expand and contract, adding and deleting subschemas in a task- and data-dependent manner. Solid lines indicate the transfer of data from one schema to another, and dashed lines indicate the transfer of activation. Crucially, then, schemas can be combined to form such *coordinated control programs* that control the phasing in and out of patterns of schema coactivation and the passing of control parameters from perceptual to motor schemas. A schema defined functionally may later be analyzed as a coordinated control program of finer schemas and so on until such time as a secure foundation of neural localization is attained (as in the example of Fig. 1b, where—unlike the model in Fig. 1a—we were able to localize some schemas to brain regions in a way that survived the test of new experiments). Moreover, perceptual and motor schemas may be embedded in coordinated control programs embracing more abstract schemas to yield accounts of cognition and language that link psychology to neuroscience. A corollary to this is that knowledge is distributed across multiple regions in the brain. A multiplicity of different representations must be linked into an integrated whole, but such linkage may be mediated by distributed processes of competition and cooperation.

Figure 1-2 clearly separates perceptual and motor schemas. But this raises the question as to why I do not combine perceptual and motor schemas into a single notion of schema that integrates sensory analysis with motor control. Indeed, there are cases where such a combination makes sense. However, recognizing an object (an apple, say) may be linked to many different courses of action (to place it in one's shopping basket; to place it in a bowl; to pick it up; to peel it; to cook with it; to eat it; to discard a rotten apple, etc.). Of course, once one has decided on a particular course of action, then specific perceptual and motor subschemas must be invoked. But note that, in the list just given, some items are apple-specific whereas others invoke generic schemas for reaching and grasping. It was considerations like this that led me to separate perceptual and motor schemas—a given action may be invoked in a wide variety of circumstances; a given perception may precede many courses of action. There is no one grand "apple schema" that links all "apple perception strategies" to "every action that involves an apple." Moreover, in the schema-theoretic approach, "apple perception" is not mere categorization—"this is an apple"—but may provide access to a range of parameters relevant to interaction with the apple at hand. Thus, this approach views the brain as encoding a varied network of perceptual and motor schemas and coordinated control programs built upon them, perhaps with the mediation of coordinating schemas. And, looking ahead, while much of our activity is routine (mustering a coordinated control program that we have already mastered), much else involves the marshaling of schemas in novel assemblages to meet the demands of novel situations.

Perception and Cooperative Computation

A schema is what is learned (or innately given) about some aspect of the world, combining knowledge with the processes for applying it. A schema *instance* is an active deployment of these processes. Each schema instance has an associated *activity level*. The activity level of a perceptual schema signals the credibility of the hypothesis that what the schema represents is indeed present, whereas other schema parameters represent other salient properties such as size, location, and motion of the perceived object. The activity level of a motor schema instance may signal its "degree of readiness" to control some course of action.

Schema instances may be combined (possibly with those of more abstract schemas, including coordinating schemas) to form schema assemblages. An expanded perspective on the assemblage of perceptual schemas came about at the University of Massachusetts at Amherst where my colleagues Ed Riseman and Allen Hanson were developing a scene-understanding system that could move from a color photograph to a recognition of the various objects contained in the scene. Their VISIONS system[5] was implemented on a serial computer but the underlying computational architecture offered useful insights into the way I believe the brain operates, via cooperative computation—the competition and cooperation of a multitude of schema instances, extending the basic style of operation exhibited in Figure 1-1b. Before the schemas can operate, low-level processes take an image of an outdoor visual scene and extract an intermediate representation, including contours and surfaces tagged with features such as color, texture, shape, size, and location. Perceptual schemas process different features of the intermediate representation to form confidence values for the presence of objects like houses, walls, and trees. The knowledge required for interpretation is stored in *long-term memory* as a network of schemas, while the state of interpretation of the particular scene unfolds in *working memory* as a network of schema instances. Note that this working memory is not defined in terms of recency (as in very short-term memory) but rather in terms of continuing relevance. An example (increasingly rare in the age of smart phones) of working memory is the ability to remember a phone number long enough to enter it, but then forgetting it once it is no longer needed.

Interpretation of a novel scene starts with the data-driven instantiation of several schemas (e.g., a certain range of color and texture might cue an instance of the foliage schema for a certain region of the image). When a schema instance is activated, it is linked with an associated area of the image and an associated set of local variables (Figure 1–3). Each schema instance in

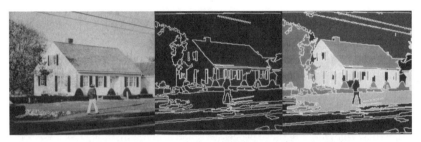

FIGURE 1-3.   Segmentation of a scene into candidate regions provides the bridge between the original image and the interpretation of a scene in VISIONS by associating regions of the image with schema instances. In this example, VISIONS classifies regions of the scene as sky, roof, wall, shutter, foliage, and grass, but it leaves other areas uninterpreted. (Figures supplied by kind courtesy of Allen Hanson.) (See color insert for full color version of this figure.)

working memory has an associated confidence level that changes on the basis of interactions with other units in working memory. The working memory network makes context explicit: Each object represents a context for further processing. Thus, once several schema instances are active, they may instantiate others in a "hypothesis-driven" way (e.g., recognizing what appears to be a roof will activate an instance of the house schema to seek confirming evidence such as the presence of walls in the region below that of the putative roof). Ensuing computation is based on the competition and cooperation of concurrently active schema instances. Once a number of schema instances have been activated, the schema network is invoked to formulate hypotheses, set goals, and then iterate the process of adjusting the activity level of schemas linked to the image until a coherent scene interpretation of (part of) the scene is obtained. Cooperation yields a pattern of "strengthened alliances" between mutually consistent schema instances that allows them to achieve high-activity levels to constitute the overall solution of a problem. As a result of competition, instances that do not meet the evolving consensus lose activity and thus are not part of this solution (though their continuing subthreshold activity may well affect later behavior). Successful instances of perceptual schemas become part of the current short-term model of the environment (Fig. 1-4).

Another system from the 1970s also embodied cooperative computation even though implemented on a serial computer. In the HEARSAY-II speech understanding system (Lesser, Fennel, Erman, & Reddy, 1975), digitized speech data provide input at the parameter level (energy in the speech signal in different frequency bands); the output at the phrasal level interprets the speech signal as a sequence of words with associated syntactic and semantic structure. Because of ambiguities in the spoken input, a variety of hypotheses must be considered. To keep track of all these hypotheses, HEARSAY uses a dynamic global data structure, called the blackboard, partitioned into various levels

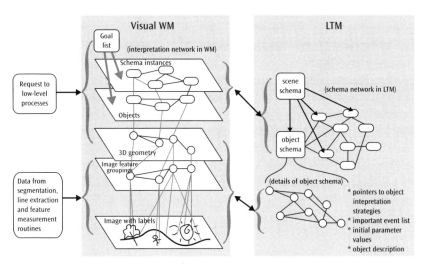

Figure 1-4.   The visual working memory (WM) of VISIONS interprets the current scene by a network of parameterized instances of schemas from long-term memory (LTM). These schema instances are linked to the visual world via the intermediate database that offers an updatable analysis of the division of the world into regions that are candidates for interpretation as agents and objects, possibly in relation with each other.

(Fig. 1-5). Processes called knowledge sources act upon hypotheses at one level to generate hypotheses at another. First, a knowledge source takes input data to hypothesize a phoneme at the surface-phonemic level. Many different phonemes may be posted as possible interpretations of the same speech segment, with different confidence levels. A lexical knowledge source takes phoneme hypotheses and finds words in its dictionary that are consistent with the phoneme data, thus posting hypotheses at the lexical level and allowing certain phoneme hypotheses to be discarded.

To obtain candidate phrases, knowledge sources embodying syntax and semantics are brought to bear.[6] Each hypothesis is annotated with a number expressing the current confidence level assigned to it. Each hypothesis is explicitly linked to those it supports at another level. Knowledge sources cooperate and compete to limit ambiguities. In addition to data-driven processing that works upward, HEARSAY also uses hypothesis-driven processing so that when a hypothesis is formed on the basis of partial data, a search may be initiated to find supporting data at lower levels. For example, confidence in the plural form of a verb may resolve uncertainty about whether or not an –s sound occurred on a preceding noun. A hypothesis activated with sufficient confidence will provide context for determination of other hypotheses. However, such an island of reliability need not survive into the final interpretation of the sentence. All we can ask is that it forwards the process that eventually yields

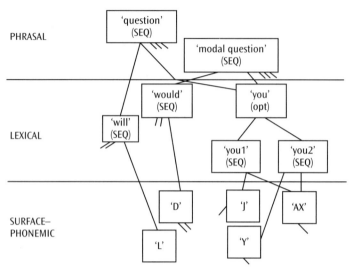

FIGURE 1-5.   At the surface-phonemic level of the HEARSAY speech understanding system, different phoneme instances are activated for particular periods of time, with confidence levels based (at first) on the spoken input for each time period. Word hypotheses are then activated at the lexical level, each with a confidence level based on the confidence levels of the various phonemes that make up the word. But phonemes that can be aggregated to form words with a high confidence level have their confidence levels strengthened in turn. Similarly, at the phrasal level, processing seeks phrases (defined by syntactic and semantic rules) that are strongly supported by hypotheses at the lexical level and the high-confidence phrases can support word hypotheses in turn. Thus, cooperative computation proceeds both bottom-up and top-down until one high-confidence phrase or sentence is accepted as the interpretation of the spoken input. (Lesser et al., 1975, © 1975 IEEE.)

this interpretation. Arbib and Caplan (1979) discussed how the knowledge sources of HEARSAY, which were scheduled serially, might be replaced by schemas distributed across the brain to capture the spirit of "distributed localization" of Luria (e.g., 1973). Today, advances in the understanding of distributed computation and the flood of brain imaging data make the time ripe for a new push at a neurolinguistics informed by the understanding of cooperative computation.

Schema Theory in Historical Perspective

The decision to call the components of the frog model of Figure 1-1 "schemas" was prompted by my friend Richard Reiss because he noted that my action-oriented view of the organism that seeks from the world the information it needs to pursue its chosen course of action has resonances with that of Jean Piaget who argued that all human knowledge is connected with action—and who used the term *schemas* (or *schemes*, depending on the translation from the French) to ground his analysis. Given the adoption of this term, it is worth a brief detour to note a few other classic uses of the word in describing human cognition and behavior.

Piaget called himself a genetic epistemologist. Just as embryology seeks to understand the genesis of the body, so Piaget sought to understand the genesis of the mind in the construction of reality in a child (Piaget, 1954). He talks both of *assimilation*, the ability to make sense of a situation in terms of the current stock of schemas, and of *accommodation*, the process by which the stock of schemas may change over time as the expectations based on assimilation to current schemas are not met. Acting on the basis of an action schema usually entails the expectation of certain consequences. "[T]o know an object or a happening is to make use of it by assimilation into an action schema ... [namely] whatever there is in common between various repetitions or superpositions of the same action." Piaget traces the cognitive development of the child from reflexive schemas through eye-hand coordination and object permanence all the way to schemas for language and abstract thought that are no longer rooted in the sensorimotor particularities.

Earlier, Head and Holmes (1911) introduced the term *schema* to the neurological literature, speaking of the *body schema*: "Anything which participates in the conscious movement of our bodies is added to the model of ourselves and becomes part of those schemata: a woman's power of localization may extend to the feather of her hat." A person with unilateral damage to the parietal lobe may lose awareness that the body on the opposite side actually belonged to her—not only ignoring painful stimuli but even neglecting to dress that half of the body. Damage to thalamus and somatosensory system may also produce disorders of the body schema.

Bartlett (1932) carried the schema idea from neurology into cognitive psychology, with a schema being "an active organization of past reactions [or] experiences, which must always be supposed to be operating in any well-adapted organic response." He stressed the constructive character of remembering. When people try to recall a story, they reconstitute it in their own terms, relating what they experience to a familiar set of schemas, rather than by rote memorization of details. Instead of thinking of ideas as impressions of sense data, schema theory posits an active and selective process of schema formation (recall Piaget's notion of assimilation), which in some sense constructs reality as much as it embodies it. More generally, cognitive psychology views schemas as cognitive structures built up in the course of interaction with the environment to represent organized experience, ranging from discrete features to general categories. Not only is input from the environment coded in terms of the schemas currently operating, but that input also selects relevant schemas, as a chair activates not only the "chair schema" but also the more general schemas such as "furniture" and inhibits other competing schemas.

Schemas and their connections with each other change through the processes of accommodation. These processes adjust the network of schemas so that over time they become able to better handle a wide range of situations. Through learning, a complex schema network arises that can mediate first the child's, and then the adult's, reality. Through being rooted in such a network, schemas are interdependent, so that each finds meaning only in relation to others. For example, a house is defined in terms of parts such as a roof, yet a roof may be recognized because it is part of a house recognized on the basis of other criteria such as "people live there." Each schema enriches and is defined by the others (and may change when a formal linguistic system allows explicit, though partial, definitions). Though processes of schema change may affect only a few schemas at any time, such changes may cohere to yield dramatic changes in the overall pattern of mental organization. There is change yet continuity, with many schemas held in common yet changed because they must now be used in the context of the new network.

The Self as "Schema Encyclopedia"

The second lamppost differs from the first in that it provides new ways in which schema theory can illuminate the mechanisms of human cognition, while at the same time offering the promise of discovering evolutionary continuities between humans and their common ancestors with other species. The discussion of HEARSAY, suggesting how we interpret language through schemas, is completely human specific. When we turn to vision, we suggest that VISIONS provides a good framework for thinking about human visual perception, but it is far more sophisticated that the mechanisms of the frog's action-oriented perception. Let me close this discussion of the second lamppost by briefly sketching (no more than that) how it may illuminate the examination of human individuality.

Each of us is defined by a multitude of schemas. We each have only one body to act with and thus can carry out a limited set of actions at any one time. Thus, there has to be a channeling from the richness of understanding of a current situation and associated memories and plans to the well-focused choice, not necessarily conscious, of a course of action. Schemas interact, compete, and cooperate to yield a relatively well-focused plan of action that will commit the organism. This combination of many schemas within one body suggests a continuity of behavior by the one individual in similar situations but also, as this repertoire builds up over time, the possibility that the schemas may eventually cohere in new ways, so that what had been an expected behavior in a certain set of situations may eventually give way, through new patterns of schema interaction, to new courses of behavior. Each individual has sets of schemas with some sort of coherence between them (this is not to claim that all of an individual's schemas are coherent); and the style of such a set of schemas can change over time to provide some sort of unity. There are perhaps tens of thousands of schemas corresponding to the totality of what a human knows, with perhaps hundreds of these active at any time to subserve the current interaction of the organism with its environment.

Who we are is the totality of these schemas, yet the self we present to the world depends very much on the circumstances. I have had many social roles—son, husband, father, professor, tourist, theatregoer—and my behavior varies greatly depending on my current role. Again, I have learned how to behave in many different contexts—at home, at the university, at the shops, at a restaurant—and even there the schemas that I deploy can be even more finely graded, so that my behavior varies greatly depending on whether I am in the bedroom, bathroom, kitchen, or study. My various roles are played out through my ability to deploy appropriate schemas, respecting current circumstances to set expectations and meet goals.

Filling these roles is a function not only of my own action patterns but also of my internal models of the behavior of others, whether people are known to me as individuals or only by their roles, such as airline attendant or supermarket cashier. My sense of self depends in part on my ability to fill my roles in these varied contexts in a way which meets my expectations. I may recognize individuals by physical characteristics such as face, comportment, gesture, voice...or even a name tag. Furthermore, I have come to know certain patterns of behavior or a style of personality for individuals as well as of those playing certain social roles. My knowledge of other individuals can be strengthened by shared memories.

Part of "me" is unconscious as a result of the role- and context-dependent deployment of perceptual and motor schemas. Part of "me" is declarative—reflection on these schemas, knowing something of my style and the limitations of my skills (not necessarily the same characterization as that given by others) and memory of specific episodes. These are knit into a spatiotemporal framework and may be indexed spatially (where they occurred), temporally (when they occurred), and by a host of other associations. Indexing may be relatively absolute (in Sydney; early in 1964) or not (somewhere between Paris and Italy; just after we got married).

A continuing challenge (more often implicit than explicit in what follows) will be to understand to what extent the human genome prepares the human to develop in ways shared with other animals and in ways more or less unique to humans; and to what extent each human self is shaped by language (the embodied neurolinguistics of the next lamppost) and by the regularities we perceive in our social worlds (the social schemas of the fourth lamppost).

My Third Lamppost: Embodied Neurolinguistics

As a schoolboy, I became interested in the history of English, of how Norman French influenced the transition from Old English (Anglo-Saxon; from the 400s through 1066) to Middle English (from 1066 to about the 1400s) and the further changes that followed to yield Modern English (from the late 1400s onward), and of how different countries and even different classes put their own stamp on the language. I also read about the discovery by William Jones in Calcutta in 1786 that not only Greek and Latin but also Sanskrit, the classical language of India, shared so many similarities in both grammatical structure and vocabulary that they appeared to have emerged through history from a common ancestral language—what is called Proto-Indo-European.

I thus became fascinated by historical linguistics. In high school, I studied Latin, French, and some German, but I never became fluent in any one of them, though my reading knowledge in French was tolerable. In the years since, I have dabbled in many languages—Spanish, Russian, Japanese, and Chinese, for example—to get some appreciation of the grammar and vocabulary of each language but have never matched even my limited competence in French, except in Spanish. In other words, I am no linguist in either sense of the term; I neither have facility in many languages nor have made the deep analysis of specific languages my academic specialty. Rather, I "visit" languages the way a tourist might visit the great cities of the world, marveling at the most famous sites but easily lost when leaving the center of town. Nonetheless, all this has instilled in me a love of the variety of human languages, and a sense of the history that has forged both similarities and dramatic differences.

I met a very different view of language when I came to MIT, where each semester I would visit a young professor of linguistics named Noam Chomsky and ask, "What's new in linguistics?" At that time he was not yet *the* Noam Chomsky, arguably the most influential linguist of the 20th century (but known now to an even wider audience for his fluent political polemics). Rather, he had at that stage made a discovery that appealed very much to my mathematical mind. He suggested that we step back from the meaning of words in a sentence and just look at their categories—for example, forget what "The cat sat on the mat" might mean, but instead just look at the fact that it is a sequence of "non-terminals" of the form Det N V Prep Det N (where Det stands for a determiner, N for a noun, V for a verb, and Prep for a preposition). He then asked how might we mathematically categorize those strings of nonterminals that correspond to actual sentences of the language as against those strings—like Det Det NV, as in "A the cat sat"—that are not. He defined various classes of grammars and showed that for each class of grammars there was a corresponding class of automata. He also showed that a particular class of languages—called the context-free languages (we need not worry about the definition here)—could yield many of the grammatical properties of English and other languages but could not explain all the differences between sentences and nonsentences. In subsequent years Chomsky has presented a sequence of grand theories about "autonomous syntax," showing what we can learn about the structure of language without having to worry about how language is actually used for successful communication. Whole armies of linguists, the so-called Generative Linguists, have followed Chomsky's lead and revealed many patterns that are shared across languages whose syntax might at first seem very different. This is heady stuff, and I enjoyed the ride. Nonetheless, I will argue in later chapters that Chomsky's influence has in many ways been counter-productive when we leave the abstract study of grammatical structure. It has distorted many researchers' views of how language is used and how children acquire language and, if followed too strictly, blocks meaningful research into the evolution of language and the brain mechanisms that support it.

In any case, despite learning a great deal from Chomsky about the formal properties of language, and enjoying proving theorems about various mathematically defined families of languages, my work on neural networks and schemas in the brains of animals engaged in action-oriented perception and perception-oriented action led me to consider to what extent one could understand language performance in terms of brain function. Of course, the human brain is far more complex than a frog's brain, and the mechanisms supporting a human's use of language are orders of magnitude more complex than those supporting the frog's approach/avoid behavior. It is the task of this book to suggest how the gap may have been bridged, while still understanding language within a broader framework of the evolution of brain and behavior.

My attempt to think about language in action-oriented terms came to a head (so to speak) in the late 1970s and early-to-mid 1980s, starting with my sabbatical at the University of Edinburgh where I talked at length with the linguist Jimmy Thorne and the neurologist John Marshall and others about how to view language in terms of the computations involved in perceiving and producing it. Then at the University of Massachusetts at Amherst (UMass), I produced a paper called "Neurolinguistics Must Be Computational"[7] with a visiting scholar, David Caplan, now a highly regarded researcher on aphasia. All this led to the building of my third lamppost, "Embodied Neurolinguistics," which lets us find a key to language in a schema–theoretic approach to the brain mechanisms linking action and perception. But this is not just a program for applying the first lamppost to illuminate language—the schemas required for using language are very different from those employed for frog-level action and perception. However, the insights into schema theory offered by the second lamppost are indeed relevant. A first pass in this direction was established in the early to mid-1980s with four PhD students: With Jane Hill, I developed a schema-theoretic approach to language acquisition in the 2-year-old child (more on this in Chapter 11). Since it offered a very different view of the child from that presented by Chomsky, I sent him a copy of our theory with the request that he assess how our two theories compared. Chomsky's reply was memorable: He said he would not read the paper since he knew it was wrong, but then kindly typed a page or so explaining "the truth"—namely his theory! Note that this anecdote is completely neutral as to which approach to language acquisition is correct, but it does suggest an unfortunate attitude to the relation between data and theory. I will say more about Chomsky's notion of an innate Universal Grammar. With Helen Gigley, I investigated a formalism for grammar (categorial grammar) in the form of interacting units somewhat like neurons or schemas, and then showed how simulated lesions to the network of these grammar units could mimic certain properties of aphasia. Jeff Conklin's thesis addressed language production. He provided a computational account of how, given a visual scene, one decides what is salient about the scene, and then puts together a sentence to describe those salient aspects of the scene. And, finally, Bipin Indurkhya developed a computational account of metaphor—and we shall see that metaphor accounts for much of the way in which language can expand to express new meanings. The work of the first three students is explored in the volume *From Schema Theory to Language* (Arbib, Conklin, & Hill, 1987), while Bipin published an expansion of his thesis under the title *Metaphor and Cognition* (Indurkhya, 1992).

Another important perspective on language, learning something of the richness of sign language, came when I spent the academic year of 1985–86 on sabbatical at the University of California at San Diego. During that year, I paid several visits to the laboratory of Ursula Bellugi at the Salk Institute, just across the road from UCSD in La Jolla. I had met Ursula years earlier when she was studying how children acquired language, but now she had a new passion: American Sign Language (ASL). She had, with her husband Ed Klima, published the first linguistic study of ASL (Klima & Bellugi, 1979), and now her group studied not only the linguistics of ASL but also how strokes affecting brain areas often linked to spoken language could yield deficits in ASL signers akin to the well-known aphasias seen in speech. This work led to a fascinating book called *What the Hands Reveal About the Brain* (Poizner, Klima, & Bellugi, 1987). Through this experience, I became very much attuned to the fact that ASL was a fully expressive human language (this was reinforced by seeing the play *Children of a Lesser God*), and to the challenge of linking its study to my interest in brain mechanisms for the control of hand movement. However, when I moved to the University of Southern California in 1986, my work on language went into abeyance, and my commitment to Embodied Linguistics was put on hold until mirror neurons were discovered in the macaques of Parma.

My Fourth Lamppost: Social Schemas

In 1980, Mary Hesse, then professor of history and philosophy of science at Cambridge University, and I were invited to prepare the Gifford Lectures in Natural Theology to be given at the University of Edinburgh in 1983. We met three times over the next 3 years and corresponded at great length to put together our 10 lectures on *The Construction of Reality.*[8] A major part of our effort (apart from our friendly but marked differences over theological issues and free will) was the reconciliation and integration of my epistemology based on mental schemas and brain mechanisms "in the head" with Mary's epistemology addressing the creation of social schemas by a community. Mary had been actively engaged in understanding how, given a plethora of data, a group of scientists could come to agree on which data were most important, and on the structure of a theory that could make sense of these data and lead on to novel predictions about the world. Thus, where I looked at how the brain constructs the individual's reality (i.e., her understanding of the external world), Mary focused on how a community creates a social reality, a shared understanding.

This collaboration led me to try to understand brain mechanisms within the context of the animal's or human's social interactions. However, the bulk of my computational modeling of the brain continued to focus on sensorimotor coordination, on how the brain may extract parameters from sensory stimulation to shape the organism's behavior. Indeed, the bulk of research on neuroscience—and cognitive science more generally—at that time focused either on components of the brain, or on the behavior of an isolated animal or human, rather than on how creatures engaged in social interactions. It was in reaction to work of this kind that Leslie Brothers published her book, *Friday's Footprint: How Society Shapes the Human Mind* (Brothers, 1997), to stress the vital role of social interaction in the evolution and function of animal and human brains. The book built on Leslie's experience both as a neurophysiologist recording from the brains of monkeys observing "social stimuli" and as a psychiatrist interacting with her patients. Brothers noted that the image of Robinson Crusoe as an isolated individual alone on a desert island embodies the "isolated mind metaphor" then typical of neuroscience, but she then stressed that it is a mistake to view Crusoe as truly isolated before he saw Friday's footprint in the sand, since it ignored the history of socialization he brought with him to his exile and the extensive socialization that produces organized thought and behavior in every human being. Going further, Brothers asserted that the human brain has inborn mechanisms for generating and perceiving a "person," a construct that assigns subjectivity to individuals, just as we are biologically prepared to learn a language:

> The network of meanings we call culture arises from the joint activities of human brains. This network forms the living content of the mind, so that the mind is communal in its very nature: It cannot be derived from any single brain in isolation.

Brothers offers data from primates for this biological substrate. In addition, cultural evolution provides subtle and diverse variations on this biological theme. Brothers wrote her book in the mid-1990s. A decade later, the scene had changed drastically, in no small part because of the discovery of the mirror neurons, which are central to this book. All these ideas contribute to the development of cognitive social neuroscience.[9]

Each of us has very different life experiences on the basis of which our personal schemas (recall *The Self as "Schema Encyclopedia"*) change over time and so each of us has our knowledge embodied within a different schema network. Thus, each of us has constructed a different worldview that we take for reality. This observation is very important as we try to reconcile the schemas of individual and society. A network of schemas—be it an individual personality, a scientific paradigm, an ideology, or a religious symbol system—can itself constitute a schema at a higher level. Such a great schema can certainly be analyzed in term of its constituent schemas but—and this is the crucial point—once we have the overall network, these constituents can find their full meaning only in terms of this network of which they are a part.

The key distinction here is between the individual's schemas about the society that the individual "holds" in his own head, schemas that embody his knowledge of his relations with and within society; and what Hesse and I call a *social schema*, a schema that is held by the society en masse, and that is in some sense an external reality for the individual. The primary sense of "schema" was as a unit of mental function, which neural schema theory then seeks to relate to distributed patterns of neural interaction. A schema "in the head" can be looked at either from the inside (the mechanisms internal to the brain that support the schema) or from the outside (the external patterns of behavior evidenced by an animal or human perceiving and acting according to the designated schema). We can then bring in the social dimension by noting that related schemas in the heads of individuals create patterns of behavior across a community that can provide the environment in which a new member may perceive skills that define a member of the community.

The notion of "social schema" is an addition to that schema theory. It addresses the fact that entities like "The Law" or "Presbyterianism" or "The English Language" are not exhausted by any one individual's stock of schemas but are constituted by a "collective representation" (to adapt a term from Durkheim, 1915), which is experienced by each individual as an external reality constituted by patterns of behavior exhibited by many individuals as well as related writings and artifacts. Another related concept is that of a meme (Dawkins, 1976, from the Greek word μιμητισμός', *mimetismos*', for "something imitated") as a unit of ideas, symbols, or practices, which can be transmitted from one mind to another through social interaction rather than via the genome. However, the social schema may refer to a more general "style of thought and behavior" rather than a discrete "package."

Consider that each of us has a somewhat different vocabulary and may disagree from time to time on whether a given string of words is a "good" sentence of English. How, then, does a young child normally acquire (her own version of) the schemas in the head that embody the social schema for the language? The child is not exposed to a language as a unified external reality but rather as part of interactions with other people that may be associated with pragmatic or emotional consequences. The child thus comes to interiorize that language as a set of schemas for words and constructions and the pragmatics of use that allow her to become a member of the community by interacting successfully with other members. The schemas so mastered may not relate to words alone but may link words to more explicitly embodied forms of communication. Indeed, the first words of the young child are normally coupled with manual gestures, of which pointing is especially important (Capirci & Volterra, 2008). A child's utterance while she points at something is like a sentence containing a word like *that* in a phrase like "that toy." One may either ascribe the latter sentence in itself a rather vague meaning (where the reference of *that* is unspecified) or refine the meaning of the overall sentence by using context to infer what it is to which *that* refers.

Hesse and I explored ways in which individuals respond to a social schema to acquire individual schemas that enable them to play a role in society, whether as conformists or as rebels who reject and possibly change the social schemas that define society. Such change may involve a process of critique, whereby individual experience and social schemas are engaged in a process of accommodation in which either or both classes of schema may change. Note, too, that no individual's schemas need exhaust the social schema. In the case of "The English Language," we each know words and grammatical turns that others do not know. As the child comes to internalize the language, she too creates internal schemas that constitute an idiolect as she learns not only general lexical and syntactico-semantic patterns from those around her but also picks up some idiosyncrasies but not others.

We can thus distinguish three flavors of schema theory:

Basic schema theory: Studies schemas as dynamical, interacting systems that underlie mental and overt behavior (and not just conscious processes). Basic schema theory is defined at a functional level that associates schemas with specific perceptual, motor, and cognitive abilities and then stresses how our mental life results from the dynamic interaction—the competition and cooperation—of many schema instances. It refines and extends an overly phenomenological account of the "mental level."

Neural schema theory: The "downward" extension of schema theory seeks to understand how schemas and their interactions may indeed be played out over neural circuitry—a move from psychology and cognitive science as classically conceived (viewing the mind "from the outside") to cognitive *neuro*science. Neural schema theory analyzes data from neurophysiology, lesion studies, and brain imaging to see how schemas may be restructured to relate to distributed neural mechanisms.

Social schema theory: The "upward" extension of schema theory seeks to understand how "social schemas" constituted by collective patterns of behavior in a society may provide an external reality for a person's acquisition of schemas "in the head" in the sense of basic schema theory. The collective effect of behaviors that express schemas within the heads of many individuals constitutes, and changes, this social reality. Social schemas represent the collective effect of behavior—whether related to everyday events, language, religion, ideology, myth, or scientific society—governed by related schemas (in the sense of basic schema theory) in the individuals of a community.

Two levels of schema theory are like the separate "worlds" of Popper and Eccles (1977):

World 1: the world of physical objects and events, including biological entities
World 2: the world of mental objects and events
World 3: the world of the products of the human mind such as scientific theories, stories, myths, tools, social institutions, and works of art

World 2 is akin to basic schema theory—with neural schema theory being realized in brains, physical entities in World 1—whereas the entities of World 3 are akin to social schemas. For Popper and Eccles, World 3 is partially autonomous. For example, the development of scientific theories in World 3 leads to mental activity (World 2) that would not otherwise occur. However, the way we have defined social schema theory stresses that World 3 in the sense of Popper and Eccles is to be seen as thoroughly embedded within the social interactions of individuals (World 2) and the artifacts they produce, such as a book or a painting or a liturgical practice that exists in World 1 but can only be interpreted by humans whose schemas in the head internalize the relevant social schemas.

And So We Come to Mirror Neurons and the Mirror System Hypothesis

A scientific career can depend not only on the ability to follow through on well-laid plans but also on being able to seize unexpected opportunities as well. Years after the Brandeis meeting and the development of Figure 1-2, I was at a conference run by IBM Japan where I met the Japanese neurophysiologist Hideo Sakata. Hideo told me that he and Marc Jeannerod were teaming up with Giacomo Rizzolatti from Parma in Italy to request funding from the Human Frontier Science Program for an international collaboration. As a result of that conversation I was invited to join the consortium—the other member was the cognitive scientist Michael Jordan, then of MIT—that proved very productive. A major breakthrough occurred in Parma when it was discovered that some of the neurons in an area of premotor cortex called F5 (this terminology will be explained in some detail in Chapters 4 and 5; here the point is just to convey the general ideas) fire not only when the monkey executes a specific range of grasps *but also when the monkey observes a human or other monkey execute a more-or-less similar grasp.* These are now known in the literature as *mirror neurons* (Rizzolatti, Fadiga, Gallese, & Fogassi, 1996). Thus, macaque F5 contains a "mirror system for grasping" that employs a similar neural code for executed and observed manual actions. F5 also contains other types of neurons, including canonical neurons that are active for execution of specific grasps but not for observation of the grasps of others. The location of F5 and its relation to other brain regions will be discussed at length in Chapters 4 and 5. For now all that matters is the mantra that *mirror neurons were first found in area F5 of the macaque brain and these were related to various hand movements, but F5 contains canonical neurons as well as mirror neurons.*

This immediately raises the question: Does the human brain also have mirror neurons for manual actions? Rather than using single cell-recording to see whether individual neurons in the human brain had the mirror property, a somewhat different question was answered using human brain imaging:

"Does the human brain contain a mirror system for grasping, in the sense of a brain region active for both execution and observation of grasping as compared to a baseline task such as simply observing an object?" By that time, Scott Grafton, an expert on brain imaging, had joined the USC part of the consortium and so we were able to use positron emission tomography (PET) to look for evidence of a mirror system for grasping in the human brain. We found such areas (Grafton, Arbib, Fadiga, & Rizzolatti, 1996; Rizzolatti, Fadiga, Matelli et al., 1996) and the part of the mirror system so found in frontal cortex proved to be in or near Broca's area, an area that had traditionally been most associated with speech production.[10] What could be the connection between these two characterizations? The answer was inspired in part by the findings, discussed earlier, of Ursula Bellugi's group that damage to Broca's area could affect deaf users of signed languages (Poizner, Klima, & Bellugi, 1987), not just users of spoken language. Giacomo Rizzolatti and I (Arbib & Rizzolatti, 1997; Rizzolatti & Arbib, 1998) thus suggested that Broca's area

- evolved atop (and was thus not restricted to) a mirror system for grasping that had already been present in our common ancestor with macaques, and
- served to support the *parity property* of language—that what is intended by the speaker is (more or less) understood by the hearer, including the case where "speaker" and "hearer" are using a signed language.

This Mirror System Hypothesis provided a neural "missing link" for those theories that argue that communication based on manual gesture played a crucial role in human language evolution (e.g., Armstrong, Stokoe, & Wilcox, 1995; Armstrong & Wilcox, 2007; Corballis, 2002; Hewes, 1973).

Many linguists see "generativity" as the hallmark of language, that is, its ability to add new words to the lexicon and then to combine them hierarchically through the constructions of the grammar to create utterances that are not only novel but can also be understood by others. This contrasts with the fixed repertoire of monkey vocalizations. However, much generativity is also present in the repertoire of behavior sequences whereby almost any animal "makes its living."[11]

And thus the combined light of the second lamppost, vision and dexterity, and the third lamppost, embodied neurolinguistics, came to illuminate some crucial pieces in the puzzle that is the evolution of language. The resultant approach to language evolution has two ingredients that differentiate it from that of some linguists: (1) I regard language perception and production as rooted in brain mechanisms that first evolved to mediate practical noncommunicative action, and (2) I ascribe a great deal of importance to manual gestures in providing scaffolding for the evolution of the language-ready brain, rather than adopting a "speech-only" view of language evolution.

But before discussing language evolution in any detail, we need first to look in more detail at language, the human ability whose evolution we seek to understand. The passage from "having mirror neurons for grasping" to "having neural systems which (can learn to) support the parity property of language" is a long one, taking perhaps 25 million years from the last common ancestor of humans and macaques to the appearance of *Homo sapiens* less than 200,000 years ago.

2

Perspectives on Human Languages

Our central concern in this book is to offer answers to the question "How did the brain get language?" Before we can offer answers later in the book, we first need to discuss what constitutes a language and how languages may be described.

Individuals Do Not Speak the Same Language

We all use language every day, whether in casual greeting or to engage in conversation, to learn about other people and the world, or to change the world around us. Language often provides a running commentary as part of our consciousness of the world; it helps us clarify our thoughts. Language is also a source of entertainment and information as well as a medium for social interaction from the pleasurable to the punitive.

But how might we characterize a particular language? Is it given by the words in the dictionary? Etymology may give us new insights into words by revealing their roots in other languages or their origin in practical and social practices that are no part of our present-day lives. But we must also specify the grammar that puts those words together. And when words are combined, what do they mean and how are they used? All these considerations and more may be relevant to our quest, but for now let us consider a somewhat narrow answer for one language.

What is English? We might say "English is a Germanic language with a French superstratum that developed in the last 950 years in England but is now used in many countries of the world." However, many speakers of English have major differences in vocabulary, and dialects of English may vary in syntax. For an example of lexical variation, consider the following excerpt from the Hobart (Australia) *Mercury* newspaper of January 1999: "Someone in Tasmania has been stirring the old banger possum again and it's got owners of old bangers on the back foot." Few readers of this book will have all three lexical items "*banger* = old car," "*possum* = an issue that had been thought to have died," and "*on the back foot* = on the defensive." Going beyond differences in vocabulary, Dąbrowska (2011) reviews evidence showing that native speakers of the same language need not share the same mental grammar. They may exhibit differences in inflectional morphology, passives, quantifiers, and more complex constructions with subordinate clauses. Her review supports the view that language learners may attend to different cues in the input and end up with different grammars. Some speakers extract only fairly specific generalizations that apply to particular subclasses of items, while others—possibly as a result of more varied linguistic experience—acquire rules that apply much more generally.

What then is "English"? We have to reconcile talk of people "speaking the same language" with the fact that each person has his or her own *idiolect*—each of us knows some words that others do not, and we each may produce the occasional sentence that seems grammatical to us yet grates on the ears of some others. Basically, the notion of language is a statistical one. A group of people speaks the same language if, more often than not, their utterances succeed in conveying the intended meaning, and it is that statistical ensemble of sentence formation and lexical usage (the social schema) that defines the shared semantic and syntactic structure of the language. By a similar analysis of a given individual, we can define the extent to which that person's syntax, semantics, and lexicon vary from the statistical norm.

Languages do not simply exist; they are acquired anew (and may be slightly modified thereby) in each generation. The relevant biological property is an inherently social one about the nature of the relationship between parent (or other caregiver) and child. The prolonged period of infant dependency that is especially pronounced in humans has coevolved with the social structures for caregiving that provide the conditions for the complex social learning that makes possible the richness of human cultures in general and of human languages in particular. The "social schema" is the pattern of regularities in the language use of a community. It provides the means for shaping the schemas (units of action, perception, and thought) that underlie the individual's ability to generate and understand sentences of the language. One job of the child's brain, then, is to perform statistical inference on the utterances of the language *in relation to the context in which it is immersed* to develop its own "language schemas" whereby it can approximate to the norm—as measured more by communicative success than by notions of grammatical correctness. In this task, language and cognition, and action and perception, are intertwined, as the child comes to match sentences to features of the current situation, including his or her current needs, various objects, his or her own actions, and the actions of those around the child. Of course, the child does not need any explicit knowledge of statistics to act like a statistical inference engine—any more than a planet needs to know differential equations to follow the path that we calculate by solving differential equations based on Newton's laws of motion. Chapter 11 will say a little more about the child's language acquisition.

The actual version of English (with or without *old banger possums*) will vary, depending on the community of language users across whom the idiolects employed by individuals are mutually intelligible. If two communities are separated in time so that the language of the early community differs from that of the later community, but whose linguistic differences can be spanned by mutual intelligibility of language between successive generations, we may speak of *historical language change*. If two communities sampled at the same time have a high but not very high level of mutual intelligibility, we may speak of *dialects* of a common language, and then seek to understand the historical processes that led to their differences. We shall say more about the dynamics of language change through history in the next section and then again through two case studies of the recent emergence of new sign languages, in Chapter 13, "How Languages Keep Changing." Such accounts must be sensitive both to social interactions between adults in the same and different language communities, and to the changes brought about in a language as each child forms his or her own "statistical regularization" in becoming a member of the language community.

What is "in the brain" that enables one to be fluent in English or any other human language? Although there are some sentences we use again and again like "Sorry I'm late" followed by "You would not believe the traffic on the freeway this morning," our knowledge of the language cannot take the form of a set of reusable sentences. A multitude of sentences (such as this one) are perfectly acceptable, even though they have never been used before. We say that the brain encodes a *grammar* and *lexicon*, so that when we hear a sentence, we "apply the rules of grammar" to *parse* the sentence, finding a grammatical structure that combines words from the lexicon to let us gather the meaning of that sentence. Similarly, when we speak, we go from the idea that we want to express to a grammatical structure with which to express the idea. Hockett (1987) provided an influential list of "design features" of language. Two of Hockett's features are *discreteness* and *combinatorial patterning*—words are discrete entities (one word does not blend into another) that combine to form phrases, and phrases combine to form larger phrases and sentences. As a result, each language has no bound on the number of expressions generated within its finite system of components and *constructions* (the latter being patterns of combination from the word level and up, linking the combination of words, morphemes, and larger forms to the combination of their meanings). What needs remarking here, though—looking ahead to the evolutionary account in later chapters—is that (as Hockett would have agreed) the features of *discreteness* and *combinatorial patterning* are not restricted to language. For example, a frog's behavior may be dissected into a set of basic motor schemas (as in Chapter 1) such as orient, jump, lunge, and snap. However, there is a crucial dimension of parameter variation in the motor schemas—for example, it's not enough to decide "approach" without determining the appropriate angle of orientation to approach the prey. What the frog lacks is the ability to analyze another's behavior in these terms and imitate them or communicate about the specific form the action takes. Despite this caveat, the crucial point is raised: When we examine design features of language, we must ask whether they reflect brain mechanisms specific to language or more general capabilities.

We shall have much more to say later about how linguists define grammars to set forth the rules whereby we can put words together to form sentences, but even if what we hear is a grammatical sentence, the longer the sentence we hear, the more likely we are to have trouble understanding its meaning, let alone its structure. Such considerations lead to the distinction between (1) *competence*, the general knowledge of grammar encoded in our heads in some fashion, not necessarily open to introspection, and (2) *performance*, the actual behavior of language use that will often produce—or comprehend—utterances that differ from any complete sentence given by an explicit grammar. Since our utterances are not always grammatical, the challenge of defining a grammar is a daunting one. In any case, it is rarely the task of a linguist to characterize the idiolect of individual speakers of a grammar. Instead, they seek to characterize the common properties shared by most speakers of a dialect or language. But what constitutes a "characterization" of a grammar? As we shall see in later sections, different linguists have adopted different frameworks for describing grammars.

However, when we speak or listen, much of what we say is ungrammatical. As we see from the transcript for Figure 2-1, there may be "ums" as we try to find the right word, and we may choose one word, then add more specificity (*disaster* → *earthquake*) or start to say one word and choose another. It seems that part of our language skill is to screen out the distractions and just make sense of what remains: So even ungrammatical utterances have some grammatical structure at their core, to support the process of production and perception.[1] The situation, though, is even more dramatic when we look at conversation. My thanks to Andrew Gargett for the following example of two train dispatchers, M and S, working together:

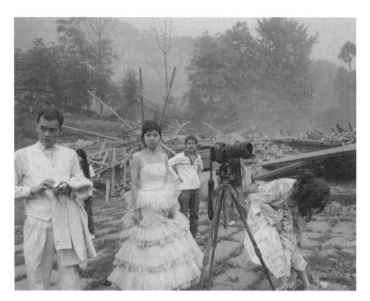

FIGURE 2-1.   An unusual wedding scene described by one viewer as follows: "uh...it looks like it was supposed to be a wedding shoot...but...um...there appears to be some sort of natural disaster...probably an earthquake of some sort um...buildings collapsed around them...they're dusty uh...the bride looks kind of shell-shocked...and...all their clothes are...ruined [laugh]...more or less...(Photo available at: http://cache.boston.com/universal/site_graphics/blogs/bigpicture/ sichuan_05_29/sichuan3.jpg)" (See color insert for full color version of this figure.)

TRAINS91, Dialogue 1.2
S: okay . . . so well say
M: +send+
S: E2 . . . I guess . . . from Elmira
M: +tshh+ . . . yeah
S: and send them . . .
M: to Corning
S: to Corning . . . okay

Here, M and S together build and express—with a mix of "wait, I'm thinking" and "yeah" noises—a shared conceptual structure: "We'll send [train] E2 from Elmira to Corning." It will not be my aim to explain this process, but the example does show the importance of turn taking and shared understanding in a prime use of language, namely conversation aimed at achieving shared goals. Here, "good grammar" lurks in the background, as it were, rather than taking center stage. The key point is that shared words and shared constructions provide the basis for language parity—the quest for shared understanding—but the formation of fully grammatical sentences is a limiting case, seen more in writing and the rehearsal of familiar stories than in the give and take of everyday language use.

Pro and Con Compositionality

Human languages are *open* in two senses:

(1) New words may be added to expand the scope of the language further and further.
(2) A full human language is generative or productive, being made up of words and grammatical markers that can be combined in diverse ways to yield an essentially unbounded stock of sentences, so that you, reading this sentence, are able to comprehend it even though you have neither seen nor heard it before. This ability to put words together in ways that allow us to freely create new meanings from old is called "compositionality." It is one of the keys to language, but not all of a language is compositional. For example, when we hear *He kicked the bucket*, the meanings of *kick* and *bucket* play no direct role in our understanding—unless we see an overturned bucket, a spill of water, and a guilty-looking boy standing nearby.

Let me offer two "case studies" that ground discussion of the extent to which language is compositional and illuminate the broad framework in which we experience language.

The Parable of the Parma Painting

While visiting the home of a friend in Parma, I was struck by a painting on her living room wall that contained the words "Emily Dickinson" and (placed horizontally) the letters

WHERE EVERY BIRD IS BOLD TO GO AND BEES ABASCHLES

It seemed that this could be segmented as

> *Where every bird is bold to go and be esabaschles*

or

> *Where every bird is bold to go and bees abaschles*

but there was no way to segment either *esabaschles* or *abaschles* into words of English—or even Italian, if the artist had decided to switch language in midstream. I thus did what my hostess had never done. I Googled "*where every bird is bold*" and thus retrieved poem 1758 by Emily Dickinson:

Where every bird is bold to go
And bees abashless play,
The foreigner before he knocks
Must thrust the tears away.

Although "abashless" was not a word in my lexicon, my knowledge of English word formation let me infer that it meant "without bashfulness."[2] The painter had made the typo (painto?) of including a "c" in *abaschles*, but what had happened to the final "s" and "play"? Well, I found the final "S" on the canvas where it had made a right angle turn stretched around the frame (my hostess had never noticed it) and then realized that some marks I had at first ignored on the canvas were a somewhat distorted and partially obscured rendering of the word *play*.

The Story of the Stairs

Whereas the first example can be seen in the context of language as comprising words arranged into sentences, the second example shows how the use of language in personal interactions may be embedded in a larger framework of *embodied communication*. At my train station, the level of the tracks is far below the street level. To get to them, one must either take an elevator or descend two long, steep flights of stairs. One morning when the elevator was not working, I found a young mother at the top of the stairs with a 2-year-old child asleep in a stroller, obviously perplexed as to how to get down the stairs, so I asked, "Would you like to carry the child while I carry the stroller?" She said, "Yes," but then proceeded to lift one end of the stroller. Rather than (compositionally) extracting the full meaning of the utterance, she had extracted an offer of help and then had signaled her idea of how that help could be rendered by grasping one end of the stroller. Receiving this nonverbal message, I chose not to correct her misinterpretation of my words since the essential offer of help had been understood, and instead showed my agreement nonverbally by lifting the other end of the stroller and then proceeding to carefully negotiate the stairs with her without dislodging the child.

The Parable of the Parma Painting was introduced to make three points:

1. Inferring the meaning of an utterance of language need not be a simple, direct translation from "syntactic form" to "semantic form" but may be an active process calling on diverse "knowledge sources" to negotiate what appears to be a satisfactory interpretation. Certainly, had I started with the poem itself and not the painting, much of this would have been avoided; but in everyday language use, what we hear may be fragmentary and distorted and so such completion processes would still apply. Moreover, we

may use our *estimate* of the overall meaning of an utterance to *guess* the meaning of a novel word therein, possibly guided by the internal structure of the word.

2. There is real compositionality at work in understanding each of the afore-mentioned four lines of poetry, both in putting words together and in pulling one word apart in search of the meaning of an item not in my lexicon.

3. Nonetheless, having a firm purchase on the meaning of each line, I cannot claim to know what Emily Dickinson intended to convey. Perhaps it was "When one encounters a place of beauty and tranquility for the first time, one cannot but be overcome by emotion"—and perhaps not. In any case it is clear that the combination of the four lines to infer the overall meaning of the poem is far from compositional.

The Story of the Stairs makes four further points:

4. What the speaker intends is not always what the hearer understands. Thus, my meaning for "Would you like to carry the child while I carry the stroller?" was essentially compositional, while the mother's interpretation was not. Indeed, that interpretation may have depended more on my posture and tone of voice in the context of her predicament than on the words themselves. Nonetheless, the success of language is based on the fact that the *parity principle* (Liberman & Mattingly, 1989)—that, more often than not, the meaning understood by the receiver is (at least approximately) the meaning intended by the sender—*usually* holds. This is crucial to the role of language as a tool for communication.

5. In its normal use, language is often embedded in a larger context of embodied communication. Such embedding is crucial to the process whereby a young child acquires the language of his or her community, and I posit that it was essential to the processes of biological and cultural evolution that led to the human ability to acquire and use language when raised in an appropriate environment. Normal face-to-face speech involves manual and facial as well as vocal gestures, while sign languages are fully developed human languages. Indeed, the core theory of this book (the Mirror System Hypothesis, briefly introduced in Chapter 1, and to be developed at length from Chapter 6 onward) gives pride of place to mirror neurons for manual actions, with language evolution built on the underpinnings provided by the evolution of brain mechanisms for so-called imitation of praxis (practical skills for, especially, manipulation of objects) and the building on that to communicate through pantomime.

6. Meaning is highly context dependent—what is the meaning of reaching for the wheels of a stroller?

7. Finally, we see that meanings may be captured not so much by some formal compositional structure (though this may be a powerful tool for analysis of some meanings) as by the far richer dimensionality of acting within the worlds of objects, actions, and social relations.

Thus, to the extent that some form of compositionality is involved in the meaning of an utterance, it may be necessary to incorporate into the utterance the bodily cues that accompany it as well as relevant properties of the immediate physical and mental worlds of the participants in a conversation. Even when we read a text, where no bodily or intonational cues are present, our interpretation of a sentence may depend on the "mental world" created by the preceding sentences of the text, as well as expectations about the author's intentions in creating the text.

Syntactic constituency determines what "pieces" the overall utterance is built from—so that "ball over" is *not* a constituent of "He hit the ball over the net," since it combines fragments of different constituents, *the ball* and *over the net*. In general, a given sentence may be ambiguous in that it can be parsed in different ways, or some of the words may have multiple meanings. There are (at least) three meanings of "row" possible in the written sentence "They had a row on the river" (though perhaps only one or two if the sentence is spoken), even though the syntactic structure does not change. Moreover, language is always used in context. A hearer may respond to the ambiguity (if he notices it) of "They had a row on the river" either by asking the speaker for clarification or by making use of context, for example, whether the speaker has been talking of people who have been having a difficult time together—though, in many cases, the nonverbal context may be what serves to tip the balance of interpretation.

We can also see the limits of compositionality in the English habit of combining two nouns to get a new noun.[3] Consider the definitions "a houseboat is a boat used as a house" and "a boathouse is a house for boats." The first definition suggests the rule "An XY is a Y used as an X," whereas the second suggests that "An XY is a Y for X's." The first definition might then suggest that "a housecoat is a coat used as a house," in other words, a tent. An attempt to save this would be to say that each XY is short for XRY, where the relation R is hidden, and that the meaning of XY can then be read compositionally from XRY. But this is unsatisfactory. Unlike the case for parsing, where the hidden relations come from a small, inferable set, here the missing R is specific to one's prior knowledge of the XY compound. Thus, the most we can say to unify these examples is "an XY is a Y (possibly in a somewhat metaphorical sense) that has something to do with X's"; in other words, X and Y are like search terms limiting the meaning of XY, rather than components whose meaning can be combined in a standard way to yield the meaning of XY. It is only our experience of English usage that tells us that a *housecoat* is a coat to be worn around the house when one is clothed, and is thus distinct from a dressing gown.

In general, then, compositionality yields but a first approximation to both the meaning intended by the speaker and the meaning extracted by the hearer. In the XY examples, there is at best a "cloud" of meanings consistent with the components and it is a matter of convention which one is intended. Language offers many devices, such as metaphor and metonymy whereby a new sentence can "infect" a word with new meaning.[4] And, dramatically, a new sentence can change the meaning of a word, such as when the child is told for the first time that "A whale is a mammal, not a fish." This causes a number of conceptual changes because, until then, the child may have identified the concepts of "whale" and "very big fish." Yet, intriguingly, this very blow against compositionality—the sentence "A whale is a mammal, not a fish" is false if the child retains her original meaning of *whale*—is also a testament to the power of compositionality, its ability to redefine constituent meanings if an overall sentence is taken to be true (in this case, on parental authority).

Note, too, the difference between language use in daily interaction and the writing of essays to be read in different times and places. In the latter case, reliance on gesture is nil, while reliance on context is much reduced—thus the addition of explanatory phrases that repair potential gaps in the reader's knowledge and enhance compositionality.

Co-Speech Gestures and Sign Language

Before discussing grammar further and the way it structures, and makes possible, the open-ended use of language, freely creating new utterances to express novel meanings, we briefly discuss the way that hands may be used to complement speech, and then the way that the deaf may use the hands and face to communicate using *sign languages* that make no use of speech at all. This should help the reader appreciate why this book's approach to language is motivated in great part by the multimodal features of facial and manual gestures as opposed to the view that equates language with speech alone. McNeill (1992) has used videotape analysis to show the crucial use that people make of co-speech gestures—gestures that people often use to accentuate or expand upon what they are speaking about. Pizzuto, Capobianco, and Devescovi (2005) stress the interaction of vocalization and gesture in early language development. Deictic gestures (such as pointing) can be observed accompanying and even preceding the production of the first word or the first association of two words, and they become enriched by iconic and other meaningful gestures in the co-speech gestures of human beings throughout their lives.

Deaf children, in the absence of any teaching, develop "home sign," (more on this in Chapter 12), a rudimentary sign language outfitted with very limited syntax (Goldin-Meadow & Mylander, 1984; Goldin-Meadow, 2003). However starting from the diverse syntactic fragments of their individual home signs, if many home signers are brought together in a community, a more complex syntactic

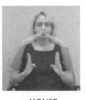

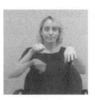

HOUSE	whole-entity CL + *loc*	BIKE	whole-entity CL + *loc*
HOUSE	located here	BIKE	located here

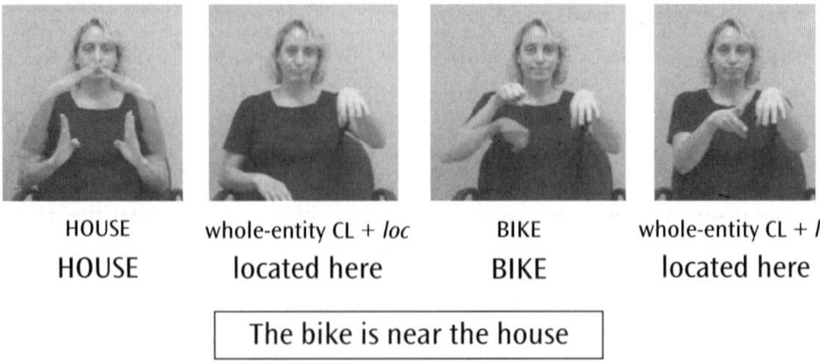

The bike is near the house

FIGURE 2-2.   This example demonstrates the way sign languages (in this case, American Sign Language) exploit space to provide syntactic cues distinct from the linear ordering of words and morphemes of speech. Here, the sign for HOUSE (the signer really has only two hands...) is followed by a classifier handshape that "places" the house in signing space; then, the sign for BIKE is made, after which a classifier handshape is made in signing space near that for HOUSE—thus conveying the overall meaning "The bike is near the house" (From Emmorey, 2002.)

system may be progressively developed by new generations, as observed in Nicaraguan deaf children (Senghas, Kita, & Özyürek, 2004) and Al-Sayyid Bedouin Sign Language (Sandler, Meir, Padden, & Aronoff, 2005). As we will see at some length in Chapter 12, in each case emergence of the sign language occurred in a community that included speakers of a full human language (Spanish and Arabic, respectively), providing a model of complex communication that could be observed though not heard, focusing our discussion on the interplay between biology and cultural milieu in the development of language.

Sign languages provide a powerful demonstration of the bridge from manual action to the open structure of language. Modern sign languages are fully expressive human languages and so must not be confused with the protosign that I will first introduce in Chapter 3 as part of the evolution *toward* language. We use signing here to denote manually based linguistic communication, as distinct from the co-speech gestures that accompany speech. The example of Figure 2-2 from American Sign Language (ASL) shows clearly both the expressiveness of sign language and the way it takes advantage of a different medium (hand movements located in the space around the signer) to structure sentences in a very different way from English. Classifier constructions use a handshape in *signing space* to represent how an object is located in "actual" space. Here, the sign for HOUSE is followed by a classifier handshape that "places" the house in signing space; then, the sign for BIKE is made, after which a classifier handshape is made in signing space near that for HOUSE—thus conveying the overall meaning "The bike is near the house."

In addition to discreteness and combinatorial patterning, Hockett also stressed *duality of patterning*, in which *meaningful* units are composed from a smaller set of *meaningless* units. Every spoken language consists of a finite set of recombinable parts that are perceived categorically, not shading one into the other. An English speaker hears either a /b/ or a /p/ even when a sound is formed intermediate between exemplars of the two. These discrete sounds combine to form words. The *phonology* of a language specifies not only the legal phonemes of the language but also how they may be combined. For example, "Krk" is the name of a Croatian island, but it is not a valid combination of phonemes in English. The letters of English approximate the phonemes of English, but there are clearly more phonemes than letters: Consider the different *a*'s in b*a*t, f*a*ther, st*a*te, and e*a*t for starters. Judging what are the phonemes of language can itself be a challenge. Furthermore, every language has conventionalized meaningful signals that are not composed of the phonemes of the language. Examples in English are the click of disapproval ("tsk"), a fast outbreath signaling relief ("phew"), a signal of disgust ("yuck"), and so on. Although these sounds really cannot be spelled out accurately, they are conventionally meaningful. Some might not count them as language, but Jackendoff (2002) sees them as primitive fossils of language precursors, surviving into a modern language.

Stokoe (1960) and Bellugi (1980) demonstrated that a sign language also has duality of patterning—meaningless handshapes, locations, and movements combine to form a large set of lexical items. Even though there are no sounds involved, we speak of the phonology of a sign language—characterizing the handshape, location, and movement elements used in the language and how they may be combined. However, Aronoff et al. (2008) find an unexpectedly high degree of intersigner variation in Al-Sayyid Bedouin Sign Language (ABSL; more on the emergence of this new sign language in Chapter 12), suggesting that linguistic proficiency *can* occur without complete adoption of duality of patterning. For example, the second generation of ABSL signers use signs for "tree" that remain close to pantomime and thus vary greatly, though the signs used by different family members may be similar.

In seeking to more carefully characterize the structure of ASL, Sandler and Lillo-Martin (2006, Chapter 5) distinguish classifier constructions from actual lexical items, arguing that the former are not "words." In classifier constructions, each formational element has meaning (is a morpheme), combining in complex predicates—an object of such-and-such a type is located *here*—while the same handshape, location, and movement elements are meaningless in words of the language. Regardless of whether one accepts this distinction, Figure 2-1 is a pretty fancy structure, combining signs (HOUSE, BICYCLE) with classifier constructions (STATIONARY-OBJECT-LOCATED-HERE, VEHICLE-LOCATED-HERE) and even disrupting the phonology by signing BICYCLE with one hand in order to maintain the location of the house in the background.

In both speech and signing, we recognize a novel utterance as in fact composed of (approximations to) known actions, namely uttering words (and we may think of many signs as forming "words") and morphemes that modify them (as adding *–ing* changes *run* to *running* in English). Crucially, the stock of words is open ended. However, sign language achieves this by an approach very different from speech. Signing exploits the fact that the signer has a very rich repertoire of arm, hand, and face movements, and thus—as we see from Figure 2-2—builds up vocabulary by variations on this multidimensional theme (move a handshape [or two] along a trajectory to a particular position while making appropriate facial gestures). Manual control is under visual feedback, providing a wide range of hand movements available for the inspection of others even in the absence of intended communication. By contrast, the use of orofacial and vocal articulators has few visual correlates, and so their use for vocalization requires a dramatically different mode of control. Moreover, speech employs a system of articulators for which there is no rich behavioral repertoire of sound producing movements to build upon. Instead, cultural evolution of speech "went particulate," so that the spoken word is built (to a first approximation) from a language-specific stock of "particles" such as phonemes, actions defined by the coordinated movement of one or more articulators but with only the goal of "sounding different from other phonemes" rather than conveying meaning in themselves.[5] This is the duality of patterning we met earlier.

The brain imaging of Figure 2-3 shows the very different sensory (visual versus auditory) and motor (manual versus vocal) systems for signed and spoken languages, yet—as we saw in discussing sign language aphasia in Chapter 1—they share central brain mechanisms. We next distinguish (signed)

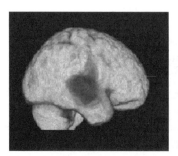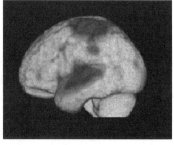

FIGURE 2-3.   This figure is based on brain imaging of people who have mastered both English and ASL. It shows in purple those parts of the brain that are more active for speaking than for signing, and in red those areas that are more active for signing. Much of the purple area is related to hearing, while much of the red area is related to the spatial structuring of action. By contrast, areas like Broca's area implicated in less peripheral aspects of language processing are used equally in both spoken and sign language, and thus they do not show up in the comparison. (Adapted, with permission, from a slide prepared by Karen Emmorey. See Emmorey et al., 2002; Emmorey, McCullough, Mehta, Ponto, & Grabowski, 2011, for related data.) (See color insert for full color version of this figure.)

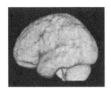 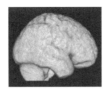

BRUSH-HAIR   READ

Figure 2-4.   Whereas pantomime and signing dissociate with left hemisphere damage, there is no difference in brain activation between "pantomimic" and nonpantomimic *signs*. (Adapted, with permission, from a slide prepared by Karen Emmorey.) (See color insert for full color version of this figure.)

language from pantomime. The signs for HOUSE and BIKE are clearly *iconic* (Fig. 2-2) in the sense that that they bear a strong resemblance to the shape of the object (for HOUSE) or an action with the object (pedaling for BIKE). By contrast, the ASL sign for BLUE is not iconic at all—it is a reduced form of the finger spelling of B, the first letter of "bleu," the French for "blue." Of course, B is also the first letter of "blue," but the fact is that ASL is derived from a sign language introduced from France. Thus, ASL is similar to French Sign Language, but it is very different from British Sign Language—the etymology of most signs has nothing to do with the forms used in the dominant spoken language of the country in which a sign language is used. BLUE in ASL is an exception. As Figure 2-4 shows, brain imaging of someone using signs of ASL shows no significant different in activity whether the signs do or do not appear iconic. Moreover, although signs like BIKE and HOUSE in ASL seem to have an iconic "etymology," it would be a mistake to think they are pantomimes; instead, they are conventionalized signs agreed upon by the Deaf community. Indeed, there is neurological evidence that the neural representation of signed gestures is independent of whether the sign resembles a pantomime. Corina et al. (1992) demonstrated the dissociation of pantomime from signing in a lesioned ASL signer, WL. For example, WL could no longer make the ASL sign for FLY but would instead spread out his arms like the wings of a plane and pantomime the plane's flying. Similarly, Jane Marshall et al. (2004) described a British Sign Language (BSL) signer for whom production of pantomime-like gestures was superior to sign production even when the forms of the signs and gestures were similar.

From Phrase Structure to Universal Grammar

But let's return to spoken languages. The *autonomous syntax framework* separates a *competence grammar* from the mechanisms that use it to produce or perceive sentences. It then ascribes differences between speaker judgments related to the grammar to limitations of these processing mechanisms—without calling into question the hypothesis that the competence grammar really is encoded "in the head." Espousing such a framework, Noam Chomsky (e.g., 1972) has asserted that syntax is the *essence* of language, and that the central data to which a linguist should attend concern whether a string of words—such as Lewis Carroll's famous sentence *"Twas brillig and the slithy toves did gyre and gimble in the wabe"* from his poem *Jabberwocky*—is grammatically correct, rather than whether or how it conveys meaning, or how it may be used in social situations. From this point of view, the job of the linguist in analyzing a given language has two parts:

1. To gather data on which strings (sequences) of words of a language are *well-formed sentences*, that is, which ones would be judged by speakers of the language as being "structurally correct" sentences, regardless of whether they are meaningful. (At a lower level of analysis, each word must be analyzed as a sequence of *phonemes*.)
2. To develop a *formal grammar*, a set of explicit grammatical rules that characterize just which strings are indeed well formed for that language. For example, in English we might look for rules that (a) tell us which noun is the subject of a verb, (b) tell us how to mark nouns and verbs as singular and plural, and (c) require us to ensure that subject and verb agree, that is, are both singular or both plural.

Here is a fragment of what is called a *context-free grammar*—so-called because it shows how to generate a set of strings of a language by replacing each grammatical symbol by a string of other symbols without checking on the context in which the symbol occurs. The fragment has the following *productions* or *rewriting* rules: Our first rule is

1. S → NP VP

that is, a sentence (S) may comprise a noun phrase (NP) followed by a verb phrase (VP). Of course, a full grammar of English (or any other language) would add a variety of other ways to build sentences, but here our aim is just to establish a base level for understanding an autonomous syntax in which a sentence is built up by paying attention to only the syntactic categories of words (e.g., whether they are adjectives, verbs, nouns, or prepositions) without paying attention to the meaning of the words themselves. In our second rule

2. NP → N | (Adj) NP (PP) (S)

the vertical line | is an "or" sign—we can replace the left-hand symbol with any of the choices separated by the |s, while the parentheses indicate that inclusion of an item is optional. (2) says that a noun phrase (NP) can either comprise a single noun (N) or can be formed by putting an adjective (Adj) in front of another noun phrase and/or following a given noun phrase with a prepositional phrase (PP, see later) and/or a sentence (S) of a certain form, as in "tall women in long dresses who wear lots of jewelry."

Rule (2) illustrates the fact that language is *recursive* in that the rules used to build a constituent may also be used to build a larger constituent of the same type of which the first constituent is part. For example, (2) shows that, among other possible structures, a noun phrase can comprise a single noun or an adjective followed by a noun phrase. This supports forming "rose," then "blue rose," and then "wilted blue rose." One noun phrase (whether just a noun or already built up using adjectives) can be a constituent of a larger noun phrase, and this provides our basic example of recursion. Similarly, a verb phrase (VP) may contain just a verb (V) or can be augmented as follows:

3. VP → V | VP (NP) (PP) (S).

The next rule says that a prepositional phrase (PP),

4. PP → Prep NP

consists of a preposition followed by a noun phrase.

While we have these productions in front of us, it will be useful to set out some general terminology from linguistics: The *head* of a phrase is the key word that determines the properties of the phrase. So in a phrase such as *delicious raw food*, the head of the phrase is the noun *food*, and consequently the phrase is a noun phrase. This corresponds to applying two of the aforementioned productions: NP → Adj NP → Adj [Adj N]. A noun phrase can occupy typical positions associated with nouns, as in *John eats delicious raw food*. The *complement* of a head word is an expression that is directly merged with it, thereby projecting the head into a larger structure of essentially the same kind—so in our previous example, *delicious raw* is the complement of *food*. In *close the door*, the NP *the door* is the complement of the verb *close*, exemplifying the production VP → V NP. A head-first structure is one in which the head of an expression is positioned before its complement(s); a head-last structure is one in which the head of an expression is positioned after its complement(s). In a sentence such as *He never doubted that she would win*, the clause *that she would win* serves as the complement of the verb *doubted*.

Returning to our simple grammar (too simple, as we shall later see), we close with the rules that specify what actual words (the so-called *terminals*) belong to a given category:

Noun → door | food | balloon | ...
V → hit | eat | close | ...
Adj → raw | delicious | ...
Prep → in | on | within | ...

and so on. In this way, sentences can equally well be generated that are meaningful or (because the chosen words are implausible together) meaningless.

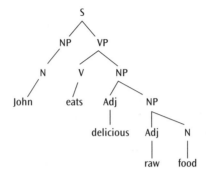

FIGURE 2-5.   A parse tree revealing the hierarchical structure of the constituents of the sentence *John eats delicious raw food* using our simple grammar. In general, syntax is more subtle than shown here, and the structure of the derivation increases in complexity accordingly.

Figure 2-5 shows the hierarchical structure obtained by deriving *John eats delicious raw food* by repeated application of the rules of our simple grammar starting from S and ending up with terminals on all the leaves of this upside-down tree.

What we have seen here is a simple (and partial) example of a *generative grammar*. The idea is two-fold: First, a sentence is made up of *constituents* (like verb phrases, noun phrases, and prepositional phrases); and, second, there is a set of rules that will *generate* just those strings of words that are members of a class of constituents. Moreover, the constituents of a particular sentences are just those sets of words that can be read off by starting with one symbol in the tree and working out to the leaves of the subtree for which it is a root.

Before proceeding further, we need to ponder the notion of a *well-formed sentence.* I defined such a sentence earlier as one that would be judged by speakers of the language to be a "structurally correct" sentence, regardless of whether it is meaningful. Having already noted that individuals speak somewhat different languages, we see that two speakers of English, or any other widespread language, may well quibble over the status of some sentences, but here I want to raise another issue. While a string could be called well-formed because speakers intuitively find it to be a "real" sentence of the language, a person who takes a prescriptive view of language might only accept a sentence if it can be constructed according to the rules of some grammar. Of course, some disagreement may occur if a grammar is not "good enough," but another disagreement has been quite influential in modern linguistics. Simply put, most grammatical rules do not limit the length of a sentence. For example, in English we rarely put more than two adjectives in front of a noun, but we would not want to make it a rule of English grammar that the number of adjectives be capped at a certain number. We would not want to decree that *I hate that bad brown dog* would be an English sentence, whereas *I hate that noisy bad brown spotted dog* would not. The result, of course, is that we can write sentences that are so long that we cannot be sure at a single hearing whether they are grammatically correct. Yet, if we could go through them time and again, grammar book in hand, we might come up with the verdict, "Yes, it's grammatically correct, but it's really too long to be useful." This is somewhat strange, for it says that when your immediate judgment of whether a string of words is an English sentence fails you, you should put aside your intuition in favor of the dictates of theory, namely the "calculations" made using a particular grammar for English—even though you know that the grammar is probably incomplete, no matter how well it describes the structure of a wide range of English sentences. In other words, limitations in immediate performance may throw into question hypotheses about what indeed constitutes competence.

Note that the claim for autonomy of syntax implies that syntax is but one of several levels. We have already mentioned *phonology*—this can provide not only rules for how phonemes are allowed to fit together into a pronounceable sequence but may specify other rules, such as when it is correct to use *a* versus *an* before the following word. *Morphology* determines the appropriate form of a word when it is employed in different syntactic contexts, as in handling the agreement between subject and verb—*eat* should be *eats* in the sentence *John eats bagels for breakfast*. And, of course, there is the Jabberwocky point: No matter how close this syntax comes to defining a fragment of English as far as "grammatical correctness" is concerned, it does nothing to ensure that the sentence is meaningful. That's the job of *semantics*.

The point at issue here is not whether one needs to consider phonology, morphology, syntax, and semantics in defining the structure of a language. The issue is to what extent they can and should be processed autonomously. Analysis in the style of Chomsky bundles the use of a generative grammar with the idea of autonomy of syntax. On this account, analyzing a sentence is a two-pass process: The syntactic pass checks whether and how the words of the sentence could be generated by the rules of the grammar. The subsequent semantic pass then applies *compositional semantics* to derive the meaning (if any) of the result of assembling the constituents in the specified way. Later, I will instead advocate Construction Grammar as an approach in which *some* elements of semantics are integrated into the syntactic structure. The problematic element will be to suggest what that use of the word "some" entails.

Universal Grammar or Unidentified Gadgets?

For Chomsky, the challenge of syntactic theory is far greater than to write grammars one by one for each language. Rather, his Holy Grail is a Universal

Grammar from which the particular grammar of each and every actual or possible human language can be obtained (e.g., Chomsky, 1981). The aim is not simply to look for different formal descriptions of the grammatical particularities of one language at a time—so-called *descriptive adequacy*—but rather to seek a single *Universal Grammar* that can be specialized to yield a principled account of at least the core structure of the grammar of each language. Different descriptions of a given language are then to be compared with respect to this single evaluative framework. The notion is that to the extent that a grammar falls into this universal framework, then to that extent is it a better explanation of the observed structure of the language. Chomsky speaks here of *explanatory adequacy.*

Many linguists accept all or most of this program. Others like myself learn from the various formalizations that it offers even while rejecting the autonomy of syntax. In particular, if one is concerned with neurolinguistics, one must give primary attention to the brain mechanisms for the actual perception and production of language.

However, Chomsky goes beyond the quest for explanatory adequacy. He claims that Universal Grammar is not simply a useful touchstone for linguistic research but is in fact a *biological property* of humans fixed in the ancestral genome of *Homo sapiens.* Some authors use the term "Universal Grammar" as a synonym for whatever mechanism it is that allows children to acquire language, but I think this strategy renders good words meaningless. Let us reserve "grammar" for a mental representation that underlies our ability to combine words to convey or understand meaning, or for the systematic description of the commonalities of individual grammars of the members of a community. Then let us distinguish between having an innate grammar and an innate ability to acquire grammar. The thesis of this book is that human brains are "language ready" (and the brains of other species are not) in the sense that children do have an innate ability to acquire grammar, but they do not have any rules of syntax prespecified in the genome (see Chapter 11).

Chomsky's view of language structure, and thus of what constitutes the Universal Grammar, has changed over the years. *Syntactic Structures* (Chomsky, 1956) developed a notion of grammar that could be characterized in a mathematically rigorous way. He showed that such grammars could capture some, but by no means all, features of the syntax of English. Chomsky's early work was very important for computer science as well as linguistics, for while it showed that, for example, the important class of context-free grammars did not have descriptive adequacy for human languages, computer scientists found such grammars very useful for the formal definition of computer languages. However, Chomsky's importance for linguistics did not become fully clear until the publication of *Aspects of the Theory of Syntax* (Chomsky, 1965) in which he emphasized the notion of *transformations* as the key for understanding grammar. For example, in English, we can recognize "John hit Mary," "Mary was hit by John," and even "Did John hit Mary?" as being in some sense the same. The idea, then, was that the three sentences shared a common "deep structure" (D-structure) but had different "surface structures" (S-structures), and that these were related by transformations, such as those that could change an active sentence into a passive sentence or even a question. The autonomy of syntax approach was exemplified by the fact that these transformations acted on the derivation tree (parsing diagram) with no regard for the meaning that the corresponding sentence was meant to convey. By contrast, other linguists offered a counter-theory, called *generative semantics*, which started from *thematic relations* such as Action (Agent, Object), for which Hit (John, Mary) would be a special case, as expressing meaning separate from its expression in a specific sentence, and sought to explain how sentences could be derived to express the meanings of compounds of such relations.

Chomsky is not only a most influential linguist but also an ardent polemicist (many people know him for his political tracts expressing his strong condemnation of US foreign policy and know nothing of his work on language), and he turned these polemical skills to rubbishing work, such as that of the generative semanticists, contrary to his own. Yet even as he argued vehemently that his own published views were the one true approach to the study of language, he was simultaneously developing a radical new approach to Universal Grammar that might better meet the demands of descriptive adequacy. And, thus, when he published "LGB," *Lectures on Government and Binding: The Pisa Lectures* (Chomsky, 1981), not only had most specific transformations (such as passivization and question formation) been thrown out of Universal Grammar to make way for more abstract processes, but the hitherto derided Thematic Relations became a crucial component of what constituted a grammar. Ten years later, a further recasting of Universal Grammar occurred under the banner of the Minimalist Program (MP: Chomsky, 1992, 1995), which built upon LGB but also made radical changes, even moving D-structure and S-structure out of the grammar.

The Minimalist Program's approach to linguistic *competence* characterizes which strings of lexical items are "grammatically correct" as follows (Fig. 2-6): A set of lexical items is taken at random, the computational system then sees whether legal derivations can be built, each of which combines all and only these elements. *Spell-Out* occurs when one of the legal derivations, if any, is chosen on the basis of some optimality criteria. The Computational System then transforms the result into two different forms, the *Phonological Form*, the actual sequence of sounds that constitutes the utterance, and the *Logical Form*, which provides an abstract semantics of the sentence in the style of mathematical

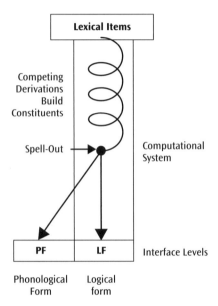

FIGURE 2-6.   Derivations and the Computational System in the Minimalist Program.
Derivation processes seek to determine whether, and if so how, a specific bag of words can
be combined in a grammatical way. If a successful, possibly optimal, derivation is found, the
result is spelled out in two ways to provide both its phonological form and logical form.

logic. The Minimalist Program thus posits an "articulatory-perceptual interface" that links the language faculty to the perceptual-motor system and
recasts the semantic component as a "conceptual-intentional interface," which
links the language faculty to other human conceptual activity. At first glance,
the emphasis of Chomsky's Minimalism on an "articulatory-perceptual interface" and a "conceptual-intentional interface" seems compatible with a performance view of language within a broader framework of action and perception.
However, closer inspection shows that the Minimalist Program is far removed
from a *performance* model of the speaker or hearer using language. There is no
attempt here to model actual sentence production, going from a meaning to
an utterance which expresses it—the process starts with words chosen at random and only at the end do we see whether they can be arranged in some way
whose spell-out yields a semantic structure.

From one point of view, the fact that Chomsky has built on new research in
linguistics to provide a modified theoretical framework every decade or so is
admirable. A new version of Universal Grammar is published. Many scholars
try to describe a range of languages using the current version. Many ad hoc
patches are required to explain new data, and so a new decade sees a radically
different version of Universal Grammar, hopefully with increased explanatory

adequacy. Since the definition of Universal Grammar has changed so radically over the years, it is clear that whatever was done to argue that the Universal Grammar of the 1960s was genetically encoded actually militates against the claim that an LGB- or Minimalist-style Universal Grammar would be genetically encoded (see Chapter 11). But might it be countered that my argument is wrong-headed because the trend of work on Universal Grammar has been such as to make the demands on genetic encoding and the complexity of learning a specific language less demanding with each innovation? That this is not so seems to be convincingly argued by the following extract. The reader need not worry about the technical jargon. The overall implication is clear.

> One of the motivations of the X-bar-theoretic program [a key component of the LGB approach] was the elimination of the stipulativeness of phrase structure grammars in favor of a few phrase structure parameters whose values could be acquired on the basis of simple and overt evidence....the LGB system with its beautiful elegance seemed to come close to this ideal but...more and more evidence has been presented in recent years that it is too restrictive in many ways to be descriptively adequate. Functional head theory [a key feature of the Minimalist Program] with its new devices holds the promise of overcoming these difficulties but at the same time brings into focus the tension between descriptive phrase structure parameters and explanatory adequacy....
>
> [Consider the problem of learning whether a language employs SVO word order.] In a phrase structure grammar, a language learner will only postulate categories that can be filled by overt constituents...To capture the order of elements, typically no more than two rules will be necessary: S → NP VP and VP → V NP [for SVO versus VP → NP V for SOV]. In a minimalist grammar, the following decisions have to be made:
>
> - Do Agr_s, T, Agr_o, and V precede or follow their complements?
> - Do the specifiers of these heads precede or follow their sister?
> - Are the head features of these heads weak or strong?
> - Are the Spec features of these heads weak or strong?
> - Is the functional head morpho-phonologically overt or covert?

The new descriptive devices thus bring with them many additional decisions to be made by language learners (Webelhuth, 1995, pp. 83–85).

Fairness dictates that I warn the reader that the way I am using Webelhuth's comments might be seen to carry a whiff of anti-intellectualism, one that I wish to disown. What I have just said *might* be paraphrased as follows: "Everybody can speak or sign in a human language. Therefore, any complicated theory of language must be wrong—since we certainly do not use fancy theoretical constructs when we hold a conversation or read our e-mail." But that is not what I intend at all. Compare the linguists' careful and explicit description of a language and the neuroscientists' careful and explicit description of the supporting brain mechanisms to the engineers' careful and explicit specifications of a Boeing 747. The former, just like the latter, is going to be very complex—though the former is still being developed by scientists, while the latter has been completed by engineers. The design of the 747 is only made possible because of basic principles of materials science, aerodynamics, electronics, and so on that are inaccessible to the average airplane traveler. Similarly, the function of the brain rests on basic principles that govern its anatomy, electrophysiology, and plasticity. In either case, the principles involved are subtle and complex, building on the cumulative insights of centuries of scientific research.

However, the general principles are only part of the story. For the 747, the specs are complete and explicit. For the human, the genome is crucial in setting the *initial conditions* for the growth of the brain and the disposition of its connections and memory structures. One crucial role of the genome is to control development, rather than directly specifying the adult structure of body and brain. The adult system reflects the results of subtle interactions of genetic prescriptions and constraints with experience shaped by the nature of both the physical world *and* the social world. The real issue, then, is not a debate over the complexity of a "Universal Grammar" that provides all the tools necessary to describe all human languages. It is rather over the issue of how to apportion that complexity between what is provided by the genome and what—like most of the specifications of the 747—is the fruit of human innovations and is thus a cultural rather than a biological product.

In my view, Universal Grammar is at best tenable only as a descriptive umbrella for the immense variety of human languages, not as a "genetic reality" or "neural reality" that implausibly contains all possible grammatical structures in embryo—and, even then, it is problematic how much of the "core" that one can discern across broad families of languages needs to be supplemented by more specific features as one turns to specific languages or special families of languages. What is universal is the need for expression, not the choice of linguistic structure for meeting those needs. The evolution of language from protolanguage is part of the *history*, not the biology, of *Homo sapiens*. (Chapter 11 offers a brief introduction to the study of how languages change.)

Evans (2003) supports this view by surveying a series of linguistic structures reflecting kinship structures common in the Australian culture area but unknown elsewhere. Pronouns reflecting moiety-type categories, subsections, moiety lects, and systems of triangular kin terms are embedded in the grammar, rather than being expressed merely by adding words to the lexicon. Other examples of the variety of languages across the world may add to the impression that the range of syntactic devices may reflect separate paths of cultural evolution. Certain grammatical categories are found in all languages, but they are realized in different ways (Dixon, 1997, Chapter 9). Consider first the marking of past, present, and future. Biblical Hebrew, for instance, had no tenses, but it did distinguish the perfective aspect (an action with a temporal end, e.g., "John sang a hymn") from the imperfective (an action with no temporal end specified, e.g., "John sang"). In Fijian there are past and future tense markers, but these are optional. The Bushman language !Xu has no grammatical marking for tense or aspect, although it does have temporal adverbs such as *now, long ago, yesterday, finally, then*, and *will*. And the most common tense system has just two choices, past and nonpast, as found in Sinhalese, whereas the language spoken in the Western Islands of the Torres Strait has four past tenses (*last night, yesterday, near past*, and *remote past*) and three futures (*immediate, near*, and *remote future*).

An intriguing grammatical specification absent in the most widely spoken languages is *evidentiality*. This is an obligatory grammatical specification of the kind of evidence on which a statement is based, for example, whether the speaker observed it himself, or someone told him, or he inferred it, or assumed it. In a language with evidentiality, you cannot say, "The dog ate the fish" without including one of the evidentiality markers: *visual* would be used if you saw the dog eat the fish; *nonvisual* if you had other immediate sensory data such as hearing (but not seeing) the dog in the kitchen or smelling fish on the dog's breath; *apparent* could be used if there were fish bones on the floor around the dog, which looked satisfied; *reported* if someone told you that the dog ate the fish; and *assumed* if the fish was raw and people don't eat raw fish so it must have been the dog that ate it. Dixon reports that a grammatical category of evidentiality developed independently at least six different times in the Amazon basin and comments that if linguists had not gone out to the Amazon jungle to study these languages, we would have no idea that the grammar of a human language could include complex systems of evidentiality. Different languages that mark evidentiality in their grammar may do so in different ways—as with tense, there is great variety in the categories represented.

Such examples strengthen the claim that linguistic structures are historical products reflecting the impact of various processes of "cultural selection" on emerging structure. There is *no* plausible scenario for bundling these special features into a genetically based Universal Grammar. If the proponent of Universal Grammar as an innate reality objects that, for example, Evans's examples of grammaticalization of kinship structures simply proves that these are peripheral features of Australian grammars, and not part of the core grammar that Universal Grammar can cover, he has embarked on a slippery slope in which more and more "language devices" are conceded to be cultural products that are learnable without the support of Universal Grammar. When it comes to "UG," we should not put our faith in Universal Grammar but rather seek to identify the hitherto Unidentified Gadgets (a coinage of the late Jean-Roger Vergnaud) that make human use of language possible.

What I have tried to make explicit here is that Universal Grammar is a protean concept and that there are no hard data to support the view that a Universal Grammar in any interesting sense (to be discussed in Chapter 11) is innately specified in a way that reduces the demands on learning mechanisms that enable the child to master the lexicon, periphery, and conventions of his or her language. I further reject the view that language is something to be learned explicitly as a formal manipulation of abstract strings of symbols (i.e., as autonomous syntax) rather than implicitly and iteratively through the effective use of initially very simple utterances. Nonetheless, the notion of autonomy of syntax is attractive. As we saw from Lewis Carroll's *Jabberwocky*, we can enjoy the form of language even if it sacrifices meaning so long as it preserves some orderliness of grammatical structure and prosody in a way that a mere list of random nonwords can rarely accomplish.[6] It is thus certainly fruitful to have *some* linguists try to understand grammatical structure abstracted from the assemblage of meaningful words into meaningful utterances. However, I do not think that syntax evolved as an autonomous part of the mind or that the child acquires syntax in isolation from its meaning. The use of pictures in children's books to help connect patterns of words with meaning gets at the essence of language. On the other hand, the importance of songs and nursery rhymes for children hints at roots of language that complement syntax and semantics but lie in a different direction.

Language in an Action-Oriented Framework

The characterization of linguistic competence as an abstract set of syntactic rules is a useful abstraction, but I doubt that this is the essence of the brain's ability to support language. The Minimalist Program (Fig. 2-6), which is a model of Competence within the framework of autonomous syntax, seeks to define grammars that characterize which strings of words and morphemes do or do not belong to a given language. This may be compared to the way in which Kepler used "conic sections" to *describe* planetary motion. In contrast, Newton's laws of motion, including the inverse square law of gravitation, provided a *dynamical explanation* of planetary motion. My aim now is to turn from a minimalist view to an attempt to situate language within a more general framework provided by action, perception, and social interaction that challenges us to understand how our brains implement two quasi-inverse processes: the production and the perception of utterances of a language.

Recall the discussion of schema theory for basic neuroethology in Chapter 1. Figure 1-1 showed how perceptual schemas activated by a moving object could trigger motor schemas for approach or avoidance in the frog brain. Figure 1-2 showed how a number of perceptual schemas simultaneously activated to characterize properties of an object could activate motor schemas for the coordinated control of reaching for and grasping the object. Here an important point was that the set of activated motor schemas would change as the coordinated actions progress. Figure 1-4 emphasized that visual perception may do more than characterize a single object: it showed how visual input could invoke knowledge coded as a network of schemas in long-term memory to create an assemblage of schema instances that represented aspects of the visual environment.

Figure 2-7 integrates these observations into a single perspective, the *action-perception cycle*. At any time our current perception of the world combines with our current goals, plans, and motivations to activate certain combinations of motor schemas that determine our actions. Each action may change the world and/or our relationship with the world (contrast opening a door versus turning the head, which just shifts the focus of attention). Thus, the input available about the world at any time will change, both because of our actions and because the world may be changing anyway. As a result, the assemblage of currently active schemas will be updated (and will include perceptions of actions and other relationships, as well as objects and their properties or parameters). The rotating arrows at center left indicate that memory structures are invoked in updating our perceptions and our plan of action (further variables relate to the motion and internal state of the body), but they also indicate that each time we perceive the consequences of our actions or simply observe correlated changes in the external world so may both our working memory and long-term memory be modified.

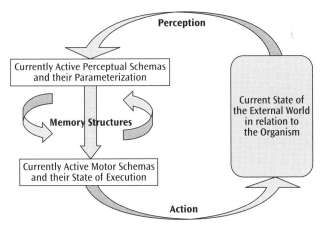

FIGURE 2-7. The Action-Perception Cycle. What we perceive depends on our current plans and actions.

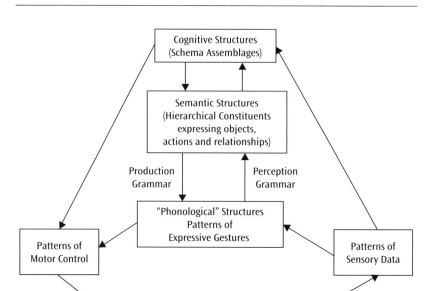

FIGURE 2-8.   The figure places production and perception of language within a framework of action and perception considered more generically. Language production and perception are viewed as the linkage of Semantic Form and Phonological Form, where the "phonology" may involve vocal or manual gestures, or just one of these, with or without the accompaniment of facial gestures.

The three examples of Figures 1-1, 1-2, and 1-4 all relate to our interaction with the physical world. But what of communication with conspecifics, the generation and perception of *communicative actions?* Figure 2-8 creates a framework for approaching language within this enlarged framework. The outer loop Cognitive Structures → Motor Control → External World → Sensory Data → Cognitive Structures is meant to correspond to the action-perception cycle of Figure 2-7. I hypothesize that when we are about to say something, we have extracted certain aspects of the current cognitive structure for expression. I call the result a "semantic structure." For example, in seeing an athlete playing baseball, we may perceive his stance, his uniform, his face, and the pattern of his motion yet abstract from that just his name and his action upon the ball. This might be summarized as Hit (Jim Gromwich, ball, hard). Though the neural coding of this "action frame" would be very different from this sequence of letters, the point here is that what is encoded is stripped bare of details irrelevant to finding the words to express it. It is the job of the *Production Grammar* to then combine semantic, syntactic, and phonological processing to convert this into a sequence of patterns of expressive gestures that command motor control to produce an appropriate utterance in audible or visible form. Conversely, the utterance of a conspecific yields patterns of sensory data that can be recognized, first, as expressive gestures and then "decoded" by the *Perception Grammar*, exploiting cues at various levels, to extract the semantic structure of the utterance that can then modify current cognitive structures, affecting the state of working memory and, possibly, leading to changes in long-term memory structures as well.

I warn the reader that computer scientists and linguists may mean very different things by "semantic structure," so I emphasize that what I mean here is not "logical form" but rather something that is coupled with world knowledge. Thus, for example, a perception might incorporate the knowledge that Hit (Jim Gromwich, ball, hard) is more likely than Bit (Jim Gromwich, ball, hard) to disambiguate a poorly enunciated word that could be heard as a "hit" or "bit." Our discussion of HEARSAY (Figure 1-5) indicated how such a process might operate within a schema-theoretic framework in which schemas compete and cooperate at multiple levels to yield an overall interpretation of an utterance.

Putting this in other terms, at any time we might have much that we could possibly talk about, represented as cognitive structures (*Cognitive Form*; schema assemblages) from which some aspects are selected for possible expression. In most linguistic models of *production*, it is assumed that a semantic structure is given in some "internal code" and that this must be translated into well-formed sentences. However, in an ongoing conversation, our current mental state and our view of the mental state of our listeners create a richness that our next sentence can only sample, and the generation of that sentence may reflect many factors that change our thoughts even as we express them in attempting to reach some communicative goal. To borrow the terminology of motor control, a sentence is not so much a preplanned trajectory as a more or less elegant attempt to hit a moving and ill-identified target. From a "conventional" linguistic viewpoint, a sentence like "Serve the handsome young man on the left" would be analyzed using syntactic rules to parse this specific string of words. But let us look at the sentence not as a structure to be parsed but rather as the result of the attempt by the manager of a restaurant to achieve a *communicative goal*: to get a waiter to serve the intended customer (Arbib, 2006a). His *sentence planning strategy* repeats the "loop" of adding more specifics until (he thinks) referential vagueness is resolved:

(1) Serve the young man.
    Still too vague?
(2) Serve the young man on the left.
    Still too vague?

(3) Serve the handsome young man on the left.

Still too vague? Apparently not. So the manager "executes the plan" and says, "Serve the handsome young man on the left" to the waiter.

Here, a noun phrase NP may be expanded by adding a prepositional phrase PP after it [as in expanding (1) to (2)] or an adjective Adj before it [as in expanding (2) to (3)]. The suggestion is that syntactic rules of English, which I approximate by NP → NP PP and NP → Adj NP, are abstracted in part from procedures that serve to reduce referential vagueness in reaching a communicative goal. This example concentrates on a noun phrase—and thus exemplifies ways in which reaching a communicative goal (identifying the right person or object) may yield an unfolding of word structures in a way that may clarify the early rise of syntactic structures. How the word structures unfold certainly depends on a range of possible syntactic structures from which the manager (or anyone else) could choose. He would not say "handsome the on the left serve man young." But my point (contra checking that a bunch of words can be combined grammatically) is that we generate sentences to achieve a communicative goal, so that cognition, semantics, and syntax all play their role *in an integrated way*. In terms of Figure 2-8, the manager has already perceived the customer he wants the waiter to serve, but he keeps updating the fragment of that structure to be expressed as he assesses whether the semantic structure he is about to employ will indeed serve its purpose. If not, the semantic structure and its phonological expression are unfurled by processes that will, to a greater or lesser extent (recall Fig. 2-1), respect the syntactic constraints of the language employed.

Of course, the syntactic structure of noun phrases reflects a long history of English (and will have a different history and more or less different form in other languages), and so it no doubt has "evolved" to satisfy, more or less adequately, a range of sometimes conflicting criteria. This is *cultural* evolution, which varies from one language community to another. This *Serve the handsome young man on the left* example could be translated into Japanese, and the Japanese restaurant manager's utterance would have pretty much the same communicative goal as that of the English-speaking restaurant manager, but the lexicon and grammar of Japanese would yield a very different phonological expression. My claim, then, is that when we find commonalities in syntax across languages, it is because they evolved culturally to reach shared communicative goals, not because they reflect a single genetically encoded Universal Grammar.

In summary, I see the sentence not as a static structure but rather as the result of adapting and "unfurling" a nested hierarchical structure to extract a set of actions to reach a communicative goal. Thus, while syntactic constructions can be usefully analyzed and categorized from an abstract viewpoint, the pragmatics of what one is trying to say and to whom one is trying to say it will combine with syntactic constraints to drive the goal-directed process of producing a sentence or an even simpler utterance. Conversely, the hearer has the inferential task of unfolding multiple meanings from the word stream (with selective attention) and deciding (perhaps unconsciously) which ones to meld into his or her cognitive state and narrative memory.

Cognitive Linguistics and Construction Grammar

The approach of Figure 2-8 can be seen as a variation on the general theme of Cognitive Linguistics which, as summarized by Croft and Cruse (2005), has three tenets:

1) Language is not an autonomous cognitive module, separated from non-linguistic cognitive abilities.
2) Grammar is linked to conceptual expression.
3) Knowledge of language emerges from language use rather than resting on a predefined, possibly innate, "core" of maximally abstract and general representations of grammatical form and meaning, with many grammatical and semantic phenomena assigned to the "periphery."

For Croft and Cruse (2005), the processes of language use are not fundamentally different from cognitive abilities that human beings use outside the domain of language, such as visual perception, reasoning, or motor activity. However, in this book, we take a somewhat different, though related view. In seeking to understand the evolution of brain mechanisms unique to the human that support the cultural evolution and use of human languages, we do emphasize how much is shared between the cognitive abilities involved in language use, visual perception, and motor activity. Nonetheless, we also seek to understand what extensions of the basic primate brain architecture were required to support language and the forms of reasoning that seem to demand comparable forms of cognition that go beyond the sort of "reasoning" seen in other animals.

In speech, we play variations on a word by various morphological changes that may modify internal phonemes or add new ones. In sign languages, "words" can be modified by changing the source and origin, and by various modifications to the path between. For everything else, it seems enough—for both action and language—that we can create hierarchical structures subject to a set of transformations from those already in the repertoire. For this, the brain must provide a computational medium in which already available elements can be composed to form new ones, irrespective of the "level" at which

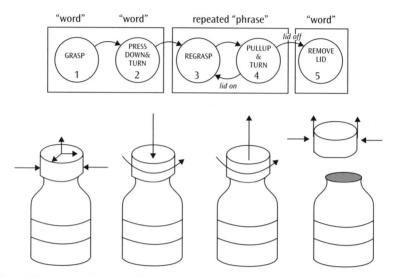

Figure 2-9.   A Motor "Sentential Form": An action such as this one of opening a childproof aspirin bottle is a "sentence" made up of "words" that are basic actions akin in complexity to "reach and grasp": a hierarchical sequence whose subsequences are not fixed in length but instead are conditioned on the achievement of goals and subgoals. (Adapted from Michelman & Allen, 1994; original © IEEE 1994.)

these elements were themselves defined. When we start with words as the elements, we may end up with compound words or phrases, other operations build from both words and phrases to yield new phrases or sentences, and so on recursively. Similarly, we may learn arbitrarily many new motor skills based on those with which we are already familiar.

In Figure 2-9, the example of opening a childproof aspirin bottle illustrates the parallel between action and language offered by a Motor "Sentential Form":

> While holding the bottle with the non-dominant hand, grasp the cap, push down and turn the cap with the dominant hand; then repeat (release cap, pull up cap and turn) until the cap comes loose; then remove the cap.

This hierarchical structure unpacks to different sequences of action on different occasions, with subsequences conditioned on the achievement of goals and subgoals. But chimpanzees can open aspirin bottles, even though they cannot compose sentences. The key challenge of Part 2 of this book will be to bridge this divide, while stressing the role of mechanisms that are shared between human and chimpanzee brains that undergird the features that make the human brain uniquely language-ready. Certainly, a key difference between opening an aspirin bottle and uttering a sentence is that the *external* state of the bottle provides ongoing affordances to guide one as to what to do next. As one utters a sentence word by word, no such guidance from the environment is available, whereas (according to the perspective in Fig. 2-8) the goals for what to say are contained in the *internal* semantic structure that extracts the communicative goals on which the production grammar operates.

Just as cognitive linguists may invoke models from cognitive psychology of memory, perception, attention, and categorization to develop linguistic models of the organization of linguistic knowledge, so too do we appeal to related models, though with more attention to the data of neuroscience, while extending schema theory from perception and action to meet the demands of linguistics. This schema-theoretic approach accords well with the second hypothesis mentioned earlier, which is based on Langacker's slogan "grammar is conceptualization" (Langacker, 1986, 1991). However, where our focus on the book is more on "what grounds the emergence of language?" cognitive linguists are, indeed, linguists—and so their emphasis is on grammatical inflections and constructions and various lexical semantic phenomena, including polysemy and metaphor (Lakoff & Johnson, 1980).

The third major hypothesis certainly accords with our views on how categories and structures in semantics, syntax, morphology, and phonology are built up from our cognition of specific utterances on specific occasions of use. The challenge, briefly touched upon later in Chapter 11 in the section "Language Acquisition and the Development of Constructions" is to show how inductive process of abstraction and schematization can yield the subtleties of grammatical constructions and word meanings that relate to communication within the social schemas of the particular language community in which the child (or the later language learner) develops.

Cognitive linguists see subtle variations in syntactic behavior and semantic interpretation as demanding a different model of grammatical representation that accommodates idiosyncratic as well as highly general patterns of linguistic behavior. For this, we now turn to Construction Grammar. The starting point is not the emergence of language so much as the way in which each modern language contains relics of its history in the form of *idioms*, which have meanings familiar to speakers of the language *even if they bear no obvious relation to the meaning of the words that make up the idiom*. Thus, the English idiom *he kicked the bucket* means *he died*. Perhaps one could give a fake etymology (maybe it's even correct) for this, as in suggesting someone standing on a bucket and attempting to hang himself would only succeed when he kicked the bucket away. But the point is that this "etymology" plays no role in understanding the phrase, and so we cannot infer its meaning by applying compositional semantics and the general rules of syntax to understand this idiom. One approach would be to think of such phrases as not being part of grammar at all, instead simply adding idiomatic expressions like *kick the bucket, shoot the breeze, take the bull by the horns* and *climb the wall* to the lexicon since, after all, no dictionary is really complete if it only contains single words and excludes all portmanteaus. This raises a problem, though. Our use of idioms is productive. We can say *He kicked the bucket* or *They'll kick the bucket if they keep messing with the drug gangs*— but perhaps not *They are kicking the bucket.* So it seems that we still need grammar "inside the idioms." Thus, rather than consider the meanings of idioms as a supplement to the general rules of syntax and semantics, Fillmore, Kay, and O'Connor (1988) suggested that the tools they used in analyzing idioms could form the basis for *construction grammar* as a new model of grammatical organization. On this view, constructions range from lexical items to idioms to rules of quite general applicability. The grammar of each language is given by a more or less language-specific set of constructions that combine *form* (how to aggregate words) with *meaning* (how the meaning of the words constrains the meaning of the whole—though I will later have to re-examine the various kinds of meaning or semantics that enter into our understanding of sentences). In the case of an idiom, *it is the construction itself, rather than the meanings of the words that comprise it, that determines the overall meaning.* This is to be contrasted with a grammar in which autonomous syntactic rules can only put words together in very general ways without regard for the meaning of the result. Linguists working within Construction Grammar, with its close relations to Cognitive Grammar, have teased out the rule-governed and productive linguistic behaviors specific to each family of constructions (Croft & Cruse, 2005). Constructions, like items in the lexicon, combine syntactic, semantic, and even in some cases phonological information. In Construction Grammar, *He kicked the bucket* is ambiguous because it has two parsings. One yields an instance of the general formula *He X'd the Y* whose overall meaning varies with the meanings of *X* and *Y*. The other yields a term in which no substitutions can be made for *kick* and *bucket* and the meaning has no relation to those of *kick* or *bucket*. As Hurford (2011, Chapter 4) notes, there is evidence that on hearing an idiom, both the overall meaning (e.g., *die*) and the meanings of the individual parts (e.g., *kick* and *bucket*) can be primed, suggesting redundant storage. This fits in with our general view of competition and cooperation of schemas, so that in this case, the initial activation of constructions for both parsings can have a priming effect even though just one wins the competition in determining our understanding of the sentence that contains the idiom.

Consider the contrast between the Active and Passive constructions yielding the two forms:

Active: John kissed Mary.
Passive: Mary was kissed by John.

In each case, the underlying action is kissing, with John the Agent and Mary the Patient of the act. But the two forms of the underlying "action-frame" Kiss (John, Mary) shift our focus of attention.

The Active form gets us to attend to what John is doing.

The Passive form emphasizes what is happening to Mary.

Another contrast between what at first seem to be equivalent ways of arranging a given set of words is that between the Dative and Ditransitive:

Dative: You gave the book to Mary.
Ditransitive: You gave Mary the book.

These seem to mean much the same thing. Consider this example:

Dative: You gave the slip to Mary.
Ditransitive: You gave Mary the slip.

These are both acceptable if *the slip* is an undergarment, but the Dative form is blocked if *giving the slip to* is used as an idiom for *eluded* or *escaped from*.

Thus, it seems that the Ditransitive adds this extra kernel of meaning to the words in a way that the Dative does not. It is keeping track of the restrictions on what can fill the slots in the constructions, as well as the need to keep track of how the construction can add its own meaning to its application that motivates the move to construction grammar. Note the analyses of an autonomous syntax:

Dative: [NP [V NP1 [to NP2]] *versus* Ditransitive: [NP [V NP2 NP1]

do not carry the extra subtleties we need for the above analyses, namely

Dative: *You gave the book to Mary* as a case of *XWY to Z* meaning
                X moved Y along path Z by means W.
                You moved the b*ook* along path *to Mary* by means *giving*
Ditransitive: *You gave Mary the book* as a case of *XWZY* meaning
                X transferred Y to Z by means W, with the restriction that Z
                can serve as an active recipient.
                You transferred *the book* to *Mary* by means of *giving*.

The rules of generative grammar have "slots" that can be filled with any item that belongs to a very broad syntactic category. By contrast, the set of fillers for given slots in a construction may comprise a single word (*bucket* cannot be replaced by *pail* in the idiom *he kicked the bucket*, though *he* can be replaced by another expression for a formerly animate person) but may vary between constructions from a specific word in one construction to a narrowly defined semantic category, to a broadly defined semantic category, to a syntactic category that cuts across semantic categories, but that may do so in a highly language-specific way (Croft, 2001). Thus, the categories in a construction grammar may be very different from those in a generative grammar. In some cases they are similar to general syntactic categories like *noun* or *verb* that cut across constructions, but in other cases they will be more semantic in nature.

Kemmerer (2000a, 2000b) was among the first to make explicit the relevance of construction grammar to neurolinguistics and has used the framework of construction grammar to present the major semantic properties of action verbs and argument structure constructions (e.g., Kemmerer, 2006). He supports the view that grammatical categories like noun, verb, and adjective gradually emerged over the course of hundreds or thousands of generations of historical language transmission and change and became increasingly complex, perhaps according to well-known processes of grammaticalization (Givón, 1998; Heine, Claudi, & Hünnemeyer, 1991; Tomasello, 2003b; see Chapter 13). But what constitutes a noun, a verb, or an adjective may differ radically for different languages. The criteria used for grammatical categories in some languages are either completely absent in others or are employed in ways that seem bizarre for those brought up on English. Nouns are often marked for case, number, gender, size, shape, definiteness, and possession/alienability; verbs are often marked for tense, aspect, mood, modality, transitivity, and agreement; and adjectives are often marked for comparative, superlative, intensive, and approximative. However, some languages, like Vietnamese, lack all inflection, while other languages have inflection but employ it in a surprising manner, as exemplified by Makah, the language of a group of Native Americans of the American Northwest, which applies aspect and mood markers not only to words for actions that are translated into English as verbs but also to words for things and properties that are translated into English as nouns and adjectives.

For such reasons, Croft (e.g., 2001) rejects the claim for innate, universal grammatical categories and instead seeks to identify the grammatical categories of an individual language according to the constructions the language employs. *This does not preclude cross-linguistically identifying prototypical nouns as specifying objects and prototypical verbs as specifying actions.* But a word classified as a nonprototypical verb in one language may correspond to a different category in another language. On this account, human languages contain an open-ended spectrum of historically shaped, constructionally based, hierarchically organized, and distributionally learned grammatical categories. This is very much consistent with the notion espoused in this book that languages evolved culturally as the collectivity of many properties through *bricolage*, that is, a process of "tinkering" that added, combined, and modified constructions, not just modifying the lexicon. This process occurred in diverse ways across many communities and with diffusion between communities rather than Language-with-a-capital-L evolving as a biological unity (Dixon, 1997; Lass, 1997).

A Visually Grounded Version of Construction Grammar

In discussing the sentence *Serve the handsome young man on the left*, we suggested that the production of a sentence could be interpreted as involving planning of how to reach a communicative goal. In terms of Figure 2-8, then, the manager has a rather elaborate task: His cognitive structures include representations of certain relevant aspects of the current situation, some aspects of a desired situation (a particular customer gets served straight away), and some appreciation of the "mental state" of the waiter, i.e., what he knows and thus what he needs to be told (were the customer a regular, the manager might instead say *Serve Larry Zhang*, assuming the waiter recalled the young man's name). Before going on, let me ask the reader to ponder the structure and meaning of the two previous sentences. They are more formally structured than they would have been had I sought to convey the same idea during spontaneous speech, but they too required a (very complex) cognitive structure that combined my understanding of what I wanted to tell you with my estimate of what you knew at this stage of reading the book, and where it might be appropriate to jog your memory. A full computational account of how this can be achieved in such complexity, let alone a deep analysis of the neural mechanisms involved, is currently beyond the state of the art. Instead, I devote this section to a much simpler case: the generation of an utterance that describes a visual scene. The hope is that this special case, despite its obvious limitations in addressing the phenomena involved in producing the sentences of this paragraph, will lay a firm groundwork for future exploration.

Inspired by the VISIONS system that deploys a set of perceptual schemas to label objects in a static visual scene (Chapter 1), Arbib and Lee (2007, 2008) introduced SemRep as a hierarchical graph-like "semantic representation" of a visual scene, whether static or dynamically extended over time (an episode). In terms of Figure 2-8, the schema assemblage of VISIONS provides the example of a Cognitive Structure while a SemRep provides the example of a Semantic structure. As we will see shortly, the production grammar employed is Template Construction Grammar.

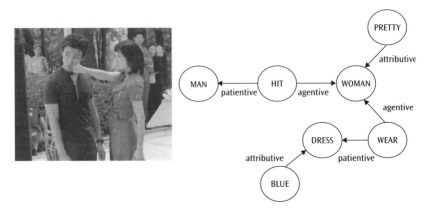

Figure 2-10.   (*Left*) A picture of a woman hitting a man (original image from "Invisible Man Jangsu Choi," Korean Broadcasting System). (*Right*) A SemRep graph that could be generated for the picture. Arbib and Lee (2007, 2008) describe how Template Construction Grammar may operate on this to yield the sentence "A pretty woman in blue hits a man." (See color insert for full color version of this figure.)

Consider the specific scene shown on the left of Figure 2-10. The visual system may initially recognize a variety of aspects of the scene centered around the central figures of the man and woman, while ignoring other aspects of the scene—a given scene may be perceived in many different ways. This analysis may combine activation of a number of schema instances together with activity in the visual system that could be used to support further schema analysis, but it has not yet done so. SemRep then abstracts from this pattern of schema activation a set of nodes and relations that constitute one possible semantic structure for the current scene. The properties of a recognized object are attached to the node for that instance of the object, and the semantics of an action are attached to another node with specific edges linking it to nodes representing agents and objects that play specific roles in that action. The attached concepts will later be translated into words by the language system. However, the SemRep graph is not labeled with words but with more abstract descriptors, allowing the same graph to be expressed in multiple ways within a given language. Thus, the concept YOUNG FEMALE could yield a variety of phonological forms such as "girl," "woman," or even "kid" and the action concept HITTING WITH HAND could be expressed as "hit," "punch," or "slap." Again, the visual configuration where object A is placed vertically higher than B can be expressed as "A is above B," "B is below A," "A is on B," and so on. The suggestion is that each SemRep expresses semantic relations but with no commitment to word choice, and it can thus be the basis for description in any language once the appropriate grammar and lexicon are deployed. (But, of course, the SemRep does reflect the viewer's development within a particular community, and thus it reflects the interaction of visual experience with the use of a particular language in shaping the viewer's perceptual schemas.)

A single scene can have many SemReps. Each SemRep encompasses one analysis that captures a subset of the agents, objects, actions, and relationships that may be present in the one (temporally extended) visual scene. For example, the initial perception of the scene might be expanded to take into account more and more of the objects and figures in the background. SemRep may be viewed as an abstraction from the assemblages of schema instances in the working memory of VISIONS, but with the crucial addition of actions and events extended in time. Note that dynamic scene analysis takes us beyond the analysis of single images. If we see a picture of a man with a woman's hand flat against his cheek, and we have no cues from his facial expression, we cannot tell whether the scene is "woman slapping man" or "woman stroking man's cheek" unless we can see the temporal sequence of which this is part.

A schema instance may be associated with a number of parameters (in the sense of characterizing an object)—some of which (such as size, shape, orientation, and location) may be relevant to possible interactions with an object that the schema represents (cf. the reach to grasp of Fig. 1-2 in Chapter 1) and yet not be included in a verbal expression concerning the object. We thus postulate that SemRep needs to explicitly represent very few parameters of the observed objects and actions, and can direct requests to Visual Working Memory when the information is needed for explicit cognitive processing or verbal expression. Each parameter that *does* get made explicit at the SemRep level is considered an attribute and given its own node to be linked to the node for the parameterized schema. For example, the color blue might be used "subconsciously" to conduct the segmentation of the visual scene that separates the figure of the woman from the background, but this does not guarantee that the color is noticed consciously. Figure 2-10 represents the case where it has been, so that the color BLUE is an attribute of the object DRESS.

One more observation. VISIONS proceeds with scene analysis by the setting and updating of "confidence levels," indicating the weight of evidence for a specific schema instance to interpret a given region of a scene, based on the state of competition and cooperation within the network. Similarly—but the two values are different—in SemRep, each node may be assigned a value representing "discourse importance." Thus, if we are talking about John, then John has greater discourse importance than Mary, and we might say, "John loves Mary"; but if the focus (higher significance value) is given to Mary, we might instead say, "Mary is loved by John."

Template Construction Grammar (Arbib & Lee, 2008) adopts two major policies of conventional construction grammar: Each construction specifies the mapping between form and meaning, and the systematic combination of constructions yields the whole grammatical structure. However, in Template Construction Grammar, the semantic structure of an utterance is given as a SemRep graph (with suitable extensions to be provided in further work).

A *construction* is defined by a triple (name, class, template) where:

- *Name* is the name of the construction. It is not involved in the language process—it is only there for reference purposes.
- *Class* specifies the "category" of the result of applying the construction. It determines for which other constructions the result of applying this construction could serve as an input. In the examples considered here the class is the conventional syntactic category, such as NOUN or VERB, for the head of the phrase, which is returned on applying the construction. In general, though, the class of a construction will have to define a more-or-less subtle combination of syntactic and semantic information.
- The *template* defines the form-meaning pair of a construction and has two components:
- *Sem-Frame* (SemRep frame) defines the meaning part of the construction. Its meaning is defined by the part of a SemRep graph that the construction will "cover." Each element of this graph is attached to a concept and an activation value as is a typical SemRep graph element. Added to that, Sem-Frame also specifies the "head" element, which acts as a representative element of the whole construction when forming hierarchy with other constructions.
- *Lex-Seq* (lexical sequence) defines the form part of the construction. It is a string of words, morphemes, and empty slots. Each slot can be filled with the output of other constructions. Each empty slot specifies the class of a construction that will fill it and the link to the element of Sem-Frame connected to the slot.

The lexical constructions at the top of Figure 2-11 exemplify the way in which the concept associated with a single node of the SemRep can ground the selection of a word to express that concept. The constructions at the bottom of Figure 2-11 move expression up the hierarchy to cover larger and larger parts of the SemRep. Thus, the IN_DRESS construction has the interesting property that it must recognize a node like FROCK but only uses it to license the construction that yields *pretty woman in blue*, where the nodes for WOMAN and PRETTY have already been covered by another construction to yield the phrase *pretty woman* to fill the NP slot in IN_DRESS.

A SemRep may yield one or more utterances as Template Construction Grammar finds ways to "cover" the relevant portion of the given SemRep with a set of "small" subgraphs, where each is chosen such that a construction is available which expresses that subgraph in the given language. In production mode, the template acts to match constraints for selecting proper

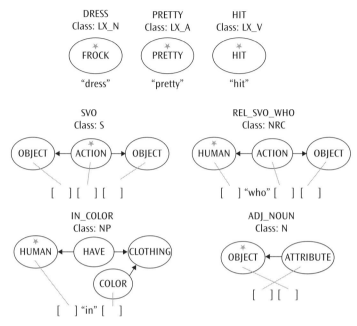

FIGURE 2-11.   (*Top*) Examples of constructions that correspond to elements in the lexicon. (*Bottom*) Higher level constructions used to encode grammatical information. Each construction is a SemRep-like graph with either generic or specific labels on the edges and nodes, with each linked to a text or an empty slot. For each slot there may be restrictions as to what can serve as slot fillers. The star singles out the head of each construction.

constructions by being superimposed on the SemRep graph. The semantic constraint of each construction is considered to be encoded in the template since the template specifies concepts as well as the topology of a SemRep graph. Thus, constructions are applied recursively, by starting with lexical constructions, which have no variables (Fig. 2-11 top), and then by applying higher level constructions (Fig. 2-11 bottom) in such a way that slots are matched to the results of earlier application of constructions whose category matches that of the slot. In this way, the scheme of VISIONS may be lifted to a similar structure (Fig. 2-12) in which the Linguistic Working Memory for the state of applying construction to the current SemRep provides the workspace for the operation of construction selection and attachment, thus providing a dynamic set of extended SemReps with varying degrees of confidence.

Figure 2-12 shows two systems running basically in parallel. During production of a description, a number of constructions are activated simultaneously to build upon the unfolding SemRep. Constructions cooperate and compete with each other in order to produce a verbal description of a scene.

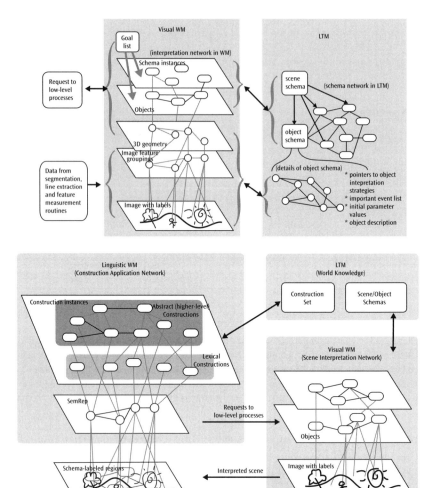

FIGURE 2-12.   (*Top*) The VISIONS system (this is just Fig. 1-4). Visual Working Memory (Visual WM) provides a segmentation of the image, associated with instances of perceptual schemas that cover various regions. (*Bottom*) The structure of our model of scene description. It echoes the interaction of Visual WM and Long-Term Memory (LTM) in VISIONS, but here the input is the spatial array of schema instances provided by Visual WM. Based on visual attention and communicative goals, the system extracts a SemRep to capture key aspects of the scene. TCG then can apply lexical constructions to associate nodes with words, and higher level constructions to build on nodes that are either in SemRep or have already been formed as the result of earlier application of constructions. The current Linguistic Working Memory holds a hierarchical covering of the current SemRep by iterated application of constructions from Long-Term Memory—it provides not only Working Memory for Construction Applications but also allows an utterance to be read off at any time. Just as VISIONS allows Visual WM to request more data from low-level processes, so does our model link Linguistic WM to the visual system via the Visual WM when completion of an utterance requires further attention to the visual scene.

The language system, which develops the Linguistic Working Memory (WM), applies constructions on SemRep hierarchically and reads off the formed sentence or sentence fragments that result. The vision system concurrently interprets the scene and updates the SemRep. As Spivey et al. (2005) note, the visual environment can be treated as an external memory with eye movements being the typical access method. Sometimes the language system may generate requests for more details from the vision system. Constructions are applied based on the "current" SemRep, and on the WM, where there are a number of partially (or fully) created construction structures. The system produces utterances as soon as some threshold is reached. A speaker with a low threshold may produce "sentence fragments," while one with a high threshold may tend to talk in complete sentences. The sentence-forming process is both incremental since new constructions are constantly being applied according to the current conceptual representation, SemRep, and hierarchical since constructions may be applied atop other constructions to form a hierarchical organization above those attached directly to the SemRep.

By making explicit how mechanisms for describing a scene in words are similar to those for recognizing what is in the scene, Figure 2-12 illustrates the earlier claim that "we do emphasize how much is shared between the cognitive abilities involved in language use, visual perception, and motor activity...[but] we also seek to understand what extensions of the basic primate brain architecture were required to support language." The general thesis here is that language processing should not be analyzed in terms of abstract processing of strings or trees of symbols (though this is, for some purposes, a useful abstraction), but rather should be seen as "lifting" more general processes whereby spatiotemporal patterns of sensory data are converted into one of many possible courses of action. In the present case, construction applications are accumulated with varying degrees of confidence, with sequences of words read out from time to time from composites of recent, high-confidence applications of constructions in linguistic working memory.

3

Vocalization and Gesture in Monkey and Ape

All animals have ways of communicating with members of their own species. Ants live in social societies coordinated by the secretion and sensing of chemical signals. Bees returning to the hive after foraging dance a waggle dance that signals the direction and distance of a food source they have discovered. Chickens have a variety of calls, and some songbirds learn their own distinctive songs to defend their territory and attract mates. And primates—including the great apes and monkeys—can, to degrees that vary from species to species, communicate by vocal calls and by facial and manual gestures. Yet none of these communication systems constitutes a language in the sense in which English or Thai or Swahili is a language—possessing both an open-ended vocabulary or lexicon, and the syntax supporting a compositional semantics for combining the words of that lexicon into novel, meaningful, and possibly quite complex, sentences as the occasion demands.[1]

Our concern in Part 2 of this book will be to understand how the human brain evolved to enable us to learn and use language whereas other creatures cannot. To maintain focus, we will say little more about the birds[2] and nothing about the bees, but we will focus on the communication systems of monkeys and apes. This will suggest something of the state of the last common ancestors of humans and monkeys and of humans and apes. One estimate suggests that the human evolutionary line diverged from that of monkeys some 25 million years ago, from the gorillas 7 million years ago, and from chimpanzees, our closest extant nonhuman relatives, some 5 to 7 million years ago.[3] Figure 3-1 provides a gallery of the monkeys and the apes (including humans!) we will meet in the following pages.

Vocalization

Nonhuman primates—including the great apes and monkeys—share to some extent an overall body plan with humans, but we lack tails and there are other

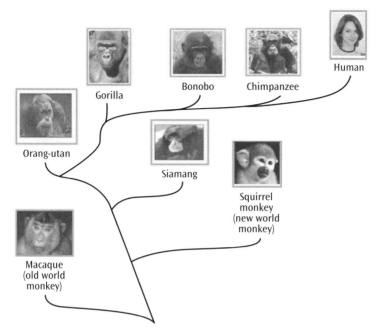

F<small>IGURE</small> 3-1.　An evolutionary gallery of primates, including humans. (Photographs by courtesy of Katja Liebal; expanded from a figure in Arbib, Liebal, & Pika, 2008.)

differences, such as in our degree of dexterity and in our brains and behaviors. Humans are more dexterous, can learn to speak, and can walk on two legs far better than other primates can. The monkey's communication system is *closed* in the sense that it is restricted to a small repertoire. By contrast, human languages are *open* both as to the creation of new vocabulary and the ability to combine words and grammatical markers in diverse ways to yield an essentially unbounded stock of sentences whose meanings are new yet understandable.

"Birds fly" is a useful generalization, but there are particular species of birds—such as penguins, kiwis, and ostriches—to which it does not apply. Similarly, there are many different species of monkey, and different species have different sets of communicative gestures. Thus, when I talk of "*the* monkey," I am offering rather large generalizations, which will from time to time be qualified by data on a particular species. In particular, when it comes to brain mechanisms in the next chapter, we will focus primarily on the macaque monkey and, to a lesser extent, the squirrel monkey. Monkeys exhibit a call system (a limited set of species-specific calls) and an orofacial (mouth and face) gesture system with some of these expressive of emotion, while others vary depending on the social hierarchy (Maestripieri, 1999). The linkage between the face and voice reminds us that communication is inherently multimodal— requiring both auditory and visual perception, at the very least, as well as the ability to control a range of different effector systems.

Perhaps the most famous monkey calls are the three alarm calls of vervet monkeys—one each to distinctively signal the presence of leopards, eagles, and snakes (Cheney & Seyfarth, 1990). The meaning of the *leopard alarm call* can be *approximated* in English by "There is a leopard nearby. Danger! Danger! Repeat the call. Run up a tree to escape." The first monkey to see the leopard utters the call; the call is then contagious, as (depending to some extent upon context) other monkeys both utter the call and seek to escape by running up a tree.

Here's an example of the type of study that has been conducted with monkeys to show that the calls have much the same behavioral impact as the actual cry or growl of the predator, even though these sound quite different from the alarm call. If, say, the eagle call is played back again and again in the absence of an eagle, the monkeys habituate— that is, they respond less each time. The same is true for repeated playback of the actual shriek of an eagle. The crucial observation is that if the monkey is habituating to the eagle alarm call and the eagle shriek is then played, the habituation carries over, even though the vervet's call and the eagle's shriek are completely different acoustically. In other words, the monkey has habituated to the semantics of the call, not its sound (Zuberbühler, Cheney, & Seyfarth, 1999).

Primate calls do exhibit an *audience effect*—vervet alarm calls are given usually in the presence of conspecifics who would react to them (see Cheney & Seyfarth, 1990, Chapter 5). For example, vervet monkeys do not always call when a predator appears, but the likelihood of their calling will increase in the presence of close kin. Learning does not seem to play a role in acquiring the vocal patterns for these calls, but it does play a role in knowing precisely when to use these signals and how to respond to them when they are produced by others (Seyfarth & Cheney, 2002). Infant vervet monkeys often make mistakes by giving an eagle alarm call to other moving things in the sky, not just eagles. Only later do they learn to confine these to adult-like contexts.

Vocalizations seem not to be used intentionally to influence the behavior of specific others. For example, chimpanzees seem unable to suppress food grunts, although these may inform higher ranking group members about the presence of food so that as a result the grunting chimpanzee loses access (Goodall, 1986). Such communication indicates how the animal feels or what the animal wants. Topics for nonhuman primate communication include play, nursing, grooming, travel, willingness (or otherwise) to mate, defending territory, aggression or appeasement directed toward a conspecific, keeping in contact with other members of the group, or alarm calls that warn of the approach of predators. Thus, nonhuman primate vocal communication may not involve the caller's assessment of the recipient's knowledge but simply the recipients' presence or absence. However, Byrne and Whiten (1988) report that monkeys will give alarm calls when they are being attacked by other monkeys or when they wish to keep some food for themselves. If indeed the latter is a case of genuine "deception," then perhaps some aspect of the voluntary does enter the picture.

Units of primate communication systems almost never combine to yield additional meanings. This contrasts with human language, which is based essentially on the combination of words and other units. Where most monkey calls are emitted with no particular order but rather as the context demands, there is some evidence for limited combinations in monkey vocal utterances. Male Campbell's monkeys give acoustically distinct alarm calls to leopards and crowned-hawk eagles. In situations that seem less dangerous, Campbell's monkeys precede their alarm calls with a pair of low, resounding "boom" calls. In a playback experiment, Zuberbühler (2002) established that wild Diana monkeys respond to Campbell's monkey alarm calls with their own corresponding alarm calls. But if he played back Campbell's monkey alarm calls to Diana monkeys with the alarm call immediately preceded by Campbell's monkey booms, these compound calls no longer elicited alarm calls in Diana monkeys, indicating that the booms had affected the semantic specificity of the subsequent alarm calls—the meaning of the alarm call was altered by another call that acted as a modifier. Interestingly, when the booms preceded the alarm calls of Diana monkeys (rather than those of Campbell's monkeys), however, they were no longer effective as "semantic modifiers." But let us try to speculate about the semantics involved. We may think of the boom as a specific message "The alarm that I (a Campbell monkey) am about to sound is not serious." If this "don't worry" is given by a Campbell monkey, it has no force if given before a Diana alarm call. Interestingly, then, a Diana monkey in this experiment is not simply responding to a sequence of calls but recognizes the source of the calls and responds accordingly.

In a later related study, Arnold and Zuberbühler (2006a, 2006b) found that male putty-nosed monkeys regularly combine "pyow" and "hack" calls into "pyow-hack" sequences, which usually consist of one, two, or three pyows followed by up to four hacks. They further demonstrated that this combination is linked to specific external events, such as the imminent movement of the group. They argue that "combining existing calls into meaningful sequences increases the variety of messages that can be generated." This is true, but Arnold and Zuberbühler (2006b) seemed to be claiming more when the first sentence of their abstract reads, "Syntax sets human language apart from other natural communication systems, although its evolutionary origins are obscure." Even though they never mention "syntax" or "evolution" in the body of the article, it is worth debating whether the pyow-hack sequences should be seen as a precursor of syntax. Human language has two essential properties: (a) syntax combines words and morphemes into an open-ended set of new utterances, and (b) syntax is linked to a *compositional semantics* that (in most cases) exploits the structure of an utterance to infer an overall meaning based on the meaning of its components. Having one set of sequences with a single meaning does not qualify as a precursor for syntax with compositional semantics. The distinction is between a novel combination being understood as something different and the combination being understood as one of a set of combinations formed according to some general constructions that allow the meaning of even novel combinations to be understood so long as they fall under that already shared construction. If a newcomer to Australia could correctly use the word "Good" to signify approval and the phrase "Good morning" as a greeting, and had no other words or phrases in English, one would be hard put to know whether the newcomer was on his or her way to using English as a language rather than being restricted to a small set of useful but stereotyped vocalizations.

A useful comparison point is provided by birdsong. It is common to say that a song-learning bird must learn "syllables" and how to combine those syllables, possibly hierarchically, to be able to reproduce the song. Some birds may learn a single song; a nightingale may have a repertoire of 200 songs. Some researchers refer to the putting together of syllables and phrases as a "syntax." For example, Okanoya (2004) found in Bengalese finches that lesions of NIf, a higher order song control nucleus of the bird brain, yielded a simplified "syntax" of the bird's song. Moreover, he found that females stimulated with complex songs had higher estradiol levels and carried more nesting material than those stimulated with the simpler song. However, the patterning of birdsong has no attendant compositional semantics for inferring a meaning from the assembly of its parts, and the latter is essential for language.

Just as the calls of chickens are qualitatively different from the songs of songbirds and these in turn lack the compositional semantics of language, so are primate calls qualitatively different from human speech. For example, the separation calls of a squirrel monkey, a macaque monkey, and a human are similar, and the normal crying pattern of human infants conforms to the general primate form. Intriguingly, though, Philip Lieberman (1991) has argued that the pattern of human crying has been adapted for language, though not in relation to its syntax and semantics. Instead, he suggests, it provides the breathing in and out that segments the flow of speech into sentences.[4] This supports the view that human language involves cooperative control by "old" areas (see the section *Auditory Systems and Vocalization* in Chapter 4) and "new" areas specific to the integration of phonology, syntax, and semantics in the use of language.

Facial Expressions

Facial expressions are sometimes considered a type of gesture. We may speak of orofacial gestures if we emphasize particular mouth movements as is the case for a monkey's teeth chatter or lipsmacks (Ferrari, Gallese, Rizzolatti, & Fogassi, 2003). Some facial expressions are closely linked to the production of vocalizations such as horizontal pout face in chimpanzees (linked to whimpering) or full open grin (linked to scream) (Goodall, 1986). They are difficult to measure, though recent work has developed Facial Action Coding Schemes (FACS) for chimpanzees (Vick, Waller, Parr, Smith Pasqualini, & Bard, 2007), rhesus macaques (Parr, Waller, Burrows, Gothard, & Vick, 2010), and other primates. Conversely, differing affective states—such as sexual ecstasy and pain—may result in similar facial expressions. Staring is an example of a facial gesture neither orofacial nor linked to vocalizations.[5]

As is the case for vocalizations, many facial expressions are closely linked to the affective expressions of emotional states. But some do appear to be under voluntary control and therefore can be defined as intentional signals. Great apes like orangutans and chimpanzees use a play-face when approaching the recipient to make sure that he perceives a hitting gesture or wrestling as invitation to play and not as aggression, whereas siamangs (a species of gibbon) frequently use a play-face during solitary play but do not direct it toward a particular recipient. Tanner and Byrne (1993) described a gorilla female who tried to hide her play-face by covering it with her hand, an apparent attempt to control an involuntarily displayed facial expression. Peters and Ploog (1973) report that some human patients with brain damage will produce affective facial expressions reflecting their emotional state but cannot voluntarily move the face. This suggests that the motor systems controlling affective facial expressions are different from those controlling voluntary facial movements.

A variety of facial expressions have been described for Old World monkeys such as macaques and baboons. Since rhesus macaques reared in isolation still produce their species-specific facial expressions, there may be a very strong genetic component to nonhuman facial expressions. Certain facial expressions can be found in both monkeys and apes and are used in a number of different functional contexts, such as aggressive encounters, submissive behavior, grooming, and mother–infant interactions. Differences between species may become obvious not only in the repertoire of facial expressions but also in frequency of use. For example, although both orangutans and siamangs use a few facial expressions, orangutans perform them much less than siamangs do (Liebal, Pika, & Tomasello, 2004, 2006). However, there are at present too few studies to permit us to generalize about systematic differences in the use of facial expressions between great apes, gibbons, and monkeys.

Manual Gesture

Famously, C.S. Peirce saw the trichotomy of *icons*, *indexes*, and *symbols* as the most fundamental division of signs. He differentiated these three as follows:

> ...every sign is determined by its object, either first, by partaking in the characters of the object, when I call the sign an *Icon*; secondly, by being really and in its individual existence connected with the individual object, when I call the sign an *Index*; thirdly, by more or less approximate certainty that it will be interpreted as denoting the object, in consequence of a habit..., when I call the sign a *Symbol*. (Peirce, 1931–58, volume 4, p. 531)

For example, the sign ☼ is an icon for the sun, the spoken utterance *bow-wow* is an index for a dog, but the word *horse* is neither an icon nor an index for the four-legged animal that it denotes. However, we will find it useful to employ the term *symbol* for any sign whose use is sanctioned by convention, and thus allow the notion of *iconic* symbols.[6] This makes sense because—looking ahead to language—it seems unhelpful to say a word is not a symbol if it resembles what it represents (e.g., "burble" for the sound of a brook), or that a sign of sign language is not a symbol if it is a conventionalization of a pantomime (recall Fig. 2-4 in Chapter 2). We can extend the term *symbol* to some animal calls and gestures—though if they are innate, we will not call them symbols but can nonetheless seek to determine what they refer to or what they mean to the animal that emits them and the animal that perceives them. Alarm calls are not iconic, since they do not share the form of the noises made by the relevant predators. When we turn from calls to ape gestures, however, we find that the latter often are iconic: Lowering the head or presentation of the rump may indicate submission, while high-pitched squeaky sounds also indicate submission, with deep rasping sounds indicating dominance. In either case, length, pitch, or intensity of a call or communicative gesture may vary with the degree of emotion expressed.

Apes use their gestures flexibly across a number of different functional contexts and adjust their gestures depending on the recipient's behavior. These features are characteristics of intentional communication—the sender adjusts its communicative means by augmentation, addition, or substitution of the signal until the social goal is obtained (Bates, Benigni, Bretherton, Camaioni, & Volterra, 1979). The majority of ape gestures performed in interactions with conspecifics are used dyadically for imperative purposes to attract the attention of others and to request actions from others (Pika, Liebal, Call, & Tomasello, 2005). By *dyadic*, we mean that the gesture refers only to the direct interaction between the two apes (the dyad). However, some gestures are—like the vervet alarm calls—triadic in that they relate the communicating agents to some external object or agent. We may call such gestures referential, with that third object or agent being the reference of the gesture (though, as in the case of the alarm call, that gesture will be freighted with meaning relevant to action, rather than a labeling of the referent). Indeed, there is limited evidence of ape gestures that are used referentially. For example, although gestures such as *directed scratches* used by chimpanzees in the wild (Pika & Mitani, 2006, 2009) differ qualitatively from symbolic gestures in human children, they might be transmitted via social learning and provide evidence that chimpanzees have an understanding of the intended meaning of the gesture.

Most gestures used by apes are imperative gestures "used to get another individual to help in attaining a goal" (Pika, Liebal, Call et al., 2005). These gestures are made with the trunk, the hands, the head, and the mouth, and they generally take place in a context of play, in a food context, or in an agonistic contexts such as grooming, sexual behavior, nursing, and submissive behavior.

Whereas the vocalizations of nonhuman primate calls seem to be genetically specified, the set of gestures used by apes vary between groups. Some seem to express an essential component of genetic influence; for example, human-raised gorillas that never saw a conspecific would still produce the chest beat (Redshaw & Locke, 1976). However, idiosyncratic gestures have been seen in great apes. Some were shared by several members of a group. Others were used only by single individuals—as such it seems unlikely that they were genetically determined or socially learned—and yet they were used to achieve a certain social goal such as play and most often caused a response of the recipient (Pika, Liebal, & Tomasello, 2003). Tomasello and Call (1997) argue that such group-specific gestures are learned via an individual learning process, *ontogenetic ritualization*, wherein a communicative signal is created by two individuals shaping each other's behavior in repeated instances of an interaction. The general form of this type of learning is as follows:

- Individual A performs behavior X.
- Individual B reacts consistently with behavior Y.
- Subsequently B anticipates A's performance of the complete behavior X by performing Y after observing only some initial segment X' of X.

• Finally, A anticipates B's anticipation and produces the initial step in a ritualized form X^R (waiting for a response) *in order to* elicit Y.

Here is an example from the interaction of a caregiver with a mobile human infant. At first, to get the child to come closer, the adult will grasp the child and gently pull her toward himself to initiate the child's approach. As time passes, it is enough to extend the hand toward the child for the child to come closer. Eventually, the reaching-to-pull movement may be truncated to a simple beckoning with the index finger. This example is instructive in two ways. First, consistently with the view of Tomasello and Call (1997), this gesture *may* emerge through ontogenetic ritualization. However, where they put the primary emphasis on the signal as created by two individuals shaping each other's behavior, we see here the case where the caregiver already knows the beckoning gesture and what it means, and so the process of ontogenetic ritualization is itself shaped by social learning controlled by the form of a gesture already shared within the community—the caregiver is staging the child's experience so he will eventually come to share the meaning of a gesture that is already in the caregiver's repertoire.

Returning to the apes: Play hitting is an important part of the rough-and-tumble play of chimpanzees, and many individuals come to use a stylized *arm raise* to indicate that they are about to hit the other and thus initiate play (Goodall, 1986). Thus, a behavior that was not at first a communicative signal would become one over time. In orangutans, infants suck on the mother's lips while she is eating to obtain food pieces from her (Bard, 1990). Only later, at about 2.5 years of age, do they start to produce gestures such as approaching the mother's face to beg for food without actually touching her mouth (Liebal et al., 2006).

While ontogenetic ritualization may establish a conventional signal between two individuals, other mechanisms may be involved if it is to spread to the rest of the community or help in a ratcheting-up process whereby a group-wide system evolves. And, indeed, there *are* also group-specific gestures that are performed by the majority of individuals of one group of chimpanzees but not observed in another (Goodall, 1986), in apparent contradiction of the idea that ontogenetic ritualization is the only process of gesture acquisition. For example, the gesture *offer arm with food pieces* has been observed only in one of two different orangutan groups in two different zoos, while *arm shake* and *chuck up* were specific to a single gorilla group (Liebal et al., 2006). Furthermore, gestural signals such as the gesture *leaf clipping* and the *grooming hand clasp* in chimpanzees, and *somersault* in bonobos provide further evidence that social learning might play an important role for the acquisition of some gestures in great apes in the wild and captivity (Nishida, 1980; Pika, Liebal, Call et al., 2005; Whiten et al., 2001).

If a gesture has a high probability of being formed by ontogenetic rituali-zation, then each group member may acquire it independently within a dyad. However, once this gesture is established, it may spread by social learning in addition to its "rediscovery" by dyads forming it independently through their own interaction.[7]

Tomasello and Call (1997) argue that social learning is not the *major* pro-cess involved in gesture acquisition in apes. They hold that, were social learn-ing widespread in a group, the group's repertoire would be more uniform, and more distinct from the repertoires of other groups, than has been observed. However, social learning does not imply that all group members must learn the same gestures—any more than it implies that parents and teenagers in a human family can understand every word the other uses. In any case, the data provide evidence that at least some ape gestures are not genetically deter-mined and that development of a multifaceted gestural repertoire depends on the social and physical environment and on exchanges between group members.

A very important class of human communicative gestures consists of attention-directing gestures (so called *deictic* gestures). Chimpanzees may use eye contact, physical contact, and even vocalizations to capture the atten-tion of the audience. However, *pointing*—that most basic of human deictic gestures, using the index finger or extended hand—has only been observed in chimpanzees interacting with their human experimenters (e.g., Leavens, Hopkins, & Bard, 1996; 2005) as well as in human-raised or language-trained apes (e.g., Gardner & Gardner, 1969; Patterson, 1978; Woodruff & Premack, 1979), and it is only rarely reported between conspecifics (Vea & Sabater-Pi, 1998). Since both captive and wild chimpanzees share the same gene pool, Leavens et al. (2005) argued that the occurrence of pointing in captive apes is attributable to environmental influences on their communicative develop-ment. A related suggestion is that apes do not point for conspecifics because the observing ape will not be motivated to help or inform others or to share attention and information (Liebal & Call, 2011; Tomasello, Carpenter, Call, Behne, & Moll, 2005). One hypothesis that I find attractive is this: A chimpan-zee reaches through the bars to get a banana but cannot reach it. However, a human does something another chimpanzee would not do—recognizing the ape's intention, the keeper gives him the banana. As a result, the ape soon learns that a point (i.e., the failed reach) is enough to get the pointed-to object without the exertion of trying to complete an unsuccessful reach. This is a variation on ontogenetic ritualization that depends on the fact that humans provide an environment which is far more responsive than that provided by conspecifics in the wild:

- Individual A *attempts* to perform behavior X to achieve goal G, but fails— achieving only a prefix X'.
- Individual B, a human, infers goal G from this behavior and performs an action that achieves the goal G for A.
- In due course, A produces X' in a ritualized form X^R to get B to perform an action that achieves G for A.

This depends crucially on B behaving in a way that is very human, but very rare among chimpanzees. Let me call this *human-supported ritualization.* Intriguingly, it is far more widespread than just for apes. The cats in my house have developed a rich system of communication with my wife and me. "Stand outside a door and meow" means "let me in"; "stand inside a door" will, depending on posture, signal "just looking through the glass" versus "let me out." A tentative motion down the hall toward the room with the food dishes means "feed me." And so on. Generally, then, the main forms of communication are vocalizations that attract attention and "motion prefixes" where the cat begins a performance with the intention that the human recognize the prefix and do what is necessary to enable the action to proceed to completion. Such performances succeed only because *humans*, not the cats, have evolved a form of cooperative behavior that responds to such signals.

Thus, the discordance of behavior between wild and captive chimpanzees may be explained by the impossibility, for captive chimpanzees, of reaching directly for the object of their interest, instead being obliged to develop deictic pointing gestures to signify their need to a mediator (a human or a congener) who is closer to the object or can move toward it. This hypothesis finds support in the observation that pointing in human babies occurs primarily toward targets that are clearly out of reach (Butterworth, 2003). The particularly immature state of the locomotion system of humans at birth may have driven the species to develop a deictic pointing behavior. The ability of apes (but not monkeys) in captivity to produce a similar behavior reveals some form of brain readiness for a set of communicative gestures beyond those exhibited in the wild. This relates to the general view developed in this volume that biological substrate and "cultural opportunity" are intertwined in supporting the human readiness for language.

In conclusion, it should be noted that there are not many reports of gesture use in monkeys. This could mean either that they use gestures rarely or that they are not as well researched as apes. Among the exceptions, Laidre (2011) reports a gesture unique to a single community of mandrills (*Mandrillus sphinx*) among 19 studied across North America, Africa, and Europe. The mandrills covered their eyes with their hands for periods that could exceed 30 minutes, often while simultaneously raising their elbow prominently into the air. The gesture might function over a distance to inhibit interruptions in the way a "do not disturb" sign operates. In any case, for now, the evidence does point to flexibility of manual gesture versus innateness of vocalizations as a key contrast in the communicative repertoires of nonhuman primates.

Teaching "Language" to Apes

As we share 98.8% of our DNA with the chimpanzee (Sakaki et al., 2002), our closest relative, it is of interest to track the extent to which language has appeared in apes. The quotes around "language" in the title of this section are to highlight the fact that nonhuman primate communication is very different from human language, and that even apes raised by humans can develop only a small vocabulary and seem incapable of mastering syntax. Before discussing this further, though, let's note that the 98.8% can still allow a great deal of difference between the two species.

Consider the hand. To specify how to make skin and bone and configure muscles and tendons to move the fingers in a somewhat dexterous way would seem to me to require a far larger amount of genetic machinery than is required to distinguish the overall shape and relative placement of the fingers and opposable thumb of the human from that of the chimpanzee. Similarly, we shall see in the next chapter that many features in the overall layout of the human brain are already present in the brain of the macaque (and indeed, much is common to all vertebrates, and even more is common to all mammals) so that a relatively small set of changes in the genetic specification of brain structure may be enough to distinguish at least the gross features of the brains of monkeys, apes, and humans. Nonetheless, the brains are noticeably different not only in size but also in the range and relative size of brain regions, in connectivity, and even in details of cellular function.

Attempts to teach apes to talk failed repeatedly, though comprehension of spoken words has been demonstrated by apes. The conclusion is that apes lack the neural control mechanisms to control the vocal apparatus to yield even a crude approximation to the voluntary control of vowels and consonants. However, apes do have considerable dexterity, and chimpanzees and bonobos (great apes, not monkeys) can be trained to learn the use of novel hand movements to acquire a form of communication based on the use of hand signs like those used in sign language.[8] The phrasing "hand signs like those used in sign language" is to emphasize that some apes have acquired a repertoire of hand signs but have not acquired the syntactic skills of assembling those signs in the fashion characteristic of a true human signed language.

Another form of communication taught to apes is to select and place visual symbols called lexigrams, akin to moving magnetized symbols around on the door of a fridge. The resultant system approximates the complexity of the utterances of a 2-year-old human child, in that a "message" generally comprises one or two "lexemes," but with very little if anything in the way of syntax. The bonobo Kanzi mastered 256 lexigrams on his lexigram board and could arrange a few lexigrams in novel combinations—but combinations alone do not constitute syntax and Kanzi's productions do not form a language in the sense of combining elements of an open lexicon using a rich syntax with a compositional semantics to generate an open-ended set of utterances that express novel meanings.[9]

Kanzi has a perceptive vocabulary of several hundred *spoken* words. Savage-Rumbaugh et al. (1998) report that Kanzi and a 2.5-year-old girl were tested on their *comprehension* of 660 *spoken* sentences phrased as simple requests (presented once). Kanzi was able to carry out the request correctly 72% of the time, whereas the girl scored 66% on the same sentences and task. There is no evidence that, given a sentence such as "Would you please carry the straw?" Kanzi attended to words such as "would," "please," and "the" in responding. Moreover, since Kanzi can carry a straw, but a straw cannot carry Kanzi, it would seem that Kanzi can put together objects and actions "in the probable way." This seemed to mark the limits of Kanzi's abilities but was just the beginning for the human child. No nonhuman primate has exhibited any of the richness of human language that distinguishes the adult human (or, even, a typical 3-year-old human child) from the 2-year-old, suggesting a biological difference in the brain's "language readiness" between humans and other primates. This is in addition to the fact, noted earlier, that the human brain and speech apparatus together support voluntary control of vocal articulations that the bonobo's cannot—thus the use of signing or other manual-based symbols with apes.

No nonhuman primate has been seen "in the wild" to use symbols in the way that Kanzi has learned to use them. It is Kanzi's exposure to human culture that enabled him to learn to use lexigrams to communicate, but what he acquired was but a small fragment of the full richness of human language Although there is no evidence that an ape can reach the linguistic ability of a 3-year-old human, Kanzi's prowess does emphasize the difference between having a brain "endowed with language" (a built-in set of syntactic rules) and the human child's *language-ready brain* that can learn language—but only when the child is embedded in a language-rich culture that reflects the cumulative inventions of many millennia of human culture. Kanzi was "ready" for a 2-year-old child's level of language, but no more—and was only able to manifest this readiness because of the human-centered environment to which he was exposed. Of course, the human child, too, develops language only within an existing language environment, though we shall see further subtleties when we turn to the development of new sign languages in Chapter 12.

4

Human Brain, Monkey Brain, and Praxis

When I introduce students at the University of Southern California to the graduate-level core course in neuroscience, I point out the daunting fact that the annual meeting of the Society for Neuroscience attracts some 30,000 participants. "If we assume each attendee has something worth learning about, we will have to cover the work of 1,000 of them in each of our 30 lectures." Of course, the actual lectures are far more selective. However, there is always a sense of frustration in the conscious exclusion of many fascinating topics. Similarly, in writing this chapter, there was a real challenge in deciding what to include and what to omit. In the end, I decided to go somewhat beyond the bare minimum needed to support the Mirror System Hypothesis in order to provide a sense of the context in which the brain-centered work in this book is conducted. The present chapter introduces some basic facts about the brains of both macaque and human within the context of praxis (practical interaction with objects),[1] especially visual guidance of hand movements, with some added discussion of brain mechanisms involved in emotion, hearing, and vocalization.

In addition to introducing an overall anatomical framework for the macaque monkey brain as well as the human brain, this chapter will introduce some general principles of brain operation, building on the insights into cooperative computation of schemas offered in Chapter 1. The underlying mechanisms for this are complex patterns of excitation and inhibition linking huge populations of neurons in different regions. While anatomy provides the framework for these computations, it is learning from experience—mediated in part by plasticity of synapses (connection points between neurons)—that determines the details of the wiring that makes these interactions possible and constrains them. Proceeding from the micro level of synapses we move to the macro level as we develop the theme of social cognitive neuroscience in relation to social schemas—the mix of genetic and social inheritance. But all this will be done "once over lightly," supplying some extra details in later chapters but leaving even further details to the scientific literature toward which the truly neuroscience-enthused reader can turn.

A guiding principle is that the overall ground plan of the brains of different mammals has many important features in common, and even more so for humans, apes, and monkeys. Like all mammals (but also like birds and fish and frogs and crocodiles), we are *vertebrates*; we have a spine containing the mass of neurons that is known as the *spinal cord*. All sensory information from the skin, joints, and muscles of the trunk and limbs enters the central nervous system through the spinal cord; and all the motor neurons whose synapses control the muscles of the trunk and limbs have their cell bodies in the spinal cord. This is in distinction to the *cranial* nerves, for control of the head and intake of information from receptors in the head, which enter the nervous system via the brainstem.[2]

Nonetheless, brains do differ between species, not only in overall size but also in the relative size of different regions and the presence or absence or specialization of certain nuclei. Since the brains of our distant ancestors did not fossilize, our evolutionary account of the brain cannot be based on comparison of their brains with our own. Instead, we have recourse to *comparative neurobiology*—comparing our brains to those of other creatures, especially primates such as macaque and squirrel monkeys. We will then adopt the plausible hypothesis that characteristics shared by human brains and macaque brains are likely to have been shared by our last common ancestor with the macaques, thus creating a platform for the evolutionary changes that transformed that ancient brain to the brain of our last common ancestor with the chimpanzees and then on to modern brains. The overarching anatomical framework for this work is given in Figure 4-1. Visual inspection of a dissected brain allows us to identify various regions to which we may assign labels for easy reference. Further careful analyses, with the aid of microscopes and chemical and electrical techniques, allow us to refine these subdivisions. Different parts of the brain have different functions, but a given externally defined behavioral or psychological function may involve the interaction of many regions of the brain. Thus, when an area involved in a function is damaged, cooperation between other areas may yield (partial) restoration of function. From an evolutionary point of view, we find that many "old" regions of the brain survive from those of our very distant ancestors, but that newer centers add new functions in themselves and, through new connections, allow new functions to be subserved by the older regions. We will see in Chapter 5 that a very important comparison point is that an area called F5 in the premotor cortex of the macaque that contains mirror neurons for grasping is homologous to (is the evolutionary cousin of) Broca's area of the human brain, an area implicated in the production of signed languages as well as speech.[3]

Neurophysiologists have learned how to insert microelectrodes into an animal's brain in such a way that they can monitor the electrical activity of

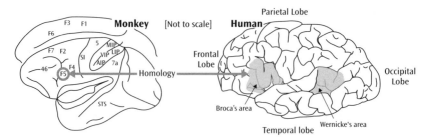

FIGURE 4-1.   Views of the monkey brain and human brain (the human brain is relatively much larger). In each case, the front of the brain is to the left, and the rear of the brain is to the right—we are looking at the left hemisphere. Here the key points are (1) that there is a region called F5 in the frontal lobe of the monkey brain (see Fig. 4-8 for explanation of some of the other labels) and it contains mirror neurons for grasping; (2) that there is a region called Broca's area in the frontal lobe of the human brain that is traditionally associated with speech production, and (3) the two regions are homologous, that is, they evolved from the same brain region of a common ancestor. The two brains are not shown to scale—the area of human cerebral cortex is approximately 10 times that of macaque visual cortex (Van Essen, 2005). As can be seen from the figure, the human cerebral cortex is more folded than that of the monkey and has a finer subdivision of anatomically and functionally discriminable regions. (Figure at left adapted from Jeannerod, Arbib, Rizzolatti, & Sakata, 1995; figure at right adapted from Williams, White, & Mace, 2007.)

single neurons. In particular, they can monitor the "firing" of an individual neuron—measuring the pattern in which the neuron sends "spikes" of electrical activity down its axon, its output line. The axon may branch again and again so that the firing of a single neuron can affect hundreds or even thousands of other neurons. Conversely, a single neuron can be affected by the firing of hundreds, even tens of thousands, of other neurons. The input to the overall network is provided by millions of *receptors* or *sensors* in our bodies that continually monitor changes in our external and internal environment. Hundreds of thousands of cells called *motor neurons* sample the activity of the neural network to control the movement of our muscles and the secretion of our glands. In between, an intricate network of billions of neurons continually combines the signals from the receptors with signals encoding past experience to barrage the motor neurons with signals that will yield adaptive interactions with the environment. This network is called the *central nervous system (CNS)*, and the brain constitutes the most headward part of this system—though we shall often speak of the brain when we really mean the CNS (the brain plus the spinal cord) as a whole.

The brain does not provide a simple stimulus-response chain from receptors to effectors (though there are such reflex paths in the spinal cord)— recall the action-perception cycle of Chapter 2, Figure 2-7. Rather, the vast network of billions upon billions of neurons is interconnected in loops and tangled chains so that signals entering the net from the receptors interact there with the billions of signals already traversing the system, both to modify activity and connectivity within the system and also to yield the signals that control the effectors. In this way, the CNS enables the current actions of the organism to depend both upon its current stimulation and upon the residue of past experience expressed in the activity and changed structure of its network. All this encodes an *internal model of the world* both in activity within the network and in the current pattern of connections that link the neurons.

Learning From Comparative Neurobiology

From the mid-19th century onward, much has been learned about the contribution of different regions of the human brain through the neurological study of lesions, whether they result from a stroke, a tumor, or neurosurgery. However, brain-damaging strokes, tumors, and other misfortunes are cruel and rare "experiments" by nature . Fortunately, there has been a revolution in the last few decades giving us new types of noninvasive brain imaging to get a large scale view of activity even in undamaged brains. These techniques can chart which parts of the brain are more active when a human performs one task as compared to another. The main technique of brain imaging using positron emission tomography (PET) or functional magnetic resonance imaging (fMRI) is to use physics and computation to make a statistical comparison of the three-dimensional distribution of blood flow in the brain when the subject executes task A as compared to task B. The idea is that a part of the brain that is more active (measured by, say, synaptic activity) in task A than B will need to extract more oxygen from the blood to support its activity during task A, and vice versa. Since the differences are minute, the comparison yields a three-dimensional map of statistical significance in the brain that has low resolution in both space and time relative to the activity of single neurons. Thus, we lose an incredible amount of detail with this approach when compared to the neurophysiology of animals, where we can get a millisecond-by-millisecond record of the activity of single cells. The plus for human brain imaging is that we can "see" the whole brain—but only at low resolution. A point on the image indicates the activity of hundreds of thousands of neurons averaged over a second or more.

Looking at brain imaging data without access to data on single neurons is somewhat akin to a news story that talks of the United States as a collection of 50 states without further regard for the differences within states and the great diversity of people within each locality, Republicans and Democrats, old and young, in sickness and in health, in jail and out, rich and poor, people of diverse religious faiths or none, and so on. The breakthrough in brain imaging lets us look at the activity of the whole human brain when people engage in the laboratory versions of everyday tasks, many of which monkeys or other animals cannot do, such as those requiring the use of language. However, while it offers a method of looking at activity in lumps of brain that correlate with tasks describable in the sort of language in which we talk about our own personal experience, it does not tell us how they are played over the detailed circuitry. We need to know much more about how to integrate the "person-level" results with the successes of molecular and microscopic neuroscience. In this chapter, we will gain a high-level view of the roles of certain regions of the human brain, then look in more detail at some neural mechanisms of the macaque brain. We will use the FARS model of how we grasp an object (Fig. 4-11) as an example of how we can proceed in cases where we have reason to believe that the brains of other creatures (in this case macaques) carry out a task in a way similar to the way humans do.

The anatomist can study slices of the brains of dead humans and monkeys under the microscope to understand how to "morph" a macaque brain into a human brain. We are confident that two regions correspond to each other if the shapes of neurons and the chemical signatures of the neurotransmitters that pass chemical messages between them are similar and the overall morphing allows us to see similar connection patterns when we look at pairs of corresponding regions. But just as no amount of plausible morphing of macaque and human bodies into each other can extend the matching of forelimbs and hindlimbs to give a human a tail, so the correspondence between the human and monkey brain that readily matches up the frontal, temporal, parietal, and occipital lobes and the cerebellum across both species can extend so far and no further. There are brain regions in the larger human brain that do not correspond directly to regions of the monkey brain. But even here, the morphing may help us by showing that a couple of regions in the human brain correspond to a single region in the monkey brain. The result then is that everything we learn about the circuitry and the neurochemistry of the region of the monkey brain gives us an excellent first approximation to what is going on in the regions of the human brain. In other words, much of this book will take the data of *comparative neurobiology*, comparing the behavior, biology, and brains of humans and other species, especially macaques and chimpanzees, to ground hypotheses about the evolutionary changes that let each species develop its own distinctive characteristics.

Introducing the Human Brain

Figure 4-2 (left) gives a medial (middle) view as it might be revealed were we to slice the head in half. The brains of mammals, and especially of humans, are distinguished from those of other species by the "explosion" of new cortex—or *neocortex*—that comes in humans to dominate the rest of the brain, as is clear in the lateral (side) view of a human brain in Figure 4-2 (right), where the outfoldings of neocortex completely hide the midbrain from view. The human cerebral cortex is only about 3 millimeters (50 to 100 neurons) in depth, but it forms a sheet of about 2,400 square centimeters in area and so must fold and fold again to fit into the space within the skull. A groove in the cortex is called a *fissure* or a *sulcus,* and the upfolded tissue between two sulci is a *gyrus.* This great expansion of forebrain comes with evolution to greatly modify circuitry in the brainstem and spinal cord.

The cerebrum is divided into four lobes, the *frontal,* which is in the region of the forehead; the *temporal,* which is to the sides in the region of the temples; the *parietal,* which is at the top where the parietal bones form part of the skull; and the *occipital* lobe, from the Latin *occipitus,* meaning back of the head. Pathways connecting regions in the two halves of the brain are called *commissures.* The largest commissure is the *corpus callosum,* which connects the two cerebral hemispheres.

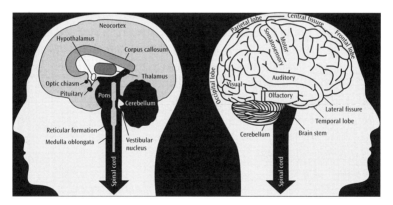

FIGURE 4-2.   Two views of the human brain as positioned in the head. The left-hand view diagrams the *medial* view—what we would see were we to slice down the middle of the head. The right-hand view diagrams the *lateral* view—what would be seen from the outside after removal of the skull. The *spinal cord* runs up through the vertebrae of the spine, receiving signals from the limbs and trunk, and contains the motor neurons that control limb and trunk muscles. The spinal cord leads into the *brainstem,* behind which is the outswelling of the *cerebellum.* Then, overshadowing all, is the great outfolding of the *neocortex* of the cerebral hemispheres. At left we can see some of the structures that are obscured by the neocortex in the lateral view. (Adapted from Arbib, 1972.)

Certain areas of cerebral cortex can be dubbed *sensory* because they primarily process information from one modality. This includes not only the area labeled *somatosensory* in Figure 4-2, which receives information relayed via the spinal cord from the body surface and joints and muscles of the limbs but also the *visual, auditory,* and *olfactory* areas (the last shown in cutaway, since it is not on the outer surface), which receive information from the distance receptors in the head. The *motor* cortex is a source of fibers that control muscular activity. Phylogenetically, somatosensory and motor cortex form a tightly coupled system, and in humans (at least) there is not only sensory representation in motor cortex (hardly surprising—cells controlling movement should be responsive to appropriate external stimuli) but there also are cells in somatosensory cortex whose axons project (i.e., form a pathway) to the motor neurons and interneurons of the spinal cord, as do those of neurons in motor cortex, thus influencing movement via at most two intervening synapses. It is thus common to refer to the regions of frontal and parietal cortex adjoining the central fissure as *sensorimotor cortex.*

The rest of the cortex is called *association* cortex, but this is a misnomer that reflects an erroneous 19th-century view that the job of these areas was simply to "associate" the different sensory inputs to provide the proper instructions to be relayed by the motor cortex. The absolutely false idea that 90% of the brain is "unused" probably arose from a layman's misinterpretation of the fact that the exact functions of many of these "association areas" were very little known until the last few decades.

Classic work in the 19th century on human brains included basic studies of localized function in relation to *aphasia* (defects in language behavior associated with brain damage). Broca (1861; see Grodzinsky & Amunts, 2006 for an English translation) described a patient with a lesion in the *anterior* region (*anterior* = in front, as opposed to *posterior* = behind) marked (b) in Figure 4-3, and which is now called *Broca's region* in his honor. Broca's aphasia seemed essentially *motoric* in that the patient was able to comprehend language but could speak only with effort and then only "telegrammatically" in short utterances, omitting most of the grammatical markers. By contrast, Wernicke (1874) described a patient with a lesion in the *posterior* region marked (a) in Figure 4-3, now called *Wernicke's region*. Wernicke's aphasia seemed essentially *sensory*, in that the patient seemed not to comprehend speech (but was not deaf to other auditory stimuli) and would speak a fluent but often meaningless stream of syllables. It should also be added that later work established that for most people (even 90% of left-handers, whose dominant hand is controlled by the right motor cortex), it is the left hemisphere that is predominantly involved in language, with lesions of the right hemisphere causing little or no aphasic symptoms but impairing speech in other ways, such as affecting

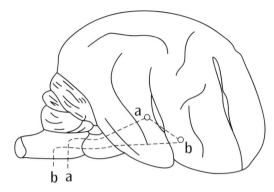

FIGURE 4-3.   Wernicke's 1864 diagram showing the principal pathways for language suggested by his and Broca's data: (a) peripheral auditory pathway→sound center for words; (b) motor center for words→peripheral motor pathways for speech. Wernicke's area (a) is more sensory and posterior, whereas Broca's area (b) is more motor and anterior. Strangely enough, Wernicke draws this diagram on the *right* hemisphere, even though for most people it is the left hemisphere that plays the dominant role in language.

prosody. It should also be stressed that it is wrong to say "Wernicke's area comprehends speech" and "Broca's area produces speech"—each has a differential role within a larger system of interacting brain regions and, indeed, people with the symptoms of Broca's aphasia usually have lesions that extend well beyond Broca's area.

Studies of vision have shown that there is really no single "visual system" in the brain but rather "many visual systems" computing such factors as depth, motion, color, and so on, even though we have the conscious experience of a single integrated visual experience. Given our concern with hand use (recall Fig. 1-2 in Chapter 1), it is particularly striking that the ability to use the size of an object to preshape the hand while grasping it can be dissociated by brain lesions from the ability to consciously recognize and describe that size.

Goodale et al. (1991) studied a patient (DF) with carbon monoxide poisoning for whom most of the damage to cortical visual areas was apparent not in area 17 (V1) but bilaterally in the adjacent areas 18 and 19 of visual cortex. This lesion still allowed signals to flow from V1 toward posterior parietal cortex (PP) but not from V1 to inferotemporal cortex (IT). In terms of Figure 4-4, the path V1→PP runs from the back of the occipital lobe up to the parietal lobe, while the path V1→IT runs from the back of the occipital lobe down to the lower end of the temporal lobe. When asked to indicate the width of a single block by means of her index finger and thumb, DF's finger separation bore no relationship to the dimensions of the object and showed considerable trial-to-trial variability. Yet when she was asked simply to reach out and pick up the block, the peak aperture (well before contact with the object) between her

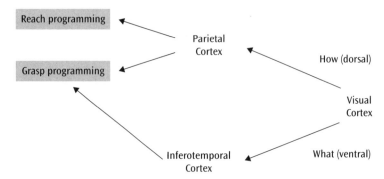

F<small>IGURE</small> 4-4.   The "what" and "how" pathways for visual information involved in successful grasping or manipulation of an object. Ungerleider and Mishkin (1982) conducted experiments with monkeys and showed that a ventral lesion would impair memory of the pattern associated with hidden food, whereas a dorsal lesion would impair memory of where the food had been hidden— and thus spoke of the "what" and "where" pathways. However, we here refer to a different paradigm—observations of the effect on reaching and grasping of lesions of the human brain. Here a ventral lesion affects the ability to describe properties of the object ("what"), whereas a dorsal lesion affects the ability to preshape for grasping or otherwise using the object ("how"). Note, of course, that knowing where the object is provides just one part of the information needed to interact with it (recall Fig. 1-2) so "how" is more than "where." It should be added that both parietal and frontal cortex involve many different subregions. Thus, the parietofrontal circuit for controlling hand movements involves different regions from the parietofrontal circuit for controlling saccades (the eye movements that can direct visual attention to an object), and the latter might well be called a "where" pathway.

index finger and thumb changed systematically with the width of the object, as in normal controls. A similar dissociation was seen in her responses to the orientation of stimuli. In other words, DF could accurately preshape her hand en route to grasping an object, even though she appeared to have no conscious appreciation (expressible either verbally or in pantomime) of the visual parameters that guided the preshape.

Jeannerod et al. (1994) report a study of impairment of grasping in a patient (AT) with a bilateral posterior parietal lesion of vascular origin that left IT and the pathway V1→IT relatively intact but grossly impaired the pathway V1→PP. This patient is the "opposite" of DF; she can use her hand to pantomime the size of a cylinder, and she can reach without deficit toward the location of such an object but cannot preshape appropriately when asked to grasp it. Instead of an adaptive preshape, she will open her hand to its fullest and only begin to close her hand when the cylinder hits the "web" between index finger and thumb. But there was a surprise! When the stimulus used for the grasp was not a cylinder (for which the "semantics" contains no information about expected size) but rather a familiar object—such as a reel of thread or a lipstick—for which the "usual" size is part of the subject's knowledge, AT showed a relatively appropriate preshape. This suggests, as indicated by the arrow at bottom left of Figure 4-4, that a pathway from inferotemporal cortex provides the parietal areas with "default values" of action-related parameters, that is, values that can serve in place of actual sensory data to, for example, represent the approximate size of a known object to help the parietofrontal system.

Figure 4-4 shows the two pathways for information from primary visual cortex V1 at the back of the brain: a dorsal path via posterior parietal cortex and a ventral pathway via inferotemporal cortex. The neuroanatomical coordinates—dorsal and ventral—refer to the orientation of the brain and spinal cord in a typical vertebrate: "dorsal" is on the upper side (think of the dorsal fin of a shark), while "ventral" refers to structures closer to the belly side of the animal.

We distinguish *praxic* action, in which the hands are used to interact physically with objects or other creatures, from *communicative* action (both manual and vocal). Waving good-bye and brushing away a cloud of flies might employ the same motion, yet they are different actions—the first communicative, the second praxic. We thus see in the AT and DF data a dissociation between parietal and inferotemporal pathways, respectively, for the praxic use of size information (which is why we call the dorsal pathway the "how" pathway) and the communicative "declaration" of that information either verbally or through pantomime (which is why we call the ventral pathway the "what" pathway).

Primary visual cortex V1 is also called area 17 or Brodmann's area 17 or BA17. (When the neuroanatomist Michael Petrides talks at conferences, he always enunciates BA as British Airways.) When we talk of areas 17, 18, and 19 here, or later say that Broca's area comprises areas 44 and 45, we are using anatomical nomenclature introduced by Brodmann (1905) to subdivide cerebral cortex of the brains of humans (Fig. 4-5), monkeys, and other species. For readers with some experience in neuroscience, these numbers will help visualize where in the cortex the area is located. Readers without this experience may simply use these numbers or the letter abbreviations like V1, IT, and PP as convenient labels to keep track of the brain areas relevant to our study. Although we will make use of very few of Brodmann's area numbers in what follows, let me note a few that may be worth remembering:

- Vision: Primary visual cortex (BA17) feeds into secondary visual cortex (BA18, BA19).
- Primary somatosensory cortex, which mediates touch and body sense (BA1), feeds into the secondary areas (BA2, BA3).

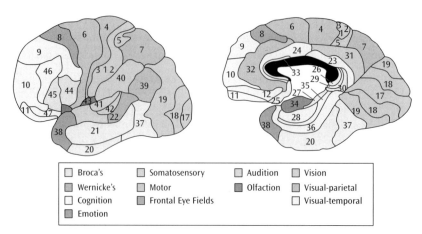

FIGURE 4-5.   Brodmann's areas in the human brain. These are all areas of cerebral cortex. There are many other regions of importance to us, including cerebellum, basal ganglia, and hippocampus. (See color insert for full color version of this figure.)

- Language areas include BA22, Wernicke's area (BA40), and Broca's area (BA44 and BA45).
- Frontal eye fields (BA8) provide a cortical outpost for the control of eye movements.

However, each region is involved in complex patterns of competition and cooperation that may vary from task to task, and each includes interaction with subcortical regions, and so one must not read too much into the functional labels of Figure 4-5.

Figure 4-6 (left) shows some areas of the human brain homologous to regions of the macaque brain we will consider in the next section. The inferior frontal gyrus (IFG) includes Broca's area but is perhaps somewhat larger than the traditional definition that comprises Brodmann areas BA44 and BA45 (see Fig. 4-5). The IFG has three parts: The pars orbitalis is an associational cortical area that is anterior (frontmost) in the IFG; the posterior part of this area may contribute (with BA44) to the production of language, while other circuits participate in prefrontal cortical networks that govern executive functions. The pars triangularis comes next, a triangular-shaped aspect of the gyral structure. The most anterior part is the pars opercularis. The superior temporal sulcus (STS) is the sulcus (groove) on the lateral surface of the temporal lobe, and it has many important circuits (e.g., for visual processing) in the banks of tissue inside the groove. And, of course, the inferior parietal lobe (IPL) is the lower part of the parietal lobe. Wernicke's area (not shown in the figure) is (approximately) the area of temporal lobe just above the STS and

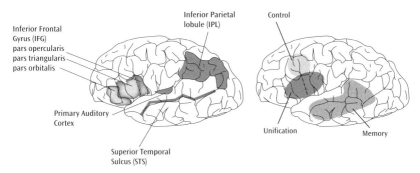

FIGURE 4-6. (*Left*) Some regions of the human brain relevant to our comparison of the human and macaque brain (adapted from Williams et al., 2007). (*Right*) The memory, unification, control (MUC) model with memory (yellow) in left temporal cortex, unification (blue) in LIFG (the left inferior frontal gyrus), and control (gray) in dorsolateral prefrontal cortex. The anterior cingulate cortex (ACC; part of the control component) is not shown. (Adapted from Hagoort, 2005.)

running back from the area contiguous to and just below the primary auditory cortex.

Figure 4-6 (right) shows how related areas are visualized by Hagoort (2005) in his scheme for language processing. Left inferior frontal gyrus (LIFG) comprises the classical Broca's area—BA44 and BA45—plus adjacent language-relevant cortex (including BA47) as well as part of premotor cortex (i.e., the area just in front of primary motor cortex), namely ventral BA6. Hagoort uses the term "semantic unification" for the integration of word meaning into an unfolding discourse representation selecting the appropriate meaning of each word so that a coherent interpretation results. He reports that, relative to a correct control sentence ("*Dutch trains are yellow and very crowded*"), exposure to sentences containing incorrect information (e.g., "*Dutch trains are white and very crowded*") or semantic oddities (e.g., "*Dutch trains are sour and very crowded*") yields an increased BOLD response in LIFG (BA47/45)—the BOLD signal is the basis for the fMRI method of brain imaging. Moreover, relative to a low-level baseline, increased activation was also seen for the correct sentences, indicating that this area is automatically recruited during semantic unification.

Hagoort suggests, then, that BA47 and BA45 are involved in semantic processing. BA45 and BA44 are said to contribute to syntactic processing, whereas BA44 and parts of BA6 have a role in phonological processing. Nonetheless, the overlap of activations (as seen in brain imaging during different tasks) for these three different types of information processing is substantial and suggests the possibility of interactive processing—hardly surprising given our emphasis (see Chapter 2) on the integration of form and meaning in the constructions of construction grammar.

Hagoort distinguishes three functional components of language processing: memory, unification, and control (MUC).

- The memory component (shown in yellow) is in the left temporal cortex. It comprises a specification of the different types of language information stored in long-term memory, as well as the retrieval operations.
- The unification component (shown in blue) is in LIFG. It refers to the integration of lexically retrieved information into a representation of multiword utterances.
- The control component (gray) is in dorsolateral prefrontal cortex but also includes the anterior cingulate cortex, which is not shown in the figure. It relates language to action, and it is invoked, for instance, when the correct target language has to be selected (in the case of bilingualism) or for handling turn taking during conversation.

This theory is by no means the last word on language processing in the human brain but does, at least, orient us to the way in which modern studies combining new concepts with the results of brain imaging are helping us move beyond the classic analysis of Broca and Wernicke (Figure 4-3).

Motivation and Emotion: The Motors of Behavior

Emotion can be analyzed under two headings:

"External" aspect of emotions: Emotional expression for communication and social coordination. If we see that someone is angry, we will interact with that person more cautiously than we would otherwise, or not at all.

"Internal" aspects of emotions: These frequently contribute to the organization of behavior (prioritization, action selection, attention, social coordination, and learning). For example, the actions one is likely to perform vary greatly depend on whether one is angry or sad.

These two aspects have coevolved. Animals need to survive and perform efficiently within their ecological niche, and in each case the patterns of coordination will greatly influence the suite of relevant emotions (if such are indeed needed) and the means whereby they are communicated. The emotional state sets the framework in which the choice (whether conscious or unconscious) of actions will unfold. But emotions, too, are embedded in the action-perception cycle, so that one's emotions may change as the consequence of one's actions become apparent—and our perception of these consequences may well rest on our perception of the emotional response of others to our behavior.

The various regions that form the "limbs" surrounding the thalamus form what is called the *limbic system*, basically the regions shown in Figure 4-7. (It has nothing to do, directly, with the control of arms and legs.) Karl Pribram (1960) quipped that the limbic system is responsible for the four Fs: feeding, fighting, fleeing, and reproduction. It is interesting that three of the four have a strong social component. In any case, the notion to be developed in this section is that the animal comes with a set of basic "drives"—for hunger, thirst, sex, self-preservation, and so on—and that these provide the basic "motor," motivation, for behavior.[4] Motivated behavior not only includes bodily behavior (as in feeding and fleeing, orofacial responses, and defensive and mating activities) but also autonomic output (e.g., heart rate and blood pressure) and visceroendocrine output (e.g., adrenaline, release of sex hormones). These lie at the heart [*sic*] of our emotional repertoire. However, the emotions that we talk about and perceive in others are both more restricted than this (how many people perceive another's cortisol level?) yet also more subtle, intertwining these basic motivations with our complex cognitions of social role and interactions, as in the cases of jealousy and pride.

To consider *briefly* the role of a number of brain regions in the support of motivation and emotion, we now turn to the brain regions of Figure 4-7. The core of the motivation system is provided by the nuclei of a deep-seated region of the brain called the *hypothalamus*. These nuclei are devoted to the elaboration and control of specific behaviors necessary for survival. Such behaviors include spontaneous locomotion, exploration, ingestive, defensive, and reproductive behaviors. Basically, the hypothalamus talks "downward" for basic behavioral control and "upward" to involve the cortex in determining when particular behaviors are appropriate. Indeed, many instances of motivated behavior—eating, drinking, grooming, attack, sleep, maternal behavior, hoarding, copulation—have been evoked by direct electrical or chemical stimulation of the hypothalamus. Animals with the hypothalamus cut off from cortex can more or less eat, drink, reproduce, and show defensive behaviors, but with no subtlety in the release of these behaviors. However, if the brain is cut below the hypothalamus, the animal displays only fragments of these behaviors, enabled by motor pattern generators in the brainstem. There are associated nuclei involved in ingestive and social (reproductive and defensive) behaviors such as sexually dimorphic behaviors, defensive responses, or controls for food and water intake. More caudal (tailward) nuclei include those involved in general foraging/exploratory behaviors. The lateral hypothalamus plays a critical role in arousal, control of behavioral state, and reward-seeking behavior. It includes what Jim Olds (1969) referred to as the "pleasure center" because rats will press a lever thousands of times per hour to deliver electrical stimulation to this region.

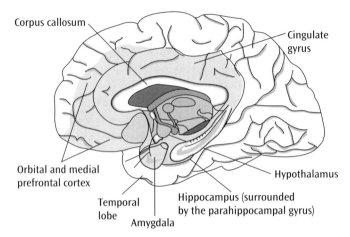

FIGURE 4-7.   A diagram of the limbic system (i.e., the brain regions "that throw their limbs" around the thalamus). Relative placement of amygdala (named for its almond shape), hippocampus (named for its sea-horse-like appearance in cross-section), cingulate gyrus, medial prefrontal cortex, and temporal lobe in the human brain. (Adapted from Williams et al., 2007.)

Joseph LeDoux (2000) argues that emotion systems evolved as sensory-motor solutions to problems of survival. He distinguishes emotions from "feelings." Such "conscious emotions" are not, he suggests, the function that emotion systems evolved to perform. He has focused on fear conditioning in the rat to define meaningful animal experiments and has been particularly concerned with the role of the amygdala in fear (see Fig. 4-7). In particular, he has studied the role of the amygdala in conditioning of fearful behavior, as an animal comes to learn that certain situations may lead to danger. The laboratory equivalent might be for a rat to learn that it will get an electric shock if it approaches a particular place in its cage. LeDoux stresses that we cannot know what feelings the rat has if it is afraid or indeed whether it has any feelings of fear. But it certainly can exhibit fearful behavior, trying to escape or, in many of LeDoux's studies, simply freezing in place. Such "freezing," a cessation of normal locomotion, is well known as a response to predators (if you don't move, the predator may not see you) and so is assumed to be a case of being too fearful to move.

In Figure 4-7 we see that the almond-shaped amygdala sits next to the hippocampus and is surrounded by the temporal lobe. Study of HM (of whom, more later) suggested that an important role of human hippocampus was to locate an event in space and time to be stored in episodic memory. Studies of spatial navigation in rats suggests that rat hippocampus provides a "you are here" function. Hippocampus thus plays a role in fear conditioning in rats, letting them use contextual cues to recognize that they are in a place "where bad things happen" and react fearfully as a result.

Regardless of whether rats have emotional feelings as well as emotional behaviors, there is no doubt that humans have feelings. How does "behavioral fear" relate to the feeling of fear or anxiety? The crucial element from an evolutionary point of view may be the set of reciprocal interactions between amygdala and cerebral cortex. Human emotions are strongly influenced by social milieu—what is embarrassing in one culture (e.g., nudity) may be regarded as perfectly normal in another The amygdala can influence cortical areas by way of feedback either from proprioceptive or visceral signals or hormones, via projections to various "arousal" networks, and through interaction with the *medial prefrontal cortex* (Fig. 4-7). This area has widespread influences on cognition and behavior and also sends connections to several amygdala regions, allowing cognitive functions organized in prefrontal regions to regulate the amygdala and its fear reactions. Connections of the amygdala with hippocampus and cerebral cortex provide the possible basis for enrichment of "behavioral emotion" by episodic memory and cognitive state.

Fellous and LeDoux (2005) suggest that medial prefrontal cortex allows cognitive information processing in prefrontal cortex to regulate emotional processing by the amygdala, whereas emotional processing by the amygdala may influence decision making and other cognitive functions of the prefrontal cortex. They then suggest that the prefrontal–amygdala interactions may be involved in the conscious feelings of fear. However, this division between the cognitive cortex and emotional amygdala strikes me as too simple to do justice to the brain's integration of widely distributed functions—both because not all parts of cortex give rise to conscious feelings and also because human emotions seem to be inextricably bound up with "cortical subtleties." The *medial prefrontal cortex* is adjacent to the orbitofrontal cortex (so-called because it is in the front of the brain just above the orbits in the skull that hold the eyes). Orbitofrontal cortex, too, is part of the emotional system. Rolls (2005) documents how damage to the caudal orbitofrontal cortex produces emotional change, which includes the tendency to respond when responses are inappropriate, including a tendency not to withhold responses to nonrewarded stimuli. Rolls sees orbitofrontal neurons as part of a mechanism that evaluates whether a reward is expected and generates a mismatch (evident as a firing of the nonreward neurons) if the reward is not obtained when it is expected. When we briefly return to a consideration of emotion in Chapter 5, we will be stressing the role of emotion in social interactions—involving not only the specific expression of emotion via facial expressions but more subtle inferences of the mental state of others—and the extent to which the recognition of another's emotional state does or does not involve feelings of empathy.

Beyond the Here and Now

In this section I use two case studies to introduce some of the brain regions that let us go in our thoughts "beyond the here and now," recalling past episodes and planning for the future, abilities that are so much a part of the human condition. First will be a study of how a man referred to in the neurological literature as HM lost the ability to form new "episodic memories"—he could not remember any events or episodes that he had been involved in since the time he had major neurosurgery. We then turn from recalling the past to planning for the future with the story of Phineas Gage, who lost the ability to plan ahead and to inhibit antisocial behavior as a result of a freak accident while working on the railroad. These stories will emphasize the roles of the hippocampus and the prefrontal cortex, respectively.

The Missing Episodes of HM

HM (1926–2008)[5] began to have grand mal epileptic seizures when he was 16 years old. By 1953, his seizures arrived with such frequency that he was unable to hold a steady job. His family thus turned to a neurosurgeon for help. The surgeon, William Scoville, reasoned that he could cure HM if he removed damaged brain tissue that provided the source of the "electrical storms" that raged through his brain during epileptic fits. Since the seizures appeared to begin in the temporal lobes on either side of the brain, Scoville opted for radical brain surgery on HM, removing large sections of his temporal lobes, including the hippocampus, the amygdala, and the entorhinal and perirhinal cortices (the latter being parts of the parahippocampal gyrus of Fig. 4-7). The consequences of the surgery were tragic for HM, but they yielded major new insights into the brain mechanisms of human memory. HM became unable to create new memories of the events of his life.[6]

One of my colleagues from my time at Stanford University, Karl Pribram, described a meeting with HM as follows (paraphrasing somewhat): "I talked to him about various things and applied a psychological test or two, and to my confusion he appeared completely normal. I was then called away to answer a phone call. When I returned several minutes later, I apologized for my absence. HM thanked me for my courtesy but had no recollection that we had met before."

The crucial concept we need in order to make sense of this anecdote is *episodic memory*—our ability to remember previous episodes from our lives, such as the time one first met a lover or the way one embarrassed oneself at a certain party. HM could remember episodes from his life before the neurosurgery but could not form new memories of any of the events of his life thereafter. We say he has *anterograde* amnesia, the inability to form new memories going *forward* in time from the surgery. More common in many patients is *retrograde* amnesia, where the loss of memory extends *back* in time from some terrible head trauma such as might be suffered in a car crash or in military combat. It is also clear that HM had *working memory*, the ability to hold in one's head information that is relevant to a current course of action but that is discarded once it is no longer useful. The classic example, as mentioned in Chapter 1, is remembering a telephone number until we dial it (or touch it, to be more contemporary).

It thus seemed that HM could form no new memories apart from working memory. Amazingly, this turned out not to be true. Here's an example of the sort of thing that provided this new insight. HM was shown a new game of moderate complexity. He expressed interest in the novelty of the game, held the rules in working memory while his attention stayed focused on the game, and played like any beginner. The next day, HM was shown the same game. He did not remember seeing it before. Again he expressed interest in the novelty of the game, and he was able to hold the rules in working memory and play according to the rules while his attention stayed focused on the game. And the next day, HM was shown the same game yet again, and he did not remember seeing it before. And so it went on, day after day, with each day the game appearing to HM to be a complete novelty—he had no memory of previous episodes in which he played the game. But here's the surprise. Although HM never remembered having seen the game before, he nonetheless became more skillful at playing the game. In other words, even though he could not add to his *episodic* memory, he was able to acquire new skills, extending his *procedural* memory. This includes memories of procedures such as how to speak English language or how to go about the routines of everyday life.

Thus, HM not only kept his old episodic memories (from more than 50 years ago by the time of his death) and was able to form and discard working memories, he could also form new *procedural memories*. So we can explain Karl Pribram's experience as follows: When Pribram talked to HM, HM could store relevant items in his working memory and call on skills from his procedural memory to respond appropriately both in talk and action. However, where most of us keep transferring data (unconsciously) about our current situation from working memory to episodic memory, HM was unable to do so. Thus, when Pribram left the room, working memory that had maintained its relevance while he was present was now no longer relevant and was then discarded—and none of it was archived in episodic memory. Thus, when Pribram returned, he seemed to HM to be someone new.

Before proceeding, let me just offer a cautionary tale about the way I have phrased things in the last paragraph. It sounds as if working memory and episodic memory are each like a set of notes written on scraps of paper, to be stored in a set of pigeonholes in the case of episodic memory or to be thrown in the trash after use in the case of working memory. Procedural memory, on the other hand, would be a drawer full of recipes or sets of instructions to be retrieved when needed. Or one could repeat this account, but with each memory stored in a set of "memory locations" in an electronic computer and processed accordingly. Either of these descriptions will serve as a first approximation, but the brain is nothing like a collection of notes scribbled on paper, or even like the highly ordered storage of an electronic computer, where "memory storage" and "processing units" are rigidly separated. Instead, memories are stored by changing the properties of neurons and the connections (synapses) between them, and the same neural network that stores the memory also processes it as patterns of neural firing that form and spread and diffuse and re-form, linking action and perception with our many kinds of memory.

Moviegoers may recognize in the case of HM the inspiration for the 2000 movie *Memento*. The hero, Leonard (Guy Pearce), is an insurance investigator whose memory loss, following a head injury received in events following his wife's murder, exhibits symptoms akin to HM's. Leonard somehow acquires the new skill of tattooing notes on himself and taking Polaroid pictures to provide a substitute for episodic memory. The plot turns on the fact that such "memory" is even more fallible than normal human memory. The movie gets its dramatic force, and its disquieting sense of Leonard's predicament, by presenting its various episodes in reverse order. Thus, when we follow any particular event in Leonard's life, we too have no episodic memory of what went before and instead have only the tattoos and pictures to frame the current situation.

Based on HM's pattern of memory loss and subsequent research on memory, researchers formed the following hypotheses:

1. Working memory involves mechanisms in a different part of the brain than does episodic memory.
2. Hippocampus is necessary for the formation of episodic memories. (Note that this goes beyond what we know about HM, since Scoville had removed several adjacent regions as well as the hippocampus.)
3. However, the fact that episodic memory from before the neurosurgery remains available shows that the hippocampus is not necessary for the long-term storage of episodic memories. We thus talk of a process of *consolidation* whereby episodic memories, shaped by the hippocampus, are eventually stored in long-lasting form elsewhere.
4. Hippocampus is *not* necessary for the formation of procedural memories. (In fact, we now think that procedural memory involves a partnership between regions of frontal cortex and other regions of the brain called the basal ganglia and the cerebellum.)

It is important for our later work to know that different parts of the brain can be involved in different types of learning, but in this book we will not need to look at the details of neuron activity and synaptic plasticity that allow the properties of neurons and their connections to change, whether in the short term or for the long term, to yield these diverse forms of learning and memory.

The Disordered Priorities of Phineas Gage

We now turn to events further in the past to gain insights about how the brain prepares for the future. Phineas Gage was the foreman of a railway construction gang working on the Rutland and Burlington Rail Road when, on September 13, 1848, an accidental explosion of a charge he had set blew his tamping iron through his head.[7] The tamping iron was 3 feet 7 inches long and had a diameter that increased from 1/4 inch at the point of the iron to the 1 1/4 inch diameter of the last 3 feet of its length. The iron went in point first under Gage's left cheekbone and exited through the top of his head, landing about 30 yards behind him. Much of the front part of the left side of his brain was destroyed. A physician named John Harlow treated him successfully, and Gage returned home 10 weeks later. Dr. Edward Williams, who examined Gage before Harlow arrived, mentioned that "the opening through the skull and integuments was not far from one and a half inch in diameter; the edges of this opening were everted, and the whole wound appeared as if some wedge-shaped body had passed from below upward." Amazingly, though, during the time Williams examined this wound, Gage "was relating the manner in which he was injured to the bystanders; he talked so rationally and was so willing to answer questions, that I directed my inquiries to him in preference to the men who were with him at the time of the accident. [N]either at that time nor on any subsequent occasion, save once, did I consider him to be other than perfectly rational."

Before the accident, Gage was a capable and efficient foreman. After his recovery, Harlow reported him to be "fitful, irreverent, indulging at times in the grossest profanity which was not previously his custom, manifesting but little deference for his fellows, impatient of restraint or advice when it conflicts with his desires, at times pertinaciously obstinate, yet capricious and vacillating, devising many plans of future operation, which are no sooner arranged than they are abandoned." He was no longer "himself."

After holding down several jobs—he seemed to have had stable employment, though the jobs did not require the responsibility he had shown as a foreman and had lost with his accident—Gage settled in San Francisco. In February 1860, he began to have epileptic seizures and died on May 21, 1860.

No studies of Phineas Gage's brain were made postmortem. Late in 1867 his body was exhumed, and his skull and the tamping iron were sent to Dr. Harlow, who published his estimate of the brain damage in 1868 in the *Proceedings of the Massachusetts Medical Society*. The skull and tamping iron are now on display at Harvard's Countway Library of Medicine.

But what was the damage to Phineas Gage's brain? There are two problems: Can the path of the tamping iron be estimated accurately from the damage to Gage's skull? And can the damage to his brain be inferred from that path? There are three places where Gage's skull is damaged, one under the cheekbone where the tamping iron entered, the second in the orbital bone of the base of the skull behind the eye socket, and the enormous exit wound. This includes an area of total bone destruction at the top of the skull, mainly to the left of the midline, and another on the lower left side. Between them there is a flap of frontal bone, and behind the main area is a second flap of parietal bone. Harlow replaced both flaps. The parietal flap reunited so successfully that it is difficult to see from outside the skull. The main problem in estimating the trajectory of the iron is to know which part of each of these areas the iron passed through.

Hanna Damasio et al. (1994) located a likely exit point at the top of the skull and identified other possible exit points around it. These points all fell within half of the tamping iron's diameter from the edges of what they called the area of total bone damage, though they excluded the rear flap. They then projected likely trajectories from these mainly right frontal points through the center of the hole in the base to the entry area under the cheekbone. All of them lie to the right of the midline and have the tamping iron emerge under the reunited frontal flap. Ten years later, Ratiu et al. (2004) compared computer-generated three-dimensional reconstructions of a thin-slice computed tomography (CAT) scan of Gage's skull with the actual skull. They observed a continuous line of fracture that began from well behind the area of bone loss on the top of the skull and ran down to the lower left side of the jaw. They also noted that the area of bone loss at the entrance and in the eye socket was about 50% smaller than the maximum diameter of the tamping iron. This convinced them that the skull had hinged open to allow the iron to enter and then been closed by the soft tissue of the head after the iron had emerged through the hole in the unhealed area at the top of the skull.

The different views on the passage of the tamping iron led to different views about which parts of Gage's brain were damaged. Where Hanna Damasio and her colleagues estimated the damage to be quite far frontal and right side, Ratiu and his colleagues concluded that the damage was limited to the left frontal lobe. To make matters worse, even if there were no such disputes over the path of the tamping iron, there would still be massive damage outside the trajectory due to hemorrhaging and the effects of the iron pushing fragments of bone through the brain. Given all these uncertainties, Macmillan concludes that "Phineas Gage's case is important for what it pointed to, rather than what we can learn in any detail from it about the relation between brain and behavior." For Antonio Damasio (1994), the significance of Phineas Gage is that the

> observance of previously acquired social convention and ethical rules could be lost as a result of brain damage, even when neither basic intellect nor language seemed compromised. Unwittingly, Gage's example indicated that something in the brain was concerned specifically with … the ability to anticipate the future and plan accordingly within a complex social environment; [and] the sense of responsibility toward the self and others.

I will not follow the argument further and assess the particular theory of emotion and decision making that Antonio Damasio has developed. But our discussion of HM and Phineas Gage will have been worthwhile if it helps the reader appreciate some of the systems that must be brought into play to situate ourselves with respect to our past experience (whether through episodic memory or the mastery of new skills) and to base our actions on the ability to temper our short-term inclinations (motivation and emotion) with a longer term view of the effect of our actions, both physical and social.

Introducing the Macaque Brain

We now build on our brief tour of the human brain to learn how to read a diagram like Figure 4-8 for the macaque brain and master some of the basic jargon used by neuroanatomists to locate where different structures and pathways occur in the brain. It may seem a bit daunting at first, but think of it in the same way you would approach your first visit to a city—you need to know the names of the main streets and some key landmarks, plus a few foreign phrases, before you can comfortably find your way around.

Figure 4-8 (left) shows the left hemisphere of the cerebral cortex of the macaque (rhesus monkey), with the front of the brain at the left and the back of the brain at the right (as did the left side of Fig. 4-1). There are many important brain regions sheltered within the cerebral cortex, and these provide the brain with pathways and processing stations that link the cortex via the midbrain to the sensory systems and muscles of the head, and via the brainstem to the spinal cord, which contains the sensory and motor neurons for the body and limbs. As in the human brain, each cerebral hemisphere is divided into four lobes. The frontal lobe is at the front, the occipital lobe is at the back (it houses the primary visual cortex, the main way station for visual signals entering cortex), the parietal lobe lies at the top of the brain between the frontal and occipital cortices, while the temporal

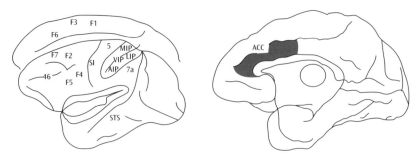

FIGURE 4-8.   (*Left*) A side view of the left hemisphere of the macaque monkey brain
dominates the figure. The central fissure is the groove separating area SI (primary
somatosensory cortex) from MI (primary motor cortex, here labeled F1). Frontal cortex is
the region in front of (in the figure, to the left of) the central sulcus, whereas parietal cortex
is behind the central sulcus. Area F5 of premotor cortex is implicated in the "abstract motor
commands" (part of the motor schemas) for grasping and other actions. The groove in the
middle of the parietal cortex, the intraparietal sulcus, is shown opened here to reveal various
areas. AIP (the anterior region of the intraparietal sulcus) processes "grasp affordances,"
visual information about objects relevant to the control of hand movements directed to those
objects. AIP is reciprocally connected with F5. (Adapted from Jeannerod et al., 1995.) (*Right*)
A glimpse of the medial view of the right hemisphere to show the anterior cingulate cortex
(ACC) involved in monkey vocalizations.

lobe lies in front of the occipital lobe but lower in the cortex. Figure 4-8 (right)
provides a medial view of the right hemisphere to show the anterior cingulate
cortex (ACC), which we will later see to be involved in monkey vocalizations.

I have labeled several areas that anatomists can distinguish by inspecting
their connections, cell structure, and chemical properties. But for now, all we
need to focus on are the areas labeled F5, in frontal cortex, and AIP, in parietal
cortex. We don't need to know all the anatomical details of these regions to
understand the Mirror System Hypothesis, but we will need to know a little bit
about how the firing of neurons in these regions correlates with perception or
behavior, and something of the pathways that link these regions to each other
and to other areas of the brain. F5 gets its label because it is the 5th region (F
for Frontal) in a numbering for areas of the macaque frontal lobe developed
by anatomist colleagues Massimo Matelli and Giuseppe Luppino of Giacomo
Rizzolatti's lab in Parma—a different labeling from that provided by Brodmann
(he mapped the macaque brain as well as the human brain). F5 lies in what is
the ventral part of premotor cortex, and *premotor cortex* gets its name because
it is the part of cerebral cortex just in front of ("pre") the primary motor cortex
shown as F1 (often denoted MI instead) in Figure 4-8. Motor information is
transferred from F5 to the primary motor cortex, to which F5 is directly connected, as well as to various subcortical centers, for movement execution.

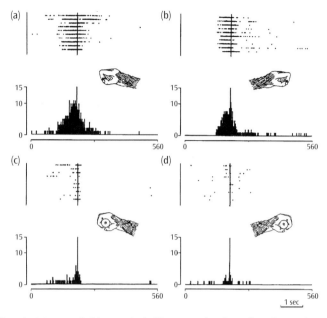

FIGURE 4-9.   Activity recorded from a single F5 neuron that fires when the monkey executes a precision pinch but not when it executes a power grasp. In each panel, we see the grasp executed by the monkey, a set of 10 patterns of the neuron's spikes when the monkey performs the indicated grasp, and a histogram summing the spike recordings to give a statistical view of the cell's response in each of the four cases. Surprisingly, although the cell "cares" about the type of grasp it does not matter which hand executes it. (From Rizzolatti et al., 1988. © Springer.)

Neurophysiologists have shown that many neurons in F5 fire when the monkey grasps an object. Importantly, the firing of these neurons can be correlated with the action that the monkey is carrying out. For example, some neurons fire when the monkey is using a "precision pinch" to grasp a small object between thumb and index finger (Fig. 4-9), while others fire more strongly when the monkey uses a "power grasp" to grab an object without fine finger movement (di Pellegrino et al., 1994; Gallese et al., 1996; Rizzolatti et al., 1996). In addition to "grasping-with-the-hand" neurons, F5 includes "grasping-with-the-hand-and-the-mouth" neurons, "holding" neurons, "manipulating" neurons, "tearing" neurons, and many more—as the monkey learns new skills, like tearing paper or breaking open peanuts, neurons can become tuned for these actions. In Chapter 5, we will introduce the *mirror neurons* of F5, which fire not only when the monkey carries out an action himself but also when he observes a human or other monkey carrying out a similar action. By contrast, the *canonical neurons* are those that fire when the monkey executes a manual action but not when he observes such actions executed by another.

The parietal area AIP is near the front (anterior end) of a groove in the parietal lobe, shown opened up in Figure 4-8, called the intraparietal sulcus (i.e., the sulcus/groove in the parietal lobe). Thus, AIP stands for *a*nterior region of the *i*ntra*p*arietal sulcus. AIP is reciprocally connected with the *canonical neurons* in F5. Taira et al. (1990) established that AIP extracts neural codes for "affordances" for grasping from the visual stream and sends these on to area F5. More generally, *affordances* (Gibson, 1979) are features of an object or the environment relevant to action, in this case to grasping, rather than aspects of identifying the object's identity. Object identity seems to be extracted in the lower, forward part of the temporal lobe, the inferotemporal cortex (IT). For example, a screwdriver may be grasped by the handle or by the shaft, and one does not have to recognize that it is a screwdriver to recognize these different affordances. However, if one wishes to *use* the screwdriver, then one has to recognize this, and this recognition will lead to selection of the handle as providing the relevant affordance. The reader may relate this to the "what" and "how" pathways of Figure 4-4.

Modeling the Grasping Brain

In this section, I sketch out the conceptual basis of a computational model of grasping—but omitting the computational details—to give the reader a deeper understanding of how information flowing through the monkey brain may yield these different forms of neural responsiveness. The FARS model (Figs. 4-10 and 4-11, named for modelers Andy Fagg and Michael Arbib and neurophysiologists Giacomo Rizzolatti and Hideo Sakata) offers an account of how various brain regions cooperate in allowing a human or a monkey to look at an object, figure out how to grasp it, and have the motor cortex send the signals to the muscles, which will cause that grasp to be performed.[8] It provides a computational account of how the AIP *affordances* are transformed to specify an appropriate grasp by the canonical neurons of F5 and offers explicit hypotheses on the interaction between the dorsal ("how") and ventral ("what") streams (Fig. 4-4). This model has been specified in great detail and implemented on computers to yield interesting simulation results (as have models of the mirror neuron system described in Chapter 5), but for our purposes we can ignore the technical details and just look at the models in conceptual terms. The aim is to gain enough understanding of the patterns of activity in the brain regions modeled here to give us the vocabulary we need in later chapters to discuss key changes that occurred in the evolution of the human language-ready brain.

The *dorsal stream* (from primary visual cortex to parietal cortex) of the FARS model (Fig. 4-10) processes visual input about an object to extract affordances.

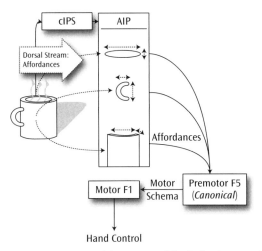

Figure 4-10. The dorsal stream part of the FARS model, which takes input from the primary visual cortex and processes it via, especially, area AIP of parietal cortex. The idea is that AIP does not "know" the identity of the object, but can only extract affordances (opportunities for grasping for the object considered as an unidentified solid) indicated here by portions of the object which are particularly graspable.

It is the part of the brain that can operate without "outside knowledge" when the goal of the monkey is to pick something up, irrespective of its use. In this case, the brain is not concerned with *what* the object is but rather with *how* to grasp the object considered as an unidentified solid, providing the mechanisms you (or a monkey) need to pick up a "nonsense object." Area cIPS (another region of the intraparietal sulcus) of the dorsal stream provides information about the position and location of patches of the surface of the observed object. These data are processed by AIP to recognize that different parts of the object can be grasped in different ways, thus extracting affordances for the grasp system, which (according to the model) are then passed on to F5. Among the important contributions of this part of the FARS model were (1) to stress the role of phase-by-phase population coding in this system, with different neurons active during different phases of interacting with an objects, and (2) to note that visual input might activate AIP codes for more than one affordance, and an affordance might activate F5 codes for more than one type of grasp, so that the circuitry had to include a winner-take-all (WTA) mechanism to select just one of the affordances encoded in AIP and/or just one of the motor schemas compatible with the selected affordance(s). This process would result in area F5 sending the code for the selected motor schema to primary motor cortex, area F1, to commit the network and thus the monkey to a single course of action. The goal has thus been narrowed from "grasp this (unspecified) object)" to "grasp this part

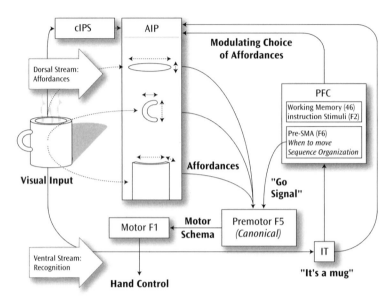

FIGURE 4-11.   Extending the FARS model by bringing in the ventral stream. We see how
the dorsal stream is integrated with the ventral stream via inferotemporal cortex (IT).
Prefrontal cortex uses the IT identification of the object, in concert with task analysis and
working memory, to help AIP select the appropriate affordance from its "menu." Given this
affordance, F5 can select an appropriate motor schema and instruct primary motor cortex to
forward its execution. (Note that the diagram only shows that IT provides inputs to prefrontal
cortex [PFC]; it does not specify the pattern of connectivity with subregions of PFC.)

of the object using this specific grasp." It was the task of F1, working in concert
with other brain regions, to command the appropriate pattern of coordinated
movement of arm and hand to achieve this goal.

The full model (Fig. 4-11) brings in the *ventral stream* (recall Fig. 4-4). It now
addresses the case where the agent has a more specific goal—for example, to
drink coffee from the mug. In contrast to the dorsal stream, the ventral stream
from primary visual cortex to inferotemporal cortex (IT) is able to recognize
what the object is. This information is passed to prefrontal cortex (PFC), which
can then, on the basis of the current goals of the organism and the recognition of the nature of the object, bias AIP to select the affordance appropriate
to the current task. For example, if we see a mug just as an obstacle in the way
of our getting hold of a magazine underneath it, we might grab the mug by
the rim to lift it out of the way; but if we plan to sip coffee from the mug, the
odds are that we will grasp it by the handle. Although there is debate over
whether prefrontal influences affect the AIP → F5 pathway at AIP or F5 or
both (Rizzolatti & Luppino, 2001, 2003), what is beyond debate is that activity
of canonical neurons in F5 is not the result of only the AIP → F5 pathway but is

modulated by activity in prefrontal cortex and inferotemporal cortex (the ventral stream).

Relevant human data come from a study by Buxbaum et al. (2006) of humans reaching to grasp an object. They distinguish shaping the hand preparatory to using an object (*use* condition) from shaping the hand prior to simply grasping the object (*grasp* condition). They provide evidence that object use but not grasping requires activation of semantic systems, with different time courses of response activation for use versus grasp. Activation for use is relatively delayed and of longer duration. Moreover, posturing the hand to use an object is significantly slower with objects such as a computer keyboard in which grasp and use postures conflict (grasp posture = clench, use posture = poke) as compared to objects such as a drinking glass in which grasp and use postures are the same (both = clench). In other words, in "conflict" objects, grasp postures compete with use postures. We again see competition and cooperation between different brain regions and pathways in committing the organism to action.

The full FARS model (Fagg & Arbib, 1998) contains further brain processes that must be coordinated with the grasp selection mechanisms we have described so far in our tour of Figure 4-11. Working memory of where you last put down the mug, encoded in one region of frontal cortex, might enable you to pick it up again even without looking at it. Even more important is that behavior involves the sequencing of actions to achieve a goal. Continuing with our mug example, reaching to grasp the handle is only part of achieving the goal of drinking from the mug: once you have a firm grip on the handle, you want to bring the mug to your mouth, then drink from it. Similarly, a monkey who grasps a raisin will, in general, then proceed to eat it. Each of the "motor schemas" for the individual actions that together make up a whole behavior needs to receive its own "go signal," and this is supplied by another region of prefrontal cortex.

Data from the laboratory of Hideo Sakata gave us a well-controlled example of a sequence of actions, observed within a laboratory setting. In what we call the *Sakata protocol*, the monkey is trained to watch an object until a go signal instructs it to reach out and grasp the object. It must then hold the object until another signal instructs it to release the object. In recording the affordance-related activity of AIP cells in a monkey trained to perform according to the Sakata protocol, Taira et al. (1990) focused their analysis on the portion of AIP cell activity correlated with the affordance of the object. However, Andy Fagg and I were able to obtain unpublished records showing the response of a variety of AIP and F5 cells (our thanks to Hideo Sakata and Giacomo Rizzolatti, respectively), which showed that different neurons might be preferentially active not only for the affordance being grasped but

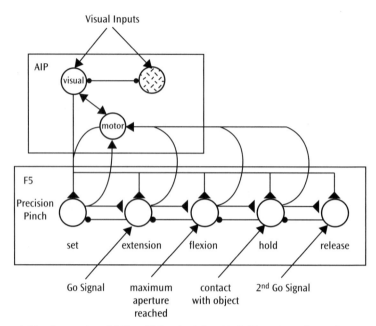

FIGURE 4-12.   Interaction of AIP and F5 in the Sakata Task. Three AIP cells are shown: a visual-related and a motor-related cell that recognize the affordance for a precision pinch, and a visual-related cell for power grasp affordances. The five F5 units participate in a common program (in this case, a precision grasp), but each cell fires during a different phase of the program, with both forward connections to prime the next action and backward connections to inhibit the previous action. (Each single cell shown here represents whole populations of related neurons in the actual brain.)

also for the phase of the overall behavior. We then developed the FARS model to address not only the affordance-based choice of a single action, using the brain regions diagrammed in Figure 4-11, but added further details to address the diversity of temporal patterns exhibited by these neurons.

Figure 4-12 gives a *preliminary* view of how the FARS model handles sequences, but we shall soon see that this view is too simplistic. Cells in AIP instruct the set cells in F5 to prepare for execution of the Sakata protocol—in this case, the recognized affordance primes grasping using a *precision pinch*. Three AIP cells are shown: a visual-related and a motor-related cell that recognizes the affordance for a precision pinch, and a visual-related cell for power grasp affordances. The five F5 units participate in a common program (in this case, a precision grasp), but each cell fires during a different phase of the program. Activation of each pool of F5 cells not only instructs the motor apparatus to carry out the appropriate activity (these connections are not shown here) but also primes the next pool of F5 neurons (i.e., brings the neurons to

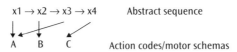

FIGURE 4-13.   A solution to the problem of serial order in behavior: Store the "action codes" A, B, C,…in one part of the brain and have another area hold "abstract sequences" and learn to pair the right action with each element of the abstract sequence.

just below threshold so they may respond quickly when they receive their own *go* signal) as well as inhibiting the F5 neurons for the previous stage of activity. From left to right, the neuron pools are as follows:

- The *set* neurons are activated by the target to prime the extension neurons.
- The neurons that control the *extension* phase of the hand shaping to grasp the object are primed by the set neurons, and they reach threshold when they receive the first *go* signal, at which time they inhibit the set neurons and prime the flexion neurons.
- The *flexion* neurons pass threshold when receiving a signal that the hand has reached its maximum aperture.
- The *hold* neurons once primed will become active when receiving a signal that contact has been made with the object.
- Having been primed, the *release* neurons will command the hand to let go of the object once they receive the code for the second go signal.

However, the problem with the diagram of Figure 4-12 is that it suggests that each action coded by F5 neurons is hardwired to determine a unique successor action—hardly appropriate for adaptive behavior. In the Sakata protocol the monkey will grasp the object, hold it, then release it. But in "real life," the monkey may grasp the object as a prelude for eating it or moving it to another location. Or consider all the possible actions that might occur immediately after you have grasped an apple. Thus, a particular action might be part of many learned sequences—as well as of many spontaneous behaviors—and so we do not expect the premotor neurons for one action to prime a single possible consequent action and thus must reject the "hard wiring" of the sequence shown in Figure 4-12.

Karl Lashley (1951) raised the problem of *serial order in behavior* in a critique of the behaviorist view that each action must be triggered by some external stimulus. If we tried to learn a sequence like A → B → A → C by reflex chaining, in which each action triggers the next, what is to stop A triggering B every time, to yield the performance A → B → A → B → A → …..?

One solution (Fig. 4-13) is to store the "action codes" (motor schemas) A, B, C,…in one part of the brain and have another area hold "abstract sequences" and learn to pair the right action with each element. In this approach, A → B → A → C would be coded as follows: One set of neurons would have connections encoding an "abstract sequence" x1→x2→x3→x4, with sequence learning then involving learning that activation of x1 triggers the neurons for A, x2 triggers B, x3 triggers A again, and x4 triggers C.

Fagg and Arbib posited that F5 holds the "action codes" (motor schemas) for grasping, while a part of the supplementary motor area called pre-SMA[9] holds the code for the abstract sequence x1→x2→x3→x4. Administration of the sequence (inhibiting extraneous actions, while priming imminent actions) is then carried out by the *basal ganglia*, which is responsible for administration of the sequence (inhibiting extraneous actions, while priming imminent actions) on the basis of its interactions with the pre-SMA.[10] The reader may best know the basal ganglia as the brain region that, when depleted of dopamine, is associated with Parkinson's disease, one deficit of which is (depending on the severity of the disease) the reduced ability or inability to sequence actions based on an "internal plan" rather than external cues. For example, a patient with severe Parkinson's disease might be unable to walk across a room unless stripes are placed on the floor, which provide external cues on where to place successive footsteps.

It is worth stressing, as noted earlier, that the FARS model and the mirror neuron system models to be described in Chapter 5 have been implemented on computers to yield interesting simulation results. It is also worth stressing that even though they are not the "final word," but rather way stations in our quest for understanding, they do provide us with key concepts we need in developing the hypotheses on the evolution of language and the brain that this book provides. There is now a range of models of all the subsystems presented earlier, including the basal ganglia, and interaction between modelers and experimentalists continues as we seek to better understand the processes of cooperative computation (supporting competition and cooperation between diverse schemas) whereby neural circuitry supports a complex range of behaviors. Finally, it is worth stressing that exhibiting a well-rehearsed sequence is just one form of behavior, and that this applies to all types of behavior, not just the manual actions we have considered here. In the example of opening an aspirin bottle (Fig. 2-8), the actual sequence executed will depend on assessment of whether certain subgoals have been achieved by the actions executed so far, and we drew parallels with the example of the manager of a restaurant planning a sentence to achieve the *communicative goal* of getting a waiter to serve the intended customer. In these cases, the action is hierarchically structured into "subroutines" that achieve different subgoals. However, in the aspirin bottle example, each step is triggered by some external condition, whereas in the more general scheme of Figure 4-13, and more general schemes for

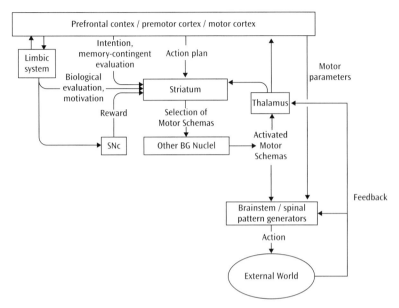

F IGURE 4-14.   A framework for considering the basal ganglia as involved in the control of cognitive as well as motor pattern generators. (Adapted from Graybiel, 1997.)

hierarchical behavior, or when we utter a sentence, we follow an internal plan, without needing such external stimuli to tell us which word to say next. The example of Figure 4-12 involves an intermediate case involving both internal and external triggers. In each case, we have evidence for the importance of the basal ganglia in interaction with other brain regions in both praxis and language (Crosson et al., 2003; Dominey & Inui, 2009; Doupe, Perkel, Reiner, & Stern, 2005; Jarvis, 2004; Kotz, Schwartze, & Schmidt-Kassow, 2009).

Finally, Figure 4-14 presents a conceptual framework (greatly adapted from Graybiel, 1997) for considering the basal ganglia (with input nucleus, the striatum, and other nuclei) as selecting motor schemas for activation on the basis of intentions, an action plan elaborated in cerebral cortex, biological motivation provided by the limbic system (Fig. 4-7), and feedback on ongoing actions. The activation of a motor schema updates, via thalamus, the state of striatum as well as cerebral cortex. It also activates motor pattern generators for both cognitive and praxic actions, with the activity in brainstem and spinal cord influenced by motor parameters from motor cortex and (not shown here) cerebellum. The SNc (substantia nigra pars reticulata) is a separate nucleus that provides dopamine input to influence learning in the striatum. Recent research has suggested that SNc does not provide a direct measure of reward so much as a measure of the error in any predictions the striatum is making as to the expected future reward based on the currently selected action (Schultz, 2006; Sutton, 1988).

Auditory Systems and Vocalization

Whereas vision is the dominant sensory modality in the control of manual action and gesture, monkeys and apes and humans, like most other creatures, depend on hearing for a wide range of information about their world that is crucial to survival. The auditory system plays the central role in many systems of animal communication, whether human speech, primate calls, birdsong, or many more. There is, however, a general consensus that animal calls and human speech are different phenomena. Among the many aspects that differentiate them, such as the strict relation of animal calls (but not of speech) with emotional and instinctive behavior, there is—as we shall see shortly— also a marked difference in the anatomical structures responsible for producing the two behaviors. Animal calls are mediated primarily by the cingulate cortex (Fig. 4-7 for humans; Fig. 4-8 for macaques) together with various subcortical structures as well as the brainstem, which bridges between the brain and the spinal cord. Speech (like language more generally) is mediated by a circuit whose main nodes include the classical Wernicke's and Broca's areas. For now, the aim is to briefly introduce brain mechanisms for hearing and vocalization.

We have seen that the visual system may be analyzed in terms of two complementary but interrelated pathways (Fig. 4-4)—the dorsal "where" pathway and the ventral "what" pathway emanating from primary visual cortex, which is in the occipital lobe. We also noted that vision involves multiple dorsal streams, so that while the what/where distinction was appropriate for a certain working memory task, the what/how distinction was more appropriate for analyzing visually directed grasping of the kind addressed in Figure 4-11.

The auditory system must also analyze both the identity and the location of the stimuli it detects: Identification of "what" can be made on the basis of input to one ear alone, but precise estimation of "where" in three-dimensional space depends on comparison of inputs to the two ears by specialized structures in the brainstem. Processing of "what" and "where" involves different structures and pathways even before the signals reach the auditory cortex. Yet cortical processing is important in both of these tasks. Research on the auditory system (Rauschecker, 1998; Romanski et al., 1999) showed that there are two auditory pathways for processing auditory input in human and nonhuman primates emanating from primary auditory cortex, which is in the temporal lobe (Fig. 4-15): The dorsal auditory stream processes spatial information, whereas the ventral auditory stream processes auditory pattern

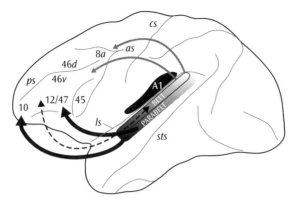

FIGURE 4-15.   The two auditory systems of the macaque start from an area called the lateral belt (the origin of the arrows in the figure, located within temporal cortex), which processes auditory information from the primary auditory cortex, area A1: The caudal ("tailward") areas on the superior temporal gyrus (the region above sts, the superior temporal sulcus) feed into parietal areas and give rise to the dorsal stream, which processes auditory spatial information. The anterior (forward) portions feed forward into the rostral superior temporal gyrus to form the ventral stream, which processes auditory pattern and object information. Both streams eventually project to the frontal cortex, which integrates both auditory spatial and object information with visual and other modalities. (From Romanski, 2007. © Oxford University Press.)

and object information. Auditory objects, including speech sounds, are identified in anterior superior temporal cortex, which projects directly to inferior frontal regions. Both streams eventually project to the frontal cortex, which integrates both auditory spatial and object information with visual and other modalities. The macaque primary auditory cortex—where auditory signals relayed via thalamus first reach cerebral cortex—has a tonotopic organization (i.e., it can be mapped in terms of the predominant frequencies of the sounds to which cells respond), whereas nonprimary auditory cortex responds to complex sounds.[11]

In humans the neocortex is involved in the voluntary control of speech (see Fig. 4-16). This is not so for other primates. Vocalizations in nonhuman primates, while complex and surprisingly sophisticated, maintain close connection to emotional drives and are only rarely under strictly volitional control. In monkeys, for example, electrical stimulation of the neocortex does not affect vocalization. Instead, stimulation of the anterior cingulate cortex elicits vocalizations, such as the isolation call, that have a volitional component, whereas stimulation of various parts of the midbrain elicits cries that are part of their fixed range of emotional displays. Experimental ablation of the areas assumed to be homologous to human Broca's area has no discernible effect whatsoever on species-typical calls in monkeys or in the chimpanzee. By contrast,

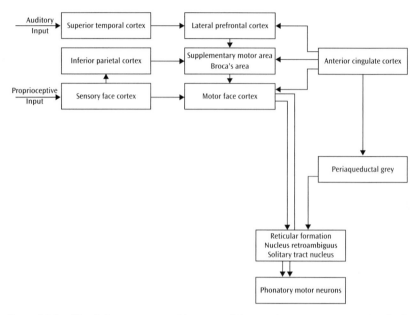

FIGURE 4-16.   Circuit diagram summarizing some of the most important structures involved in speech production. The arrows indicate anatomically verified direct connections. If there is more than one structure in a box, the arrows relate to at least one, but not necessarily all structures. The structures within a box are directly connected with each other. (Adapted from Jürgens, 2002.)

lesions in motor face cortex in humans often result in paralysis of the vocal tract, whereas ablation of the neocortical face area of the macaque produces no effect on communicative vocalizations. This suggests that not even the neural systems for motor control underlying human language and primate communication are homologous.[12]

Jürgens (2002) studied the neural mechanisms involved in species-specific communication in primates, working primarily with squirrel monkey rather than macaques. He found that voluntary control over the initiation and suppression of monkey vocalizations relies on the mediofrontal cortex, including anterior cingulate gyrus. The vocalization-eliciting substrate is an extensive system reaching from the forebrain down into the medulla and includes structures whose neurons represent primary stimulus responses as well as those where stimulation seems to elicit vocalizations as secondary reactions to stimulation-induced motivational changes. The one cortical area Jürgens links to primate vocalization is the anterior limbic cortex with the anterior cingulate gyrus being the key area for producing vocalization when stimulated. Destruction of the anterior cingulate gyrus cortex leaves spontaneous vocalizations intact but yields a severe deficit in monkeys conditioned to vocalize to get a food reward or to postpone an electric shock. Jürgens interprets such findings as suggesting that the anterior cingulate cortex is involved in the volitional initiation of vocalization. But do notice the great difference between controlling the elicitation or nonelicitation of a single call in the monkey, and the generation of diverse patterns of vocalization that the human can attune to the expression of an open-ended semantics. Jürgens found that voluntary control over the initiation and suppression of vocal utterances, in contrast to completely innate vocal reactions such as pain shrieking, relies on the mediofrontal cortex, including anterior cingulate gyrus and supplementary as well as presupplementary motor area. Voluntary control over the subcortical motor pattern generators for vocalization is carried out by the motor cortex via pyramidal/corticobulbar as well as extrapyramidal pathways. Benga (2005) argues that the evolution of vocal speech involved a shift in control from anterior cingulate cortex to Broca's area in order to include vocal elements in intentional communication. She favors the strategic view of the involvement of the anterior cingulate cortex in selection for action, suppression of automatic/routine behaviors, and error correction; however, she notes that some researchers (Paus, 2001) hold that the anterior cingulate cortex has the evaluative functions of error detection and conflict monitoring.

Rauschecker (1998), noting the capacity of humans to use minute differences in frequency, FM rate, bandwidth, and timing as a basis for speech perception suggests that enhancements relative to other primate species have occurred along those dimensions during human evolution—building on existing mechanisms that are universally available in auditory communication systems. On this basis, speech perception is thought to be possible because it combines a high-resolution system for phonological decoding with more efficient memory mechanisms and an ability for abstraction, both residing in a highly developed and expanded frontal cortex.

With this background on the brains of monkeys and humans, we can turn in the next chapter to the properties of mirror *neurons* as revealed by recording from single neurons of the macaque brain and of mirror *systems* as revealed by imaging the human brain.

5

Mirror Neurons and Mirror Systems

Introducing Mirror Neurons

The macaque brain extracts neural codes for "affordances" for grasping to provide key input for premotor area F5 (see Fig. 4-8 in Chapter 4). The breakthrough setting the stage for the Mirror System Hypothesis came with the discovery by the Parma group (di Pellegrino, Fadiga, Fogassi, Gallese, & Rizzolatti, 1992; Rizzolatti, Fadiga, Gallese, & Fogassi, 1996) that a subset of these hand-related motor neurons in F5 had the amazing property that they not only fired when the monkey carried out an action itself but also fired when the monkey observed a human or other monkey carrying out a similar action (Fig. 5-1). The Parma group called these neurons *mirror neurons* to suggest the way in which action and observation of an action mirror each other.

Mirror neurons have excited immense interest in both scientific journals and the popular press because they suggest a neural mechanism for social interaction. If a monkey can map another's action onto neurons in its own brain that are active when it executes a similar action, then it may have access to knowledge about that action that could guide its response to that action.

Mirror neurons do not discharge in response to simple presentation of objects even when held by hand by the experimenter. They require a specific action—whether observed or self-executed—to be triggered. Moreover, mirror neurons do not fire when the monkey sees the hand movement unless it can also see the object or, more subtly, if the object is not visible but is appropriately "located" in *working memory* because it has been seen recently but is now obscured (Umiltà et al., 2001). In either case, the trajectory and handshape must match the affordance of the object.

All mirror neurons show visual generalization. They fire whether the instrument of the observed action (usually a hand) is large or small, or far from or close to the monkey. They fire when the action is made by either a human or monkey hand. Some mirror neurons respond even when the object

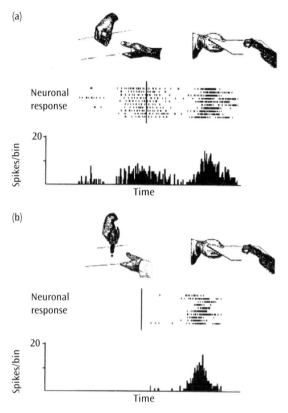

FIGURE 5-1. Example of a mirror neuron. Upper part of each panel: behavioral situations. Lower part: neuron's responses. The firing pattern of the neuron on each of a series of consecutive trials is shown above the histogram, which sums the responses from all the trials. The rasters are aligned with the moment when the food is grasped by the experimenter (vertical line). Each mark in the rasters corresponds to a spike sent down the neuron's axon to signal to other neurons. (a) From left to right: The limited firing of the resting neuron; the firing when the experimenter grasps a piece of food with his hand, then moves it toward the monkey; the firing when, at the end of the trial, the monkey grasps the food. The neuron discharges during observation of the experimenter's grasp, ceases to fire when the food is moved toward the monkey, and discharges again when the monkey grasps it. (b) When the experimenter grasps the food with an unfamiliar tool, the neuron does not respond, but the neuron again discharges when the monkey grasps the food. Recent work (Umiltà et al., 2008) has shown that monkeys can learn, after much training, to use such tools and recognize their use. (From Rizzolatti, Fadiga, Gallese, & Fogassi, 1996 © Elsevier.)

is grasped by the mouth. An important notion in the study of mirror neurons is *congruence*. The majority of mirror neurons respond selectively to one type of action. Some mirror neurons are *strictly congruent* in that the observed and executed actions that are accompanied by strong firing of the neuron must be very similar with the effective motor action (e.g., precision grip) coinciding with the action that, when seen, triggers the neuron (again precision grip, in this example). Other mirror neurons are only *broadly congruent*. For them the motor requirement (e.g., precision grip) is usually stricter than the visual requirement (e.g., seeing any type of hand grasp, but not other actions).

Such data have often been interpreted as consistent with mirror neurons coding for a single action. However, it seems more plausible to regard mirror neurons as, to the extent that their activity correlates with actions, doing so as a *population code*: In other words, the firing of a single neuron is not a "yes/no" code for whether a highly specific action is being executed or observed. Instead, each neuron expresses a "confidence level" (the higher the firing rate, the greater the confidence) that some feature of a possible action—such as the relation of thumb to forefinger, or of wrist relative to object—is present in the current action. We can then think of each neuron as casting a more or less insistent "vote" for the presence of actions with that neuron's "favorite feature"—but it is only the population of neurons that encodes the current action. Moreover, variations in the neural activity can then encode differences in the action such as the aperture and approach angle of a grasp in addition to whether it is a precision pinch, a power grasp, or some other manual action. From an evolutionary point of view, then, it seems reasonable that mirror systems evolved first to monitor feedback on actions and to support learning, with their role in social interaction being secondary.

In summary, each mirror neuron encodes a feature for characterizing an action (which may be relevant to the goal of the action, the movement of the action, or both). Since each experiment on macaque mirror neurons is conducted using only a small set of actions, the aforementioned results may be consistent with the following recasting: A single mirror neuron will be *strictly congruent with respect to a set of actions* if it encodes a feature relevant only to a specific action and those very similar thereto within that set; whereas it is *broadly congruent with respect to a set of actions* if it encodes a feature relevant to a broad class of actions within that set.

The mirror neurons linked to grasping actions constitute *the mirror system for grasping* in the monkey, and we say that these neurons provide the neural code for matching execution and observation of hand movements. Giacomo Rizzolatti (personal correspondence, 2011) has written:

> I also used the term "mirror system" for many years. I am afraid that this term is misleading. There is not such a thing as a mirror system. There are many centers in the brain of birds, monkeys and humans that are endowed with a mechanism—the mirror mechanism—that transform a sensory

representation into its motor counterpart. For example, in the inferior parietal lobule of the monkey there are two and possibly three functionally different areas that are endowed with the mirror mechanism. The term "mechanism" avoids the notion that mirror neurons have a specific behavioral function. As in the case of EPSPs [excitatory postsynaptic potentials], for example, the mirror mechanism has diverse functions (from emotion understanding to song learning in birds). [See] a recent paper (Rizzolatti & Sinigaglia, 2010) where we discuss this point.

However, I don't think the change of terminology solves the problem. (a) Yes, let's stress that there is not one unified system—which is why I wrote *the mirror system for grasping* earlier rather than *the mirror system*. (b) In the later section "Mirror Systems in the Human," I stress that each "mirror system" identified by brain imaging in humans has a lot going on that may or may not depend on mirror neurons, so calling each one a "mirror mechanism" is misleading. "Region containing a mirror mechanism" might do, but it seems verbose and so I will stick with "mirror system" as our shorthand.

We contrast mirror neurons with the so-called *canonical neurons*, which (as we saw in Chapter 4) fire when the monkey executes an action but not when it observes such actions executed by another. More subtly, canonical neurons may fire when the monkey is presented with a graspable object, irrespective of whether the monkey performs the grasp. This must depend on the extra (inferred) condition that the monkey not only sees the object but is aware, in some sense, that it might possibly grasp it (even if, in the end, it does not do so). Were it not for the caveat, canonical neurons would also fire when the monkey observed the object being grasped by another. A necessary experiment is to record mirror neurons both in the usual condition (the monkey observes another acting upon an object but is in no position to act upon the object itself) and in a situation where the observer has a chance to interact with that object—for example, by trying to grasp a piece of food that the other is reaching for. I predict that in the latter case canonical neurons would be active since the observation of the other can here prime the observer's own action.

Perrett et al. (Carey, Perrett, & Oram, 1997; Perrett, Mistlin, Harries, & Chitty, 1990) found that the rostral part of the superior temporal sulcus (STS; itself part of the temporal lobe; see Fig. 5-2) has neurons that discharge when the monkey observes such biological actions as walking, turning the head, bending the torso, and moving the arms. Of most relevance to us is that a few of these neurons discharge when the monkey observes goal-directed hand movements, such as grasping objects (Perrett et al., 1990). However, unlike mirror neurons, STS neurons seem to discharge only during movement

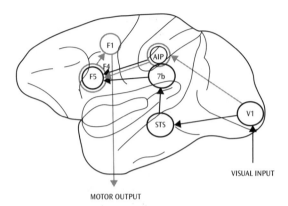

VISUAL INPUT

MOTOR OUTPUT

FIGURE 5-2.   The figure shows two of the dorsal pathways from the visual input to primary visual cortex V1 to premotor area F5. The canonical pathway (grey) runs via various other regions of visual cortex to AIP and then to the canonical neurons of F5, which are active when the monkey grasps but not when it observes others grasping. F5canonical connects to primary motor cortex F1 to help control hand movements. The mirror pathway (black) runs via various other regions of visual cortex to STS and then 7b (also known as PF) and then to the mirror neurons of F5, which are active both when the monkey grasps and when it observes others grasping.

observation, not during execution. Another brain region in the parietal cortex but outside the intraparietal sulcus, area PF (another label for Brodmann area 7b, shown just below AIP in Fig. 5-2) also contains neurons responding to the sight of goal-directed hand/arm actions and seems to provide crucial input to the F5 mirror neurons. About 40% of the visually responsive neurons in PF are active for observation of actions such as holding, placing, reaching, grasping, and bimanual interaction. Moreover, most of these action observation neurons were also active during the execution of actions similar to those for which they were "observers" and were thus called parietal (or PF) mirror neurons (Fogassi, Gallese, Fadiga, & Rizzolatti, 1998). Indeed, STS and F5 may be indirectly connected via area 7b/PF.

Fogassi et al. (2001) reversibly inactivated area F5 in monkeys trained to grasp objects of different shape, size, and orientation. During inactivation of the F5 area containing canonical neurons (buried in the bank of the arcuate sulcus), the hand shaping preceding grasping was markedly impaired and the hand posture was not appropriate for the object size and shape. The monkeys were eventually able to grasp the objects, but only after a series of corrections made under tactile control. With inactivation of the F5 area containing mirror neurons (lying on the cortical convexity of F5), motor slowing was observed but the hand shaping was preserved. Inactivation of the hand field of primary motor cortex (area F1 =, M1) produced a severe paralysis of contralateral finger movements.

My view is that canonical neurons prepare the manual action that is executed via F1, while during self-movements mirror neurons provide an important observational function. This might seem to contradict the observation by Fogassi et al. (2001) that hand shaping was preserved despite mirror neuron inactivation. However, my hypothesis is that, during self-action, the activity is not necessary when a well-rehearsed action is performed successfully. (For further discussion, see section "From Mirror Neurons to Understanding.")

Natural actions typically involve both a visual and an audio component. And, indeed, some of the neurons in area F5 of the macaque premotor cortex were found to be *audiovisual mirror neurons*. They are responsive not only for visual observation of actions associated with characteristic noises (such as peanut breaking and paper ripping) but also for the sounds of these actions (Kohler et al., 2002), and they constituted 15% of the mirror neurons Kohler et al. studied in the hand area of F5.

But there are also mirror systems for actions other than grasping. One such system involves orofacial neurons in an adjacent, indeed somewhat overlapping, area in macaque F5. About one-third of the motor neurons in F5 that discharge when the monkey executes a mouth action also discharge when the monkey observes another individual performing mouth actions. The majority of these *orofacial mirror neurons* (also known as *mouth mirror* neurons) become active during the execution and observation of mouth actions related to ingestive functions such as grasping with the mouth, or sucking or breaking food. Another population of orofacial mirror neurons also discharges during the execution of ingestive actions, but the most effective visual stimuli in triggering them are communicative mouth gestures (e.g., lip smacking). This fits with the hypothesis that neurons learn to associate related patterns of sensory data rather than being committed to learn specifically pigeonholed categories. Thus, a potential mirror neuron is in no way committed to become a mirror neuron in the strict sense, even though it may be more likely to do so than otherwise. The observed communicative actions (with the effective executed action for different "mirror neurons" in parentheses) include lip smacking (sucking and lip smacking); lips protrusion (grasping with lips, lips protrusion, lip smacking, grasping with mouth and chewing); tongue protrusion (reaching with tongue); teeth chatter (grasping with mouth); and lips/tongue protrusion (grasping with lips and reaching with tongue; grasping).

To summarize: mirror neurons for manual and orofacial actions in the macaque have been identified in F5 in premotor cortex and in PF (and the nearby area PFG) in parietal cortex (Fogassi et al., 1998; Gallese, Fogassi,

Fadiga, & Rizzolatti, 2002). The visual input to this parietal region seems to come from the STS region of the temporal lobe (Perrett et al., 1990). The activity of macaque mirror neurons is thus attributed to the pathway STS → PF → F5 (Rizzolatti & Craighero, 2004).

Four relevant observations concerning the neurons of macaque F5 are as follows:

1. There are many neurons in F5 that are neither canonical nor mirror neurons.
2. The canonical neurons lie on the bank of the sulcus containing F5; the mirror neurons lie on the crown.
3. The outflow of mirror neurons as distinct from canonical neurons has not been determined.
4. The circuitry within F5 whereby canonical, mirror, and other neurons influence each other is not known.

When the monkey observes an action that resembles one in its movement repertoire, a subset of the F5 and PF mirror neurons is activated that also discharge when a similar action is executed by the monkey itself. The crucial thing is to remember the two pathways shown in Figure 5-2:

V1 → AIP → F5canonical → F1 → motor output
V1 → STS → 7b/PF → F5mirror

In particular, we stress that parietal cortex (the "top right" part of monkey cerebral cortex in Fig. 4-8 [left] and the "top left" part of human cerebral cortex in Fig. 4-2 [right]) can be subdivided into many regions and that different parietal regions provide the input to the canonical and mirror neurons. One (AIP) is concerned with the affordances of objects, and another (7b/PF) is concerned with relations between an object and the hand that is about to grasp it.

Modeling How Mirror Neurons Learn and Function

In the general spirit of action-oriented (embodied) computation, it must be stressed that mirror neurons are as much perceptual as motor. For example, recognizing a manual action from visual observation requires, in general, recognition of the object upon which the action is to be executed and of the spatiotemporal pattern of the hand's movement relative to the object. My group's computational models of the mirror system for grasping, to which we now turn, show how neurons may *become* mirror neurons by learning to

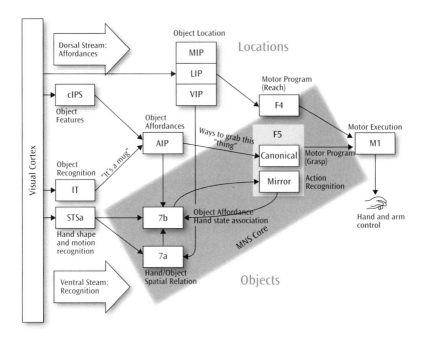

FIGURE 5-3.   A schematic view of the Mirror Neuron System (MNS) model of the mirror system for grasping. Note that visual input is processed in different streams to extract the affordances of an object and the shape and movement of a hand. The model describes mechanisms whereby particular mirror neurons come to recognize affordance-centered trajectories of the hand that correspond to specific types of grasp. It can thus equally well activate appropriate mirror neurons when the trajectory involves the hand of the self or the hand of another. Note, however, that the model does not address how attention comes to be directed to a particular hand and a particular object. (See text for a further tour of the diagram.) (From Arbib & Mundhenk, 2005; adapted from the original system figure of Oztop & Arbib, 2002.)

recognize the trajectory of the hand in an object-centered reference frame for self-execution of an action. This representation then supports recognition of the action when performed by others and, in many cases, will allow confident recognition of the action relatively early in the trajectory of the hand toward the object. Our modeling demonstrates that F5 mirror neurons lie at the end of complex processing based—at least—on inferotemporal and parietal computation.

The FARS model of the canonical system (Fig. 4-11 in Chapter 4) showed the importance of object recognition (inferotemporal cortex: IT) and "planning" (prefrontal cortex [PFC]) in modulating the selection of affordances in the determination of action. But now we want to look in more detail at the way various brain regions work together to support the activity of mirror neurons. To this end, we introduce the Mirror Neuron System (MNS) model of Oztop and Arbib (2002), which shows how the brain may learn to evaluate whether the approach of the hand to an object is an instance of a particular kind of grasp. Importantly, the model does *not* build in as innate the recognition of a specific set of grasps. Instead, the model focuses on the *learning capacities* of mirror neurons. It thus allows us to bring in the role of neural plasticity and how we employ it in models of self-organization and learning.

As shown in Figure 5-3, the MNS model can be divided into parts as follows:

- First, we look at those elements involved when the monkey itself reaches for an object as various brain regions process data on the location and affordances of an object to formulate parameters for the reach and the grasp that can be transformed by the motor cortex M1 to control the hand and the arm.

    ○ We see the pathway whereby cortex can instruct the hand muscles how to grasp. Object features computed by parietal area cIPS are processed by AIP to extract grasp affordances. These are sent on to the canonical neurons of F5 that choose a particular grasp. This corresponds to the dorsal pathway AIP → F5canonical → M1 (primary motor cortex) of the FARS model, but Figure 5-3 does not include the important role of PFC in action selection, which was highlighted in the FARS model.

    ○ We also see the pathway whereby cortex can instruct the arm muscles how to reach, transporting the hand to the object. Parietal areas MIP/LIP/VIP provide input to F4, an area of premotor cortex adjacent to F5, to complete the "canonical" portion of the MNS model. Recognizing the location of the object provides parameters to the motor programming area F4, which computes the reach.

- The rest of the figure shows the essential elements for training the mirror system, emphasized by the shading in the center of the figure. These regions provide components that can learn and apply key criteria for activating a mirror neuron, recognizing that

    ○ the preshape that the monkey is seeing corresponds to the grasp that the mirror neuron encodes;

    ○ the preshape that the observed hand is executing is appropriate to the object that the monkey sees; and

    ○ that the hand is moving on a trajectory that will bring it to grasp the object.

In the MNS model, the *hand state* is defined as a vector whose components represented the movement of the wrist relative to the location of the object and of the handshape relative to the affordances of the object. This encodes the trajectory of the relation of parts of the hand to the object rather than the visual appearance of the hand in the visual field, and provides the input to the F5 mirror neurons.

Oztop and Arbib (2002) showed that an artificial neural network corresponding to PF and F5mirror could be trained to recognize the grasp type from the *hand state trajectory*, with correct classification *often being achieved well before the hand reached the object*. The modeling assumed that the neural equivalent of a grasp being in the monkey's repertoire is that there is a pattern of activity in the F5 canonical neurons that commands that grasp.

Training occurs when the "monkey" initiates an action. The activation of the canonical neurons for that action will have two consequences:

(a) A hand-object trajectory corresponding to the canonically encoded grasps will be generated.
(b) The output of the F5 canonical neurons, acting as a code for the grasp being executed by the monkey at that time, will serve as the *training signal* for the F5 mirror neurons that they activate.

This combination enables the activated mirror neurons to increase their responsiveness to those parts of the trajectory that best correlate with the canonically encoded grasp.[1] As a result of this training, the appropriate mirror neurons come to fire in response to the appropriate trajectories even when the trajectory is not accompanied by F5 canonical firing.

Because the input to the F5 mirror neurons from area PF encodes the trajectory of the relation of parts of the hand to the object rather than the visual appearance of the hand in the visual field, this training prepares the F5 mirror neurons to respond to hand-object relational trajectories even when the hand is of the "other" rather than the "self." What makes the modeling worthwhile is that the trained network responded not only to hand state trajectories from the training set but also exhibited interesting responses to novel hand-object relationships. Such learning models, and the data they address, make clear that *mirror neurons are not restricted to recognition of an innate set of actions but can be recruited to recognize and encode an expanding repertoire of novel actions.* The modeling also shows that the trained network responded not only to hand-state trajectories from the training set but also exhibited interesting responses to novel hand-object relationships. However, the model only accepts input related to one hand and one object at a time, and so it says nothing about the "binding" of the action to the agent of that action.

A *mirror neuron*, strictly defined, is a neuron that is active both when the organism executes a limited range of actions and when it observes a strictly or broadly congruent set of actions. But if mirror neurons gain their properties as a result of learning, is a neuron in F5 to be called a mirror neuron if it fires for the recognition of an action the animal cannot perform? I would say that these are certainly mirror neurons if training has simply broadened their congruence. However, there is a deeper issue here that seems not to have been addressed in the literature. In both cases we have a set of neurons so situated that it is possible for them to become active in both the observation and execution of actions. It seems a reasonable scientific goal to understand the actual and potential capabilities of such neurons. If, even after adaptation, some of these neurons are not active for both execution and observation of similar movements, then one has a terminological choice as to whether to still call them mirror neurons. Let us introduce the following terminology:

A *potential mirror neuron* is a neuron located and subject to such learning rules that with appropriate experience of the organism it could become a mirror neuron. Depending on the course of learning, it may become active when the organism performs an action without yet firing in response to observing it (the scenario in the MNS model) or become active when the organism observes an action when the organism has yet to learn how to perform the action itself (which seems necessary when mirror neurons are involved in imitation by observation).

A *quasi-mirror neuron* extends the range of action observation beyond actions in the organism's repertoire in a very specific way: It links this observation to *somewhat* related movements that can support pantomime. For example, when I flap my arms to suggest a bird's flying, this may involve mirror neurons effective for execution only of arm flapping but for observation of both arm flapping and bird flight. I would argue that quasi-mirror neurons are crucial to the evolution of language, providing an intermediate stage which precedes the ability to abstract and perform purely symbolic gestures whose mirroring is separated from actions more iconically related to the symbolized action and object. Or perhaps we should just see these as an extended form of *broadly congruent* mirror neurons whose activation depends on rather general skills in mapping the body schema of a different species onto one's own (for further discussion, see Chapter 8). As we shall see in the next section, there are also *action recognition neurons that lie outside the mirror system*. For example, we can recognize a dog barking without activating the mirror system, but presumably the mirror system for orofacial movements would be activated if we observed the dog barking when we were preparing to imitate it.

peanut breaking

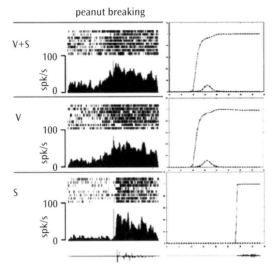

FIGURE 5-4. (*Left*) Activation of an audiovisual mirror neuron responding to (from top to bottom) the visual and audio components, visual component alone, and audio component alone of a peanut-breaking action. At the bottom is an oscillogram of the peanut breaking sound. (From Kohler et al. 2002. © Springer.) (*Right*) Simulation results from the MNS2 model showing activation of the model's external output layer when presented with a precision grasp sequence containing (from top to bottom) visual and audio, visual-only, and audio-only information. At the bottom is an oscillogram of the sound associated with the precision grasp. The experimental data and model output show anticipatory mirror neuron activity for visual-only and audiovisual conditions, but this activity is confined to the duration of the action sound in the audio-only condition. (From Bonaiuto et al., 2007.)

Now let us return to modeling. A key achievement of the MNS model was that it showed how the brain could learn to recognize "early on" the trajectory relating hand to object during a manual action. A more recent model, MNS2 (Bonaiuto, Rosta, & Arbib, 2007), has some differences in the learning model that make it more biologically plausible than MNS2, but these technicalities need not detain us. What is important here is that MNS2 augments the basic structure of the MNS model to provide circuitry that includes an audio component. Some of the mirror neurons in area F5 of the macaque premotor cortex, the so-called *audiovisual mirror neurons*, are responsive both for visual observation of a particular action, such as peanut breaking and paper ripping, which is associated with characteristic sounds and also just as responsive for those sounds (Fig. 5-4, left).

MNS2 models the processing performed by auditory cortex at an abstract level. The model learns to associate different actions with patterns of activity in the audio input units if a strong enough correlation exists between sound and action. In this way, sounds that are consistently perceived during the course of

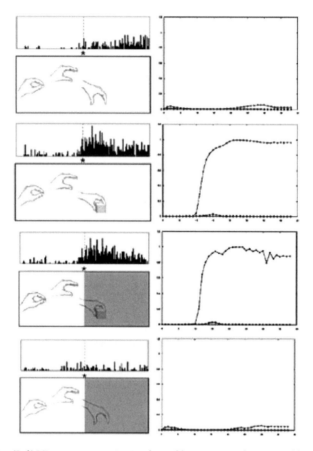

FIGURE 5-5.   (*Left*) Mirror neuron activation for visible pantomimed grasp, visible grasp, hidden grasp, and hidden pantomimed grasp conditions. (From Umiltà et al., 2001; used with permission of Elsevier.) (*Right*) Activation of the output layer of the MNS 2 model for the same conditions. The model output is in good agreement with the experimental data in that visible and hidden grasps are correctly identified, while visible and hidden pantomimed grasps elicit little or no response. (From Bonaiuto et al., 2007.)

an executed action become associated with that action and incorporated into its representation. This type of audio information is inherently actor invariant, and this allows the monkey to recognize that another individual is performing that action when the associated sound is heard. Obviously, the auditory response to observation of peanut breaking cannot start still the peanut actually breaks to emit a characteristic sound, whereas the visual response can commence earlier.

Umiltà et al. (2001, see Fig. 5-5 left) have shown that mirror neurons in the macaque monkey can "infer" the result of an action whose final portion is hidden. In these experiments, the monkey was shown an object that was then obscured by a screen. When the monkey observed the experimenter reaching behind the screen to grasp the object, the same mirror neurons responded that would respond to a visible grasp of the same object. By contrast, this neuron does not respond to a reach when no object is visible, or if the human reaches behind a screen that was not previously shown to conceal an object.

To explain this, the MNS2 model incorporates the idea of working memory—the ability to hold information while it is relevant to ongoing action. Once they are obscured behind the screen, the presence of the hand and of the object must be stored in *working memory*. The crucial difference, however, is that the working memory of the object is static, whereas the working memory of the hand must be updated continually to extrapolate the hand's position as it moves—or fails to move—toward the object. This process of updating the estimate of hand position and grasp is called *dynamic remapping*. MNS2 updates the working memory representation of wrist position by using the still-visible elbow position and the fact that the forearm is a rigid body. Before being hidden, the object position and its affordance information are stored in working memory. In this way, if the monkey observes an object that is then hidden by a screen, and then observes an experimenter make a grasp that disappears behind that screen, the wrist trajectory will be extrapolated to end at the remembered object location and the grasp will be recognized by the F5 mirror neurons.

It is not necessary for the arguments that follow to recall the details of the FARS model and the MNS models. What is important is to understand that many different neural populations must work together for the successful control of hand movements and for the successful operation of the macaque mirror system for grasping, which, as we saw from Figure 5-3, involves much more than an isolated "mirror mechanism."

Mirror Systems in the Human

Are there mirror neurons in the human brain? In humans, we cannot measure the activity of single neurons save when needed for testing during neurosurgery,[2] but we can gather data on the relative blood flow through (and thus, presumably, the neural activity of) a brain region when the human performs one task or another. We use brain imaging (e.g., positron emission tomography [PET] or functional magnetic resonance imaging [fMRI]) to test whether the human brain contains a *mirror system* for some class X of actions in the sense of a region active for both execution and observation of actions from X as compared to some baseline task.[3] As we have stressed already in our discussion of the macaque, there are different mirror systems for different X's located in different parts of the brain.

Brain imaging has revealed that the human brain has a *mirror system for grasping* (and other mirror systems as well) —regions that are more highly activated both when the subject performs a range of grasps and observes a range of grasps (Grafton, Arbib, Fadiga, & Rizzolatti, 1996; Rizzolatti, Fadiga, Matelli et al., 1996) as compared to simply looking at objects. Remarkably, activation for both the execution and observation of grasping was found in the frontal lobe of the human brain in or near Broca's area, a region that in most humans lies in the left hemisphere and is traditionally associated with speech production (Fig. 4-1 right). However, we saw at the end of Chapter 1 that it makes more sense to view Broca's area as an area for language production in a way that includes manual as well as spoken language—all in relation to a broader framework of the generation and recognition of praxic actions. Such brain imaging supports the claim for a human mirror system for grasping in the inferior parietal lobule (IPL; homologous in part to monkey PF) and the inferior frontal gyrus (IFG, including Broca's area and homologous in part to macaque F5), and one may assume a corresponding pathway STS → IPL → IFG (Fig. 5-2). The human IPL is partly specialized for language in the left hemisphere, whereas both human IPL and the macaque homolog support spatial cognition in both hemispheres.

Following this early work there have been very few papers exploring mirror neurons in the macaque or other animals,[4] and the latter primarily from the Parma group and their colleagues, but there has been an explosion of papers on the imaging of various putative human mirror systems. However, brain imaging cannot confirm whether the region contains individual mirror neurons, though this seems a reasonable hypothesis. More disturbingly, the regions whose activation is visualized in brain imaging are so large that—in light of the macaque data—we may conclude that if indeed they contain mirror neurons, they also contain canonical neurons and neurons that are neither mirror nor canonical. Indeed, this is not only a problem with fMRI resolution but rather of intrinsic organization of most association areas. For example, in the macaque IPL one can find neurons with markedly different properties in adjacent microelectrode penetrations.

Thus, although activation of a region in one condition may show mirror system properties, relatively high activation of the region in other conditions is no guarantee that the latter activation is due primarily to the firing of mirror neurons.

In other words, it is misleading to name an area for just one of the functional modes it may exhibit because such naming makes it easy to conflate those modes.[5] However, if we understand this fact, then we can avoid many of the pitfalls of using the term *mirror system*. Unfortunately, the vast majority of human studies related to mirror systems ignore this basic fact. Once a region has been found active in correlation with both observation and execution of a class of actions, it is then dubbed *the* (or *a*) Mirror Neuron System and henceforth any behavior correlated with activity in that region is said to involve, or even depend on, the activity of mirror neurons. It cannot be stressed too strongly that even if a brain region has been characterized as a mirror system for some class of actions, it must not be concluded (without further data) that activation of the region seen in a particular study is due to the activity of mirror neurons. The failure to analyze the neural circuitry implicated in the activation of a brain region in an imaging study is compounded by the predominance of "boxology" in the analysis of brain imaging data. If brain region X is more active in task A than in task B, X is often regarded as a "box" implicated in task A but not task B. However, X may be essential to both tasks, but with greater synaptic activity required in meeting the demands of A rather than B. Only through the lens of computationally testable models of detailed neural circuitry such as the FARS and MNS models can we determine whether success at a task A that involves activation of a so-called mirror neuron system rests essentially on the presence of mirror neurons in that region or is mediated by nonmirror neural circuitry.

But this seems to raise a paradox: How can there be models of detailed neural circuitry in the human brain if almost no single-cell recordings are available? The solution may lie in applying a method called *synthetic brain imaging* (Arbib, Bischoff, Fagg, & Grafton, 1994; Arbib, Fagg, & Grafton, 2002; Lee, Friston, & Horwitz, 2006; Tagamets & Horwitz, 2000; Winder, Cortes, Reggia, & Tagamets, 2007), which allows one to average over the synaptic activity of neurons in portions of a neural network model of the brain to make predictions of the relative activity that will be seen in different brain regions in actual brain imaging studies. Thus, future models will adopt the following strategy:

- For circuitry highly similar in the macaque and human brain, use a macaque model and synthetic brain imaging to directly predict results for human brain imaging, then use the empirical results to calibrate the model.
- For higher cognitive processes and language, use hypotheses about evolution of brain mechanisms to suggest how macaque circuitry is modified and expanded upon in the architecture of the human brain, then use the resultant model to make predictions for human brain imaging (Fig. 5-6).

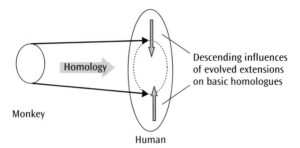

Figure 5-6.   A strategy for modeling the human brain: Use known circuitry in the macaque brain to suggest details of circuitry in homologous regions of the human brain. Extend these models using hypotheses on brain evolution. Test the result again with human brain imaging studies by the use of synthetic brain imaging.

But the details are outside the scope of the present volume.

From Mirror Neurons to Understanding

When neurophysiologists study a macaque monkey's mirror neurons (as in gaining the data of Fig. 5-1), the monkey attends to an action of the experimenter but does not respond overtly. Rather, its "reaction" is observed via microelectrodes that show which neurons active during action observation are also active when the monkey itself performs a similar action. The monkey does not imitate. What then is the adaptive value of mirror neuron activity? Most writers have noted the adaptive advantage that such a system could have for social interaction, allowing one monkey to "understand" the actions of another, and thus position itself to compete or cooperate with the other monkey more effectively. Alas, there are no data on recording mirror neurons while monkeys engage in natural social interactions, so more needs to be done to verify whether the macaque brain does indeed support "action understanding." In any case, I hypothesize that the adaptive pressure for the initial evolution of mirror neurons was *not* social. Instead, I think that the first mirror neurons for grasping served as part of a feedback system for increasingly dexterous manual control, thus yielding extraction of the hand-object relations posited in the MNS model to provide the key input to mirror neurons. But once a neural representation that could extract such relations existed, it could provide the opportunity for "social circuitry" to evolve so as to best exploit this information to more subtly delineate the behavior of conspecifics. I suggest that further evolution was required to go from mirror neurons that are part of the feedback system for motor control to having them serve as part of the circuitry that mediates understanding. Indeed, Arbib and Rizzolatti (1997) asserted that what makes a movement into an action is that (1) it is associated with a goal, and (2) initiation of the movement is accompanied by the creation of an expectation that the goal will be met: action = movement + goal. To the extent that the unfolding of the movement departs from that expectation, to that extent will an error be detected and the movement modified. In other words, the brain of an individual performing an action is able to predict its consequences and, therefore, the action representation and its consequences are associated. Thus, a "grasp" involves not only a specific cortical activation pattern for the preshape and enclosing movements of the hand but also expectations about making appropriate contact with a specific object. The expectation that the goal will be achieved may be created *before* the movement's initiation, but the point is that neurally encoding this expectation allows the brain to judge (this "judgment" need not involve conscious awareness) in due course whether the intended action was successful. This is to be distinguished from the detailed use of feedback during motor control, which can monitor any errors as they occur and provide corrective forces that may lead to successful completion of the action after all.

Despite this early discussion of expectations during self-action, almost all the attention given in the literature to the possible roles of mirror systems has focused on responding to the actions of others. To explore uses of mirror neurons active during self-action, my group has recently introduced the novel hypothesis that a mirror system may not only help in monitoring the success of a self-action but may also be activated by recognition of one's own *apparent* actions as well as efference copy from one's intended actions (Bonaiuto & Arbib, 2010). We provided a computational demonstration of a model of action sequencing, called *augmented competitive queuing* (the ACQ Model), in which action choice is based on the desirability of executable actions. The idea is this: When we start to execute an intended action within a certain context, mirror neurons can create an expectation of reaching the goal of that action. If the expectation is not satisfied, then the brain can decrease its estimate of the action's executability—of how likely it is to succeed in the given context. But if we fail to execute one action, we may nonetheless, in some cases, succeed in completing a movement and achieving a desirable goal (or taking a step toward such a goal). If so, the mirror system may "recognize" that the action looks like an action already in the repertoire. As a result, learning processes can increase the neural estimate of the desirability of carrying out that action when the animal attempts to achieve the goal in the given context. By expressing these ideas in a form that could be simulated on a computer, we showed how the "what did I just do?" function of mirror neurons can contribute to the learning of both executability and desirability, and how in certain cases this can support rapid reorganization of motor programs in the face of disruptions.

In their recent book, Rizzolatti and Sinigaglia (2008, translated from the Italian original of 2006) provide what is undoubtedly the best review of the literature on mirror neurons in the macaque brain and mirror systems in the human brain. Their account is engaging, accessible, and enriched by a broad philosophical framework. It will remain for many years the standard reference for those who wish to understand the mirror system. Nonetheless, their interpretation of the data involves some emphases that may be misconstrued with respect to the contributions the mirror system makes to human brain function. They state that the mirror neurons are *"primarily involved in the understanding of the meaning of 'motor events', i.e., of the actions performed by others"* (p. 97). I have already suggested their possible role in self-actions. However, the above statement must not be construed as implying that "the meaning of 'motor events', i.e., of the actions performed by others, is primarily accomplished by the activity in mirror neurons." Such activity *in itself* may lack the rich subjective dimensions that often accompany a human's recognition of an act or situation. Note that I am *not* denying that the monkey's recognition of action may be quite rich.[6] What I *do* deny is that the mere activity of F5 mirror neurons alone suffices to provide such richness or to constitute "understanding" the action. But what of the weaker claim that their output triggers a complex motor and sensory network similar to that activated when an individual is thinking (motor imagery) or even performing that motor act and that this similarity allows one to understand others matching their motor acts with the representation of his or her own? I think that this is acceptable if one accepts that this "thought-related network" can be activated by means other than those involving mirror neurons, while noting that activity of canonical neurons is lacking.

Consider a pattern recognition device that can be trained to classify pixel patterns from its camera into those that resemble a line drawing of a circle and those that do not (with the degree of resemblance cut off at some arbitrary threshold). I would argue that this device does not *understand* circles even if (like mirror neurons) it is linked to a device that can draw circles. However, to the extent that this recognition could be linked to circuitry for forming associations like "the outline of the sun or an orthogonal cut through a cone yields an appropriate stimulus," one might say that the larger system of which the pattern recognizer is part does exhibit understanding. Understanding is thus not a binary concept but rather a matter of degree; some things may be encoded appropriately yet not understood at all, others may be understood in great richness because their neural encoding is linked to many other behaviors and perceptions.

Figure 5-7 emphasizes that F5 (and presumably any human homolog labeled as a "mirror system") contains nonmirror neurons (here the canonical neurons are shown explicitly) but that it functions only within a larger context provided by other brain regions for understanding and planning of actions within a broader framework of scene interpretation of the kind exemplified by the VISIONS system of Chapter 1. The direct pathway (e) from mirror neurons to canonical neurons for the same action may yield "mirroring" of the observed action, but it is normally under inhibitory control. In some social circumstances, a certain amount of mirroring is appropriate, but the total lack of inhibition exhibited in *echopraxia* and *echolalia* (Roberts, 1989)—the compulsive repetition of observed actions or heard words, which in humans may accompany autism—is pathological. While it is true that mirror neuron activity correlates with *observing* an action, I have just argued that such activation is insufficient for *understanding* the movement—thus, the indication of other systems for interpretation and planning in Figure 5-7. A possible analogy might be to observing a bodily gesture in a foreign culture—one might be able to recognize much of the related movement of head, body, arms, and hands that constitute it yet be unable to understand what it means within the culture.

Rizzolatti and Sinigaglia (2008, p. 137) assert that numerous studies (e.g., Calvo-Merino, Glaser, Grezes, Passingham, & Haggard, 2005) "confirm the decisive role played by motor knowledge in understanding the meaning of the actions of others." The cited study used fMRI brain imaging to study experts in classical ballet, experts in capoeira (a Brazilian dance style), and inexpert control subjects as they viewed videos of ballet or capoeira actions. They found greater bilateral activations in various regions, including "the mirror system," when expert dancers viewed movements that they had been trained

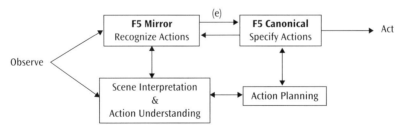

FIGURE 5-7.   The perceptuomotor coding for both observation and execution contained in F5 region for manual actions in the monkey is linked to "conceptual systems" for understanding and planning of such actions within the broader framework of scene interpretation. The interpretation and planning systems themselves do not have the mirror property save through their linkage to the actual mirror system.

to perform compared to movements they had not. Calvo-Merino et al. assert that "their results show that this 'mirror system' integrates observed actions of others with an individual's personal motor repertoire, and suggest that the human brain understands actions by motor simulation." However, nothing in the study shows that the effect of expertise is localized entirely within the mirror system. The integration they posit could well involve "indirect" influences from the prefrontal cortex such as those we studied for canonical neurons in the MNS model.

Indeed, Rizzolatti and Sinigaglia (2008, p. 137) go on to say that the role played by motor knowledge does not preclude that these actions could be "understood with other means." Buccino et al. (2004) used fMRI to study subjects viewing a video, without sound, in which individuals of different species (man, monkey, and dog) performed ingestive (biting) or communicative (talking, lip smacking, barking) acts. In the case of biting there was a clear overlap of the cortical areas that became active in watching man, monkey, and dog, including activation in areas considered to be mirror systems. However, although the sight of a man moving his lips as if he were talking induced strong "mirror system" activation in a region that corresponds to Broca's area, the activation was weak when the subjects watched the monkey lip smacking, and it disappeared completely when they watched the dog barking. Buccino conclude that actions belonging to the motor repertoire of the observer (e.g., biting and speech reading) are mapped on the observer's motor system via mirror neurons, whereas actions that do not belong to this repertoire (e.g., barking) are recognized without such mapping. However, in view of the distributed nature of brain function, I would suggest that the understanding of *all* actions involves general mechanisms that need not involve the mirror system strongly—but that for actions that are in the observer's repertoire, these general mechanisms may be complemented by activity in the mirror system that enriches that understanding by access to a network of associations linked to the observer's own performance of such actions.

Rizzolatti and Sinigaglia (2008, p. 125) assert that "the sight of acts performed by others produces an *immediate* activation [my italics] of the motor areas deputed to the organization and execution of those acts, and through this activation it is possible to decipher the meaning of the 'motor events' observed, i.e. to understand them in terms of goal-centered movements. This understanding is completely devoid of any reflexive, conceptual, and/or linguistic mediation." [I think that reflexive is used here as "requiring reflection," not as "involving a reflex."] But consider our reassessment of the Buccino et al. (2004) study, the expanded view provided by Figure 5-7, and the role of the ventral stream and prefrontal cortex in the FARS model, which augment the direct activation of mirror neurons by the dorsal path (7b/PF → F5mirror).

They bring into play conceptual processing and, in humans, provide scope for linguistic and reflective influences – as when, for example, one recognizes a smile but asks oneself "Is that person smiling at me or with me?"

In tracing the macaque neurophysiology of the mirror system (recall Fig. 5-2), we saw that neurons in the superior temporal sulcus (STS), as studied by Perrett et al., are active during movement observation though perhaps not during movement execution, and that STS and F5 may be indirectly connected via area PF, which, like F5, contains mirror neurons. As Rizzolatti et al. (2001) observe, STS is also part of a circuit that includes the amygdala and the orbitofrontal cortex—crucial components for emotional regulation in the brain (Fig. 4-7 in Chapter 4)—and so may be involved in the elaboration of affective aspects of social behavior. Although the relation of mirror neurons to emotion is peripheral to the focus of this book (but an important topic when the emphasis shifts from language to other aspects of social interaction), let's take a moment to touch briefly on the way in which human emotions are greatly influenced by our ability to empathize with the behavior of other people. We have all had moments when we felt a welling up of sadness on seeing the grief of another or smiled in response to another's smile. In *The Expression of the Emotions in Man and Animals*, Charles Darwin (1872/1965) observed that we share a range of physical expressions of emotion with many other animals. Our tendency to feel others' emotions, and the fact that certain emotions are so universal as to be shared with other mammals, have led a number of researchers to suggest that in addition to a mirror system for manual actions, we have one for the generation and recognition of physical expressions of emotion. In fact, there seem to be multiple systems involving different classes of emotions.

The suggestion is that these systems enable us to empathize with others not simply by recognizing their emotions but by experiencing them. This is related to the *simulation theory* (Gallese & Goldman, 1998), which proposes that mirror neurons support our ability to read minds by "putting ourselves in the other's shoes" and using our own minds to simulate the mental processes that are likely to be operating in the other. Other findings suggest that the ability to recognize the auditory and visual details of a person's actions may be a factor in empathy (Gazzola, Aziz-Zadeh, & Keysers, 2006). The role of a brain region called the insula in a mirror system for disgust (Wicker et al., 2003) suggests that emotional communication may involve diverse mirror systems. However, "emotion recognition" is not just a matter of empathy. If I were to see someone advancing toward me with a knife, I would recognize his anger yet feel fear. I would not empathize as I struggled to protect myself. And, indeed, much of the literature on mirror neurons does distinguish between low-level visuomotor reaction and a more comprehensive understanding of the other's emotions.

We saw motivation and emotion as the motors of behavior in Chapter 4 while in Chapter 1 we offered a schema-theoretic view of the "self" as a "schema encyclopedia," our own personal stock of schemas that guides the way we perceive and interact with the world, both physical and social. A crucial aspect of social interaction is our view of others. The term "Theory of Mind" has become widely adopted for the ability of humans to understand that other people may be like oneself yet have different knowledge and points of view. Gallese and Goldman argue that observed action sequences are represented in the observer "offline" to prevent automatic copying, as well as to facilitate further processing of this high-level social information. However, as suggested in Figure 5-7, mirror neurons alone cannot mediate understanding. Instead, understanding rests on a network of associations distributed across multiple brain regions.

This cautions us to distrust talk of "the" mirror system but rather seek to understand the roles of, and interactions between, multiple mirror systems such as those for hands and faces and—in humans—language. This book has its primary emphasis on intermediate stages in the evolution of mirror systems and the networks that support them, from the macaque-like system for grasping to those that support language. I would suggest that, similarly, a number of stages would have to intervene in the evolution of the brain mechanisms that support emotion and empathy. This raises the challenge of connecting empathy with language evolution by assessing how our ability to experience others' emotions affected the way the language-ready brain evolved. But this challenge lies outside the scope of this book.

Dapretto et al. (2006) studied children imitating facial expressions of emotion and found that *increasing* scores on measures for autism spectrum disorder (ASD) correlated with *decreasing* activation of the mirror system during the imitation task. However, the children with ASD successfully imitated the facial expressions! This suggests that normally developing children recognize the emotion and express it themselves, whereas the ASD child must reproduce the expression as a meaningless aggregate of facial movements, devoid of emotional meaning—just as we might imitate a meaningless grimace.

Another issue is this: How does mirror neuron activity related to our own actions get segregated from that involved in recognizing the action or emotional state of others? The classic version of the "binding problem" is the one addressed in studies of vision. We each have the illusion of a unitary consciousness, yet the information that makes up that consciousness is distributed across multiple brain regions. Different facets of our perceptual experience are processed separately. For example (Fig. 5-8), shape and color are processed separately in the mammalian visual system, so that when one sees a blue

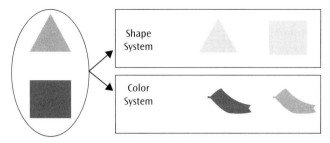

FigURE 5-8.   The classic binding problem for vision: Which color should be bound to which shape? (See color insert for full color version of this figure.)

triangle and a red square, the shape system will recognize that one is seeing a *triangle* and a *square* and the color system will recognize that one is seeing *red* and *blue*. The *binding problem* is to ensure that the appropriate attributes are bound together—triangle with blue, red with square—so that one does not mistakenly see a blue square and a red triangle.

We saw that the "Simulation Theory" proposes that we come to "read" other minds by simulating the mental processes that are likely to be operating in the other. However, one must appreciate that the other is indeed other—that is, that the "simulation" must use different "variables" from those that describe one's self. This is *the binding problem for mirror neurons*: For mirror neurons to function properly in social interaction, not only must they be simultaneously active for multiple actions and emotions, but the brain must also bind the encoding of each action and emotion (whether self or other) to the agent who is, or appears to be, experiencing it.

When two people interact, regardless of whether this interaction involves language, each builds in his (or her) brain (whether consciously or not) a representation both of his own intended actions, using internal cues like his own beliefs and desires, and the potential actions of the other agent with whom he interacts. The partial concordance of representations of actions of the self and other (including mirror neurons) are used by each agent to build a set of predictions and estimates about the social consequences of the represented actions, if and when they would be executed. An important point here is that each agent must not only register his (or her) own actions but also those of the other, and in doing so his brain must solve the "binding problem" of linking each activated set of mirror neurons encoding an action to the appropriate agent for that action as well as to the object on which the action is being performed.

To conclude our introduction to mirror neurons and mirror systems, then: Mirror neurons may play a crucial role both in self-action and in understanding the action of others. But, as sketched in Figure 5-3 (and even more sketchily in Fig. 5-7), mirror neurons do not provide understanding in and of themselves but only as part of a larger system "beyond the mirror." However, they enrich that understanding by connecting it with the motor system, going beyond mere perceptual classification, providing means to short circuit analysis of the action of others in cases where they can be integrated into the subject's own motor experience. More specifically, the MNS and ACQ models together help us understand how learning can develop mirror properties for a wide range of actions and employ them not only in contributing to the recognition of others but also (and perhaps this is prior, in evolutionary terms) in regulating one's own actions by evaluating them against the expectations generated for one's intentions.

With this understanding firmly in place, we can now restate the Mirror System Hypothesis in more detail and outline the way in which it will be developed in the rest of this book.

Part II

DEVELOPING THE HYPOTHESIS

6

Signposts. The Argument of the Book Revealed

Part 1 put in place the base of knowledge on which we will build a particular form of the Mirror System Hypothesis for the evolution of the language-ready brain. The present chapter will develop the general framework for thinking about language evolution in terms of both biological evolution and cultural evolution. We will then review the basic tenets of my version of the Hypothesis and show how they will be developed in the subsequent chapters.

The Story So Far

Chapter 1 presented the "lampposts" that have illuminated my attempts to relate language to the brain, introducing schema theory as a means of characterizing brain function in a way that complements the structural description of the brain in terms of neurons and brain regions and structures of intermediate complexity. After showing its basic relevance to neuroethology, the study of animal behavior, I went on to show how schema theory could be used for the study of vision and dexterity, establishing ways to think about cooperative computation as uniting perceptual and motor schemas in mediating our embodied interaction with the world. Social schemas then expressed patterns of social reality, collective representations such as those exhibited by people who share a common language. These patterns of behavior exhibited by a community provide an external reality that shapes the development of new schemas in the brain of a child or other newcomer whereby she comes to be a member of the community to the extent that her behavior becomes itself a contribution to that social schema.

Since our goal is to understand how language evolved, it was important in Chapter 2 to assess different frameworks for studying human languages. In modern human languages, we combine words (or words and various modifiers) to form phrases, and phrases to form sentences. Each language has a rich syntax that supports a compositional semantics whereby from the meanings of words and the constructions that combine them, we can infer the meaning of the whole phrase or sentence. This underlies our ability to create and understand an endless array of novel utterances. But composing the meanings of words does not always help—the meanings of "kick" and "bucket" do not yield the idiomatic meaning of "he kicked the bucket." Moreover, recursion plays a crucial role, in that structures formed by applying certain rules or constructions can then become units to which those same rules or constructions can again be applied.

Having gained some appreciation of how words could be combined by an autonomous syntax, we nonetheless argued that language was better understood within the framework of the action-perception cycle implicit in the work of Chapter 1, and then suggested that construction grammar—where the combination of words involves constructions that address both form and meaning—might provide a more appropriate framework for placing language in an evolutionary framework. Another important point was to rid ourselves of the view that equates language with speech. We saw that human sign languages are fully expressive human languages that, with appropriate vocabulary, can express any ideas expressed in spoken languages. We also noted that the co-speech gestures that speakers use do not form a sign language, although they can certainly enrich the spoken component of a conversation.

We used Chapter 3 to get a handle on vocalization and gesture in monkey and ape, thus providing comparison points to show how these forms of communication in nonhuman primates compare to the rich form of human communication we know as language. Each species of monkey has its own small repertoire of innate calls, whereas any group of great apes—bonobos, chimpanzees, gorillas, and orangutans—may have a limited repertoire of communicative manual gestures that in part varies from group to group. This suggests that some of their gestures have been "invented" and learned, something that is not true for monkey calls. Nonetheless, the repertoire of gestures is quite limited and shows no evidence of syntax. Moreover, when captive apes are taught to use "language," they are not really using language since their "vocabulary" is limited and they have no sense of syntax.

Having established a view of the (very limited) relation between the communication systems of nonhuman primates and human languages, we turned in Chapter 4 to the brain mechanisms of both macaque monkeys and humans as the basis for tracing in subsequent chapters the stages that the Mirror System Hypothesis posits for the evolution of the language-ready brain. We introduced the human brain and its major subdivisions, and we recalled two famous case studies of brain damage—the story of HM introduced the hippocampus, one of the brain structures that supports episodic memory (the memory of past episodes), whereas the story of Phineas Gage showed the role of prefrontal cortex in planning for the future. The brain mechanisms that they lost make "mental time travel" possible, the cognitive ability to go "beyond the here and now," which is so much part of the human condition. We then turned to an account of the macaque brain that focused particularly on the linkage of vision and action involved in manual behavior, giving a brief account of a computational model (the FARS Model) to illustrate how different parts of the brain can work together in guiding a course of action. We also looked at the auditory system of the monkey and the neural mechanisms for control of macaque vocalization, contrasting them with the cortical areas of the human brain involved in the production of speech . . . and sign languages.

We completed setting the stage with Chapter 5, Mirror Neurons and Mirror Systems. We introduced mirror neurons in some detail, looking not only at mirror neurons related to grasping but also extensions of the mirror system that bring in orofacial expressions and the sounds of actions. We used a conceptual view of a computational model, the Mirror Neuron System (MNS) model, to extend our understanding of how mirror neurons work and learn within a wider context of neural systems with which they interact. We then related mirror neurons in the macaque to mirror systems in the human brain, while stressing that a so-called mirror neuron system will contain many other neurons and that these may at times dominate its overall activity. Moreover, we were careful to distinguish the specifics of mirror neuron activity from the broader notion of understanding the action of others. The ACQ Model showed how mirror neurons could play a valuable role in the regulation of one's own actions—a role that may have preceded, in evolutionary terms, its role in recognizing the actions of others. Finally, we considered the role of mirror neurons in empathy, noting the binding problem that challenges the brain in matching emotions to the self and to others and, echoing the earlier caveat, sought to distinguish the specifics of mirror neuron activity from the broader notion of *understanding* the emotions of others.

With this, we are ready to restate the Mirror System Hypothesis in the context of a discussion of brain imaging, homologies, and a mirror system for grasping in humans. But first, let us look at the general issues posed by the study of human evolution, and then we can introduce the notion of protolanguage as a capability that our distant ancestors developed long before they had language.

Evolution Is Subtle

Darwin taught us that evolution proceeds by *natural selection*—that offspring can vary in random ways from their parents, that some changes may equip some offspring to better exploit some ecological niche and thus reproduce more successfully, and that such changes may accumulate over many generations to yield a new species. The new species may displace the ancestral species, or the two species may both survive as each is able to "make a living"—whether by using different resources from a shared environment or by migrating into different environments, with each better suited to live and reproduce in the environment that it inhabits. Subsequent research has greatly enriched this picture and added layers of subtlety. In particular, the discovery of genes and mutations established the genotype as the locus of change and the phenotype as the locus of selection. Biologists have long made the distinction between the *genotype* and *phenotype* of an individual. The *genotype* (the set of genes present in each cell of the body but expressed in different ways in different cell groups) determines how the organism develops and establishes the cellular mechanisms for how it functions, but it is the *phenotype* (which we now understand includes not only the brain and body but also the behaviors whereby the organism interacts with its world and the physical and social environment so constructed) that is the basis for making a successful living in the sense of raising offspring. What EvoDevo—the integrated study of biological evolution (Evo) and development (Devo)[1]—stresses is that genes do not create the adult phenotype directly but help channel the development of the organism (which is also responsive to environmental interactions). Moreover, genes alsp play a crucial role in the adult body, with each cell of the body *expressing* (i.e., reading out the instructions of) only some of its genes at any time. Thus, the genotype determines which genes are available and includes regulatory genes that can set constraints on how genes are transcribed and turned on or off. Particular cells will be fated to become parts of the brain, and we hold that the human genotype is unique in creating a language-ready brain. However, we now know that learning changes patterns of gene expression in neurons, as other aspects of the (internal and external) environment can change gene expression in cells more generally. Thus, the cellular architecture of the adult brain reflects not only the underlying genotype but also the social and physical milieu as refracted through individual experience, and this architecture includes not only the shape and connections of the individual cells and the larger structures they form but also the very chemistry of specific cells as differential experience changes the pattern of genes that are expressed within each one.

The emergence of the primates involved many changes that differentiate them from other mammals, including increased dexterity. Similarly, humans diverged from other primates over the course of millions of years, with many changes in both body and brain. The bodily changes include subtle changes in biochemistry, bipedal locomotion, and the resultant freeing of the hands for even greater dexterity both in practical skills and in communication, the change from fur to hair, and *neoteny* (the prolongation of infancy), to name just a few. In this book, I will take most of these bodily changes for granted, but I will be particularly concerned with the implications of increased dexterity, focusing on the evolution of the brains of hominids, the part of the primate family tree that split off from that of the great apes 5 to 7 million years ago, and of which *Homo sapiens*, the species of modern humans, is the sole survivor.[2]

There is a subtle interplay between bodily changes (including sensor organization and motor apparatus, too) and brain changes, where some of this may reflect existing mechanisms for self-organization but provide variations on which natural selection may operate to yield evolutionary changes. What needs reiterating here is that the genome does not come neatly packaged in terms of separate sets of genes for separate nuclei of the brain or each part of the body, nor does each brain nucleus control its own set of behaviors. (Caution: Biologists use "nucleus" in two senses—the nucleus of a cell is where the DNA of the genotype is stored; a brain nucleus is a grouping of tightly linked brain cells and is thus a unit in neuroanatomical analysis.) Natural selection can operate on the macromolecules from which cells are built, on crucial cellular subsystems, and on the morphology of cells themselves, as well as the connectivity of these cells and their formation into diverse brain nuclei. When we see the incredible variety of neural forms and connections in the brain, we can no longer view natural selection as a straightforward key to form and function. What is selected about a subsystem may be the impact of some change on a larger system or a smaller detail, rather than the immediate change in the subsystem itself. While portions of the genetic code control chemical processes in the cells of the adult brain, it does not specify the form of the adult brain so much as the processes of self-organization in cell assemblies that can yield "normal" connectivity in the brain of an adult raised in a normal environment (EvoDevo, again).

Hughlings Jackson, a 19th-century British neurologist, viewed the brain in terms of levels of increasing evolutionary complexity. Damage to a "higher" level of the brain disinhibited "older" brain regions from controls evolved later, to reveal evolutionarily more primitive behaviors. Evolution not only yields new brain regions connected to the old but also yields reciprocal connections that modify those older regions. After the addition of a new "hierarchical level," return pathways may provide a new context for the origin of "earlier" levels; evolutionary regression may then be exhibited under certain lesions that damage these "return pathways."

Finally, the environment that fosters adaptive self-organization may be as much social as physical in nature. Thus, for example, the brain of a literate human is different from that of someone who has never learned to read (Petersson, Reis, Askelof, Castro-Caldas, & Ingvar, 2000). As Bickerton (2009) and Iriki & Taoka (2012), among others, has emphasized, *niche construction theory* (Odling-Smee, Laland, & Feldman, 2003) is highly relevant to language evolution, focusing on the evolutionary feedback loop between genes and behavior. The basic idea is that animals modify the environments they live in and that these modified environments, in turn, select for further genetic variations. There is thus a continual feedback process wherein the animals are developing the niche and the niche is developing the species. Odling-Smee et al. (2003) list hundreds of species that, to some degree or other, engineer their own niches, including beavers, ant species like leaf-cutters that build underground fungus farms, and earthworms. Organisms may create niches that change the selective pressures for other species as well as their own. Any animal can, at least in principle, either adapt to a preexisting niche or construct a new one. A crucial aspect of language is that it greatly expanded the range of cooperation by which our ancestors could work together to construct new niches, both socially and physically.

Human Evolution: Biological and Cultural

We have seen that macaque monkeys diverged some 25 million years ago from the line that led to humans and apes, and that the line that led to modern chimpanzees diverged 5 to 7 million years ago from the hominid line that led to modern humans (recall Fig. 3-1). My concern is to hypothesize what our ancestors were like at each of these choice points. In doing so, I stress that language—as distinct from certain other forms of communication—played no role in the evolution of monkeys or apes or the common ancestors we share with them. Any changes we chart prior to the hominid line (and, perhaps, well along the hominid line) must have been selected on criteria relevant to the life of those ancient species, rather than as precursors of language—but we will be greatly interested in how the evolution of the language-ready brain built on these earlier adaptations.

The family tree for hominids has australopithecines preceding *Homo habilis*, which in turn precedes *Homo erectus* (Fig. 6-1), widely viewed as the precursor of *Homo sapiens*. New discoveries reported in 2009 suggest that we can push prehuman history back at least another million years before "Lucy" (*Australopithecus afarensis*; see the special issue of *Science*, October 2, 2009) with the discovery of much of "Ardi," a skeleton of *Ardipithecus ramidus*. It is widely agreed that *Homo erectus* evolved in Africa and expanded from there to Europe and Asia. It is also widely agreed that *Homo erectus* did not evolve into *Homo sapiens* independently in each of Africa, Europe, and Asia. Rather, *Homo sapiens* evolved in Africa and formed a second expansion out of Africa (Stringer, 2003). However, although fossil remains can tell us something of the behavior of these hominids, they reveal little about their brains beyond their overall volume and perhaps the relative size of major subdivisions as

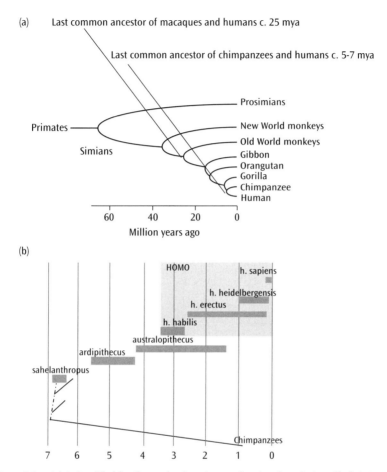

FIGURE 6-1.   (a) A simplified family tree for the primates showing the splitting off of simians from prosimians and then further divergences for monkeys, apes, and humans, with the last common ancestor of macaques and humans c. 25 million years ago and the last common ancestor of chimpanzees and humans c. 5–7 million years ago. (b) The big split in human evolution after the split from our last common ancestor with chimpanzees was between the australopithecines and the various *Homo* lineages, but the diagram also shows earlier ancient forms, *Sahelanthropus* and *Ardipithecus*. The diagram also shows some of the key species of *Homo* based on fossil evidence, as well as our own species *Homo sapiens*. A branching tree has not been inserted because it is not always clear whether an older species is ancestral to a more recent one. The time line at the bottom is in millions of years before the present; the gray bars indicate estimates of the duration of a species based on limited fossil evidence as given in the special issue of *Science* of October 2, 2009 (page 38) devoted to findings on *Ardipithecus*.

inferred from the inner surface of the skull. In this book, I will focus on comparing the brains and behaviors of living primates rather than the study of fossils in constructing a framework for assessing the evolution of the language-ready brain.

The phenotype is not only structural but also behavioral: Frogs not only have long tongues, they use them to catch prey; bees not only have the means to gather pollen, they have a dance to communicate where it came from relative to the hive. Whereas these *behavioral phenotypes* may be the result of "brain genes" acting in a relatively neutral environment, many behavioral phenotypes express both the brain's inherent organization and its shaping by the learning of the individual organism within the social and physical milieu in which the organism is raised. For many species, the "social milieu" is hard to disentangle from the biology, but for primates we can discern a variety of "rituals," "practices," and "tribal customs" that constitute a body of culture constrained by, but in no sense determined by, the biological makeup of the individuals in the social group. Patterns of tool use, for example, are "cultural" in this sense, varying from one community of apes to another (Whiten et al., 2001; Whiten, Hinde, Laland, & Stringer, 2011). Thus, as we come to analyze the evolution of the hominids, culture comes to play an important role even in biological evolution, as well as being itself subject to change and selection. As we talk about "constructed niches" for humans and their ancestors, we see an inextricable melding of culture and physical environment—as in the difference between a hunter-gatherer, a farmer, and a city dweller (and many refinements of each of these broad categories).

Another mechanism is *Baldwinian evolution* (Baldwin, 1896)—the notion that once a group has developed a useful skill by social means, the ability to perform that skill may well itself be subject to natural selection, yielding a population whose successive generations are increasingly adept at that skill. However, one should not accept the notion that every human skill has a biological basis. Consider Web surfing as an example where the rise of the skill in the population has nothing to do with biological change. Moreover, even if some biological changes were necessary, one needs to consider whether acquiring the new capability was itself the "prime mover" in selecting for the change, or whether it was some other change that made the new capability learnable once it had first been discovered. For example, one can imagine many cases where a simple increase in the ability to focus visual attention, or an increased capacity for working memory, could provide a nonspecific boost that would encourage increasing skill levels over a number of generations.

In historical linguistics, a *protolanguage for a family of human languages* is the posited ancestral language from which all languages of the family are hypothesized to descend historically with various modifications through a process of cultural evolution that need involve no genetic changes in the formation of brain and body.[3] For example, proto-Indo-European is the protolanguage for the family of Indo-European languages that ranges from Hindi to Greek and English (see the discussion of Fig. 13-1 in Chapter 13). In most of this book, however, a *protolanguage* (without further qualification) will be any system of utterances used by a particular hominid grouping (including, possibly, tribes of early humans) that we would recognize (if only we had the data) as a precursor to human language but that is not itself a "true" language (Hewes, 1973). By a *true language* I mean a system, as delineated in Chapter 2, in which novel meanings can be continuously created both by inventing new words and by assembling words "on the fly" according to some form of grammar that makes it possible to infer plausible meanings of the resulting utterance, novel though it may be. This latter process is called *compositional semantics.* Our hominid ancestors evolved a brain different from that of a monkey or an ape, one that could support protolanguage—and a protolanguage is an open-ended form of communication that is more powerful than the call and gesture systems of nonhuman primates but lacking the full richness of modern human languages. However, debate continues over what protolanguages were like—a debate to which I return in Chapter 11. Even if the nature of protolanguage were resolved, another question remains open: Did the transition from protolanguage to language require major biological evolution of brain structure to support it, or did this transition (like that from spoken language to written language) require a history of widely accepted innovations but with no necessary change in the brain's genetic plan?

It has often been observed that the human archeological record shows little trace of art, burial rituals, and other "modern" developments of human culture (as distinct from, say, hunting practices, tool making, and the use of fire) before some 50,000 to 100,000 years ago, and some have argued that this apparent transition may have occurred with the "discovery" of language (Noble & Davidson, 1996). For example, D'Errico, Henshilwood, and Nilssen (2001) report on an engraved bone fragment from c. 70,000-year-old Middle Stone Age levels at Blombos Cave, South Africa and discuss its implications for the origin of symbolism and language. Evidence of bone-working techniques was found at the site, and they argue that marks on the bone were intentionally engraved. Noting that engraved designs have also been identified on pieces of ochre from Blombos Cave, they suggest that such engraving was a symbolic act with symbolic meaning. Of course, this leaves open whether it was created by people who already had language, or indicated a growing symbolic awareness that might evolve culturally into language over the course of the following millennia.

Dating when humans first used a language (open lexicon, rich grammar) remains impossible—but the issue here is whether language was part of the genetic makeup of the earliest modern humans (*Homo sapiens*) or whether the brain of early *Homo sapiens* was "language-ready" but required tens of millennia of cultural evolution to achieve language. Let me explain this crucial distinction more fully. No one would claim that part of the biological selection that shaped the human brain more than a hundred thousand years ago was that there was a selective advantage to playing videogames. Nonetheless, the human brain was "videogame-ready": Once history had led to the invention of the appropriate technology through the accumulation and dissemination of many acts of genius, human brains had no problem acquiring the skills needed to master that technology.[4] Whether the correct figure for the emergence of true languages is 50,000 or 100,000 years is not the issue; the strong claim made in this book is that there is a real difference between protolanguage and language, and that the first *Homo sapiens* had brains that evolved biologically in part so they could support protolanguage but that they did not have language in the modern sense.

With the concept of language-readiness at hand, I phrase three pertinent questions for the study of the evolution of human language as follows:

The biological question ("biological evolution"): How did humans evolve a "language-ready" brain (and body)? This raises the ancillary questions: What is it about the human brain and body that allows humans to acquire language? How did it get to be that way? Human children can acquire language of a richness denied to nonhuman primates. However, the attributes that make this possible may not be directly related to language as distinct from protolanguage. For example, today's children can easily acquire the skills of Web surfing and videogame playing, but there are no genes that were selected for these skills.

The historical question ("cultural evolution"): What historical developments led to the wide variety of human societies and languages seen today? If one accepts the view, for which I will argue in later chapters, that the earliest *Homo sapiens* had protolanguages but did not have language in the modern sense, then one must include in this task an analysis of how languages may have emerged from earlier protolanguages (note the plural) via cultural rather than biological evolution.

The developmental question: What is the social structure that brings the child into the community using a specific language, and what neural capabilities are needed in the brains of both the child and his or her caregivers to support this process?

This last question brings us back the mindset of EvoDevo. The nature-nurture debate is dead. The development of brain and body is the result of the inextricable interactions of genetic and environmental factors, where these environmental factors range from nutrition to exercise to caregiving to social interaction. For us, in particular, the issue of what is special about the human brain goes beyond its basic structure to emphasize the processes of

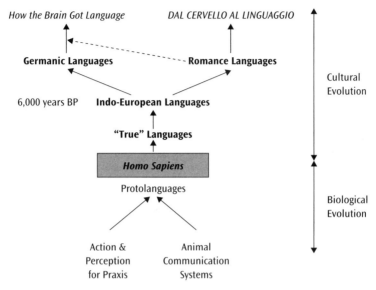

FIGURE 6-2.   When I gave a talk in Ferrara in Italy some years ago, the publicity for my talk in English gave not only the English title (How the Brain Got Language) but also an Italian title (Dal Cervello al Linguaggio—in English, From Brain to Language) that captured the spirit of the original but not its literal meaning. However, the point of the tree of language shown here is not to ponder the mysteries of translation but rather to illustrate the transition from biological to cultural evolution. Biological evolution yielded a language-ready brain and early *Homo sapiens* who had *protolanguage*, but, according to the hypotheses developed in Part 2 of this volume, it then took many tens of millennia of cultural evolution for true languages to emerge, with further historical change yielding proto-Indo-European—the ancestor of Romance and Germanic and many other language groups—perhaps only 6 thousand years ago. The same structure, could of course, be illustrated with any language family, such as the Sino-Tibetan languages, the Niger-Congo languages, the Afro-Asiatic languages, the Austronesian languages, the Dravidian languages, or any number of smaller language families.

self-organization and learning (what we refer to together as "neural plasticity") that can shape the brain's development not only in the womb but throughout life. As a result, the structure of the brain will reflect the individual's experience, though the extent to which experience can shape a given brain will depend on its "nature," the genetic mechanisms that specify the basic wiring diagram of the brain, its growth, metabolism, and plasticity. Thus, the biological and historical questions come together in the developmental question.

To close this section, let's return to cultural evolution. Italian—like Spanish, Catalan, and Romanian—is a Romance language, Roman in origin, descended from Latin. The divergence of the Romance languages from Latin took about 1,000 years. English is a Germanic language drastically restructured by overlays from Norman French, another Romance language. All Romance and Germanic languages are viewed as Indo-European languages, descended from the "proto-Indo-European" language of perhaps 6,000 years ago (Dixon, 1997). The divergence of the Indo-European languages to form the immense diversity of Hindi, German, Italian, English, and so on, occurred through processes of historical change and the interaction of many people and peoples. Given so much change in a mere 6,000 years, how can we imagine what has changed since the emergence of *Homo sapiens* some 200,000 years ago? Or in 5 million years of prior hominid evolution?

Three Key Hypotheses

Figure 6-2 summarizes the argument of this book: that biological evolution up until 100,000 or 200,000 years ago shaped the brain and body of our early *Homo sapiens* ancestors so that they could communicate in a flexible way using hands and voice but did not yet have "true" languages. It then took tens of millennia for our ancestors to progress from *protolanguages* (in the *non*-historical sense) to achieve something like true languages around 50,000 to 100,000 years ago (give or take a few tens of millennia). More specifically, the book develops three hypotheses:

Hypothesis 1. There is no innate Universal Grammar: *The human genome provides language-readiness—the capacity of the child to acquire and use language if raised in a community that already has language—rather than encoding detailed syntactic knowledge in a Universal Grammar.*

As we saw in Chapter 2, Noam Chomsky, the most influential linguist of the 20th century, showed that much could be learned about human languages by focusing on the study of syntax autonomously, that is, without emphasizing its linkage with semantics or language use.[5] The result was a sequence of frameworks (differing quite markedly from decade to decade) each seen as providing a so-called Universal Grammar rich enough to describe all the key variations in the overall structure of syntax that can be found when comparing a wide variety of human languages. However, where I part company with Chomsky is this: Not only did he offer each version of Universal Grammar as a descriptive framework for the study of syntax; he went further to assert that this machinery is actually genetically coded in the brain of every human infant, and it is essential to the operation of what he calls the Language Acquisition Device. This claim is made without reference to the empirical literature on language acquisition, but Chomsky's standing as a master linguist has given unwarranted credence to his views on language acquisition, and so they need to be addressed if one is to get a clear understanding of what the human genome must provide to develop a language-ready brain, and we shall do so in Chapter 11.

More generally, I reiterate that the human brain has the potential for amazing feats—from writing history to building cities to using computers—that played no role in biological evolution but that rested on historical developments that created societies that could develop and transmit these skills. One could then ask whether the same set of "brain operating principles" that make us language-ready also make us history-ready and city-ready and computer-ready or whether different combinations of prior properties of the "uncivilized" human brain are built upon in each of these cases. But this is outside the scope of this volume. What I shall argue is that our biological evolution yielded first a brain that gave our ancestors an ability for complex action recognition and imitation, and later yielded a brain that could use this skill for communication as well as practical action—a brain adapted for "protolanguage" rather than language in all its syntactic and semantic richness. The rest is history.

Hypothesis 2. Language-readiness is multimodal: *Language-readiness evolved as a multimodal manual/facial/vocal system with protosign (manual-based protolanguage) providing the scaffolding for protospeech (vocal-based protolanguage) to provide "neural critical mass" to allow language to emerge from protolanguage as a result of cultural innovations within the history of* Homo sapiens.

Since most humans first acquire language in the form of speech, it is natural to think that evolving a language-ready brain is the same thing as evolving a speech-ready brain. But we usually move our hands[6] and vary our facial expressions when speaking, the Deaf have sign language, and even blind persons gesture when they talk, suggesting an ancestral link between hand and language. The brain mechanisms that support language do not especially privilege auditory input and vocal output.

As deaf people have always known, but linguists only began to discover in the 1960s (Klima & Bellugi, 1979; Stokoe, 1960), sign languages are full human languages, rich in lexicon, syntax, and semantics. Moreover, not only deaf people use sign language. So do some native populations in North America (Farnell, 1995) and some aboriginal Australian tribes (Kendon, 1988). These studies suggest that we should locate language readiness in a *speech-manual-orofacial gesture complex*. During language acquisition, most people shift the major information load of language—but by no means all of it—into the speech domain, whereas for a deaf person the major information load is carried by hand and orofacial gestures. All this grounds the Mirror System Hypothesis.

The aforementioned two hypotheses do not deny that human evolution yielded genetic specification of some of the structures that *support* language. Humans have hands, speech apparatus (larynx, tongue, lips, jaw), facial mobility, and the brain mechanisms needed to learn to produce and perceive rapidly generated sequences of gestures that can be used in language. However, it does take language out of the purely vocal-auditory domain of speech, and it also distinguishes *biological evolution*, which shaped the genome for a language-ready brain (and body), from *cultural evolution*, which took us from hominids with a language-ready brain and rudimentary manual-vocal communication (protolanguage) to humans with full language capability. I will argue in later chapters that the demands of protolanguage in hominids prior to *Homo sapiens* contributed to the evolution of the human brain, whereas those features that distinguish language from protolanguage did not. This leaves open the very large questions "How is being language-ready different from having language?" and "How does protolanguage differ from language?" Chapter 10 offers partial answers.

Humans can and normally do acquire language, and monkeys and chimpanzees do not—though (as we saw in Chapter 3) chimpanzees and bonobos can be trained to acquire a use of symbols that approximates the complexity of the language precursors of a 2-year-old human child. A crucial aspect of human biological evolution has been the emergence of a vocal apparatus and control system that can support speech. But did these mechanisms arise directly from primate vocalizations? The thesis of this book is that the route was instead indirect, proceeding via a form of protosign.

Hypothesis 3. The Mirror System Hypothesis: *The mechanisms that support language in the human brain* evolved atop *a basic mechanism not originally related to communication. Instead, the* mirror system for grasping, *with its capacity to generate and recognize a set of actions, provides the evolutionary basis for* language parity—*the property that an utterance means roughly the same for both sender and receiver.*

Later in this chapter, I will spell out the way in which the Hypothesis, and the arguments for it, will be developed in the rest of this book. But first I need to say more about some of the key characteristics of protolanguage and language that will be appealed to in what follows.

Protolanguage Versus Language

In this section, I will present eleven properties that make the use of language possible. The list is by no means exhaustive, but my claim will be that the first seven were established by biological evolution that yielded the genome of the *Homo sapiens* brain and equipped early humans for the use of protolanguage, whereas the last four required no new brain mechanisms but emerged through the operation of cultural evolution on language-ready brains to yield human societies that did indeed have language. However, regardless of whether I can convince you later that protolanguage and language are on opposite sides of the divide between biology and culture, the key aim here is to encourage you to recognize that there is a divide and debate where it lies. Here, then, are the first seven properties of "language-readiness" that I see as necessary for protolanguage and also for language:

Property 1. Complex action recognition and complex imitation: *Complex action recognition* is the ability to recognize another's performance as a set of familiar movements designed to achieve specific subgoals. *Complex imitation* is the ability to use this as the basis for flexible imitation of the observed behavior. This extends to the ability to recognize that such a performance combines novel actions that can be approximated by (i.e., more or less crudely be imitated by) variants of actions already in the repertoire.

Note that this property is purely in the domain of praxis and requires more than the *mirror neuron* properties of the macaque brain: firing both when the monkey executes a specific action and when it sees a human or other monkey performing a similar action is not enough to support imitation of complex actions. The idea here is that the ability to recognize complex actions carried out by others is crucial to understanding their intentions; and that this ability becomes especially useful if it can be used for "complex imitation" to allow us to transfer new skills from one to another (Chapter 7). The evolutionary theory will then be that, although this ability evolved because of its utility for skill sharing, it established brain mechanisms that could later be adapted for language. A young child learning to speak must both recognize how basic sounds are put together and then imitate the process to add the new words to his or her vocabulary. Adults less often imitate what they hear—though we all pick up new words and catchphrases from time to time—but every time we understand a sentence we perform complex action recognition, understanding how the overall utterance is made up from the words that comprise it.

Thus, our first property is in the domain of *praxis*, the realm of practical interaction with the objects of the world, including especially manipulation. However, to get from praxis to protolanguage, our ancestors had to make the transition from voluntary actions intended to achieve practical goals to those with communicative goals—the difference between pulling your arm to bring you closer and beckoning to encourage you to approach.

Property 2. Intended communication: Here, communication is an action intended by the utterer to have a particular effect on the recipient, rather than being involuntary or a side effect of praxis.

A vervet monkey alarm call is an automatic reaction rather than an action *intended* to warn others of a dangerous predator. Again, if one monkey sees another monkey washing a potato, it may get the "message" that potato washing has some yet-to-be-discovered benefit, but the potato washer had no intention of sending this message—it was simply getting rid of some dirt before eating the potato. An intended communicative action is no longer involuntary or a side effect of a praxic action., Rather, it is intended to affect the behavior or intentions of another. The action becomes a symbol. And, of course, the symbol is of little use unless it is understood. The idea here is that complex action recognition and imitation are necessary if the next two properties, symbolization and parity, are to be available for a significantly large repertoire of symbols:

Property 3. Symbolization: The ability to associate symbols (communicative actions) with an open class of events, objects, or praxic actions.

In the section on "Manual Gesture" in Chapter 3, we reviewed C. S. Peirce's trichotomy of *icons*, *indexes*, and *symbols* as the most fundamental division of signs. However, where Peirce defined a symbol as being neither iconic nor indexical, I instead opted to use the term *symbol* for any sign whose use is sanctioned by convention, and thus I include the notion of *iconic* symbols because—looking ahead to language—it seems unhelpful to say a word is not a symbol if it resembles what it represents.

In terms of symbols that take the form of words in a human language, we are all familiar with the use of nouns to denote objects and verbs to denote actions (and other referents as well). But at first sight it may appear that languages do not employ words for events but instead put words together to describe the event, X did A to B, and so on. But if we define "eat" as "Take a substance whose ingestion is necessary for your survival, place it in your mouth, masticate it, and then swallow it," then saying "eat" is indeed a description of an event. As I will argue at length in Chapter 11, protolanguage symbols (there I will call them *protowords*) for events may in many cases have preceded the "fractionation out" of symbols for concepts that speakers of a language could use to define it.

Although it is hard to make a rigid distinction, I excluded predator-warning cries from the set of "symbols." They have the *effect* of causing evasive action among others, but it is unclear that they exhibit the monkey's intention to do so. Moreover, they are genetically precoded, rather than the result of deploying an ability to create new communicative actions and associate them with novel referents. There's a difference between an innate association as in the alarm calls, the ability to "add a few" as in ape gesture, and the open-ended semantics of human symbolization. This marks part of the evolutionary sequence we seek to understand. I shall suggest how "protolanguage symbolism" differs from "language symbolism" when we come to property 8, symbolization and compositionality, later in this chapter—and then in Chapter 10 will explore how the transition might have occurred.

Property 4. Parity: What counts for the producer of one or more symbols must count, frequently, as approximately the same for the receiver of those symbols.

The parity principle for communicative actions extends the role of the *mirror neurons* for grasping and other actions discovered in the macaque brain because they apply only to praxic actions. It serves to "lift" complex imitation from praxis to communication. A major argument of this book will be that mirror neurons provide the ancestral basis for brain mechanisms supporting parity, so that we can also call parity "the mirror property." It underlies the sharing of symbols. Parity goes beyond symbolization by ensuring that symbols not only can be created by individuals but can also be shared.

The last three protolanguage/language-readiness properties are more general, delimiting cognitive capabilities that underlie a number of the processes that eventually find their expression in language but that were, presumably, present in our distant ancestors long before they got language.

Property 5. From hierarchical structuring to temporal ordering: Animals can perceive that scenes, objects, and actions have subparts and use this to determine what actions to execute and when to execute them to achieve goals in relation to hierarchically structured scenes.

This goes back much further than hominids or even primates and is shared by a vast range of animals. For example, a frog may recognize a barrier and its prey beyond the barrier, and detour around the barrier before approaching and snapping up its prey. Thus, a basic property of language—translating a conceptual structure into a temporally ordered structure of actions—is in fact not unique to language but is apparent whenever an animal takes in the nature of its surroundings and produces appropriate behavior. However, only humans have the ability to communicate in a way that reflects these structures in as much detail as desired.

I will present the next two properties only briefly here and then later expand upon their relevance to language (properties 10 and 11).

Property 6. Beyond the here and now 1: The ability to recall past events or imagine future ones.

It may be debatable whether one sees this as necessary for protolanguage, but the possession of brain structures that can take account of specific events of the past while weighing various plans for the future is clearly a necessary prerequisite for language. This weighing of past and present clearly has independent evolutionary advantage even if the memories and plans cannot be put into words. The hippocampus helps establish episodic memory, the memory of past episodes (O'Keefe & Nadel, 1978), while the substrate for planning is provided by the prefrontal cortex (Fuster, 2004). We looked briefly at these brain mechanisms in humans in Chapter 4. Aspects of episodic memory have been seen in other species. For example, Clayton and Dickinson (1998) report that food-storing birds remember the spatial location and contents of their food caches, and they adapt their caching and recovery strategies to the perishability of the stored food. Specifically, scrub jays, allowed to recover perishable wax-moth larvae and nonperishable peanuts which they had previously cached in visuospatially distinct sites, searched preferentially for fresh wax-moth larvae, their favored food, when allowed to recover them shortly after caching. However, they rapidly learned to avoid searching for them after a longer interval during which the larvae had decayed. Note, however, the distinction between the "special purpose" episodic memory for food caching exhibited by the scrub jays and the "general purpose" episodic memory that allows humans to recall an immense diversity of prior episodes as a basis for current decision making.

Property 7. Paedomorphy and sociality: Paedomorphy is the prolonged period of infant dependency, which is especially pronounced in humans. This combines with the willingness of adults to act as caregivers and the consequent development of social structures to provide the conditions for complex social learning.

The suggestion here is that it is a rare child who can master a language without some help from loving parents or from friends, siblings, and other relatives. Probing these "social prerequisites" for language is thus an important complement to our primary focus on the brain mechanisms that support human language. Humans evolved in such a way that not only can children acquire a multitude of skills but also adults enjoy helping them acquire those skills.

Later chapters will show how the coupling of complex imitation to complex communication came together with the mirror property to evolve a language-ready brain. Let me reiterate: The hypothesis is that early *Homo sapiens* had the brain mechanisms in place that allow modern humans to learn languages—and in this sense the brain was already *language-ready*—but that it took many tens of millennia before humans *invented* language.

We now turn to four properties that, I suggest, must come into play to yield *language*, whether spoken, signed, or both, building on the brain's capabilities that underlie language-readiness—complex action recognition and complex imitation, symbolism, parity, hierarchical structuring, and temporal ordering. My claim is that brains that can support these properties can also support the additional "language properties" presented next, so long as the brain's "owner" matures in a society that possesses language in the sense so defined and nurtures the child to acquire it. Our task in Chapter 10 will be to outline how, over many generations, societies that had only a protolanguage could develop more and more complex systems of communication until finally they had what we might call a language. In this way, each generation could provide a more varied communicative environment to enrich the development of the next.

In summary, I claim that the mechanisms that underlie language-readiness are supported by the genetic encoding of brain and body and the consequent space of possible social interactions but that the genome has no additional structures specific to the four properties of language listed next.

Property 8. Symbolization and compositionality: The symbols become words in the modern sense, interchangeable and composable in the expression of meaning.

However, as we shall see in Chapter 11 the idea of what constitutes a word varies strongly between languages.

Property 9. Syntax, semantics, and recursion: The matching of syntactic to semantic structures grows in complexity, with the nesting of substructures making some form of recursion inevitable.

As we saw in Chapter 2, language is generative or productive, being made up of words and grammatical markers that can be combined in diverse ways to yield an essentially unbounded stock of sentences. The *syntax* of a language characterizes how words may be put together to make sentences. What about meaning? Many words we use, like "rose" (the noun) and "blue" (the adjective), have no meaningful parts. The letters serve to guide pronunciation of the word but mean nothing in themselves. However, the syntax of English lets us place an adjective in front of a noun phrase, and then use the meaning of the "pieces" to infer the meaning of the whole. Thus, if instructed to find a blue rose, you could do so, even if you had never seen one before. Syntax specifies how to put words together into constituents and put constituents together to form larger constituents all the way up to sentences and beyond. This ability to infer the meaning of a sentence—"Please bring me the blue rose that I left on the dining room table"—from its syntactic structure and the meanings of its words is what we have called *compositional semantics*. Of course, part of the power of language is that we have diverse means of expression that let us shade our meaning. "There's a wilted blue rose" versus "Well, I never—a *blue* rose. Anyway, the darn thing's wilted."

As we have seen, language is also *recursive* in that the rules used to build a constituent may also be used to build a larger constituent of the same type of which the first constituent is part. A famous example of a sentence built up by recursion is

> [This is [the maiden all forlorn that milked [the cow with the crumpled horn that tossed [the dog that worried [the cat that killed [the rat that ate [the malt that lay in [the house that Jack built.]]]]]]]]

and we know that the process can continue.

Symbolization and compositionality and *syntax, semantics, and recursion* are intertwined. The key transition here is the compositionality that allows cognitive structure to be reflected in symbolic structure, as when perception (not uniquely human) grounds linguistic description (uniquely human). For example, the noun phrase (NP) describing a view of an object may optionally form part of a larger NP describing the object perceived in greater detail—we first recognize a rose, then its color, then that is wilted. On this view, recursion follows from the language-readiness property, *from hierarchical structuring to temporal ordering*, once *symbolization and compositionality* becomes available.[7]

Recursion is not something that evolution had to add to compositionality; it is an immediate by-product once compositionality can be repeated to build larger communicative structures. Thus, the present approach stands in stark contrast to the claim (Hauser, Chomsky, & Fitch, 2002) that "the faculty of language in a narrow sense (FLN)" only includes recursion and is the only uniquely human component of the faculty of language. The distinction may be subtle, but what I have in mind is exemplified by our example of the wilted blue rose. The breakthrough discovery was that blue things in the world could be described by combining a symbol for "blue" with whatever symbol was required to describe the thing. Similarly, wilted things in the world could be described by combining a symbol for "wilted" with whatever symbol was required to describe the thing. Thus, if one sees a wilted rose, one can emit (the ancient equivalent of) *wilted rose*, but if one has already chosen to use the symbol *blue rose* for the rose, no extra brain power is required to say *wilted (blue rose)*—the parentheses are silent. On this view, it is the ability to freely combine two symbols to create a new symbol with a possibly novel meaning that is the crucial step in our cultural evolution—with recursion a corollary of this ability. And the corollary follows because our visual attention can hierarchically attend to properties of an object as we come to see the object more fully—a form of recursion that, it seems fair to assume, preceded the ability of language to provide the tools for communicating about these visual percepts. To put this another way, recursion in syntax is a corollary to the conceptual structure of what we want to communicate. Of course, once languages begin to gain expressive power, a virtuous circle emerges—our ability to talk about concepts allows us to extend and enrich them; our increasing conceptual mastery increases the demand not only for new words but also for new grammatical tools to express the subtlety of their composition.

We now turn to two principles that provide the linguistic counterparts of two of the conditions for language readiness, properties 6 (*Beyond the here and now*) and 7 (*Paedomorphy and sociality*), respectively:

Property 10. Beyond the here and now 2: Verb tenses or other tools express the ability to recall past events or imagine future ones.

Indeed, language involves many powerful devices that extend the range of communication. Verb tenses are mentioned here to stand in for all the devices languages have developed to communicate about other "possible worlds," including those of the imagination, that are far removed from the immediacy of current experience and action. If one took a human language and removed all reference to time, one might still want to call it a language rather than a protolanguage, even though one would agree that it was thereby greatly impoverished. Similarly, the number system of a language can be seen as a useful, but not definitive, "plug in." *Beyond the here and now 2* nonetheless suggests that the ability to talk about past and future is a central part of human languages as we understand them. However, these features of language would be meaningless (literally) without the underlying cognitive machinery hinted at in property 6 *(Beyond the here and now 1)*. Thus, the neurolinguist must seek not only to learn from the syntactician how temporal relations are expressed in a variety of languages but also to understand how these verbal structures are linked to the cognitive structures that give them meaning and thus, presumably, grounded their (cultural) evolution—irrespective of what autonomy the syntactic structures may have when severed from the contingencies of communication.

Property 11. Learnability: To qualify as a human language, much of the syntax and semantics of a human language must be learnable by most human children.

I say "much of" because it is not true that children master all the vocabulary or syntactic subtlety of a language by 5 or 7 years of age. Books written for 6-year-olds are restricted in both vocabulary and syntax compared to those in books written for adults. Language acquisition is a process that continues well into the teens (and for some of us, much much longer) as we learn more subtle syntactic expressions and a greater vocabulary to which to apply them, allowing us to achieve a richer and richer set of communicative and representational goals.[8]

The aforementioned properties, and the way the Mirror System Hypothesis addresses them, by no means exhausts the issues that have been considered by researchers working on language evolution. For example, I offer a theory that relates brain mechanisms to social learning in the use of language but do not address the issues of why humans want to communicate by engaging in frequent and lengthy conversations, and why children are interested in sharing their growing awareness of the world around them. Communication is necessary for the survival of social creatures and therefore represents a significant selection pressure, but language is a special form of communication whose particularities must be emphasized. It depends on a shared understanding of varied situations, an ability to symbolically represent an *open-ended* set of objects and actions in the environment, and the ability to use symbols in ways that allow for mutual adjustment and cooperation among members of a community in facing new situations in a flexible way that transcends the use of any animal call system—but it also can be used for gossip and for deception. Social grooming may have contributed to language (Dunbar, 1993). Darwin (1871) recognized that some evolution of hominid cognition must have occurred "before even the most imperfect form of speech could have come into use." He supported the role of social communication in language and located its origin in techniques of courtship. Social exchange in tool-using communities could also have been part of a matrix in which social and referential functions of gesture and vocalization intertwined, combining perceptual-motor skills and cultural learning. Tomasello et al. (1993) suggested that this can be tied to developmental changes in social cognition, which could have had phylogenetic counterparts (Donald, 1991, 1993), while Gamble (1994) suggests that the demands of increasing social structure to deal with long-term variations in climate and food resources were involved in the *coevolution* of increasingly subtle perceptual-motor skills involving working memory, theory of mind, planning, and language. But with this, let us turn to a brief review of what we will accomplish in the rest of this book. Then, in Chapter 7, we will plunge into the details.

Sign. posts: Expanding the Mirror System Hypothesis

As we have seen, manual "co-speech gestures" naturally accompany speech. Co-speech gestures are to be distinguished from the signs that form the elements of the signed languages employed by Deaf communities, but the latter dramatically demonstrate that the brain mechanisms that support language do not especially privilege auditory input and vocal output. The production of co-speech gestures by blind persons also highlights the ancestral link between hand and language. Thus, language use is multimodal. The question is not just "how did speech mechanisms evolve" but rather "how did the brain evolve mechanisms to support language that integrate use of hands, face, and voice?" Before offering one more preview of the answer offered by The Mirror System Hypothesis, it will be useful to note that the use of the body for communication extends far beyond language. Thus, the "secret" of language may perhaps be sought within a framework (broader than the emergence of lexicon and grammar) that marks the transition from (1) the observation of another's movements as a cue to action (e.g., a dog seeing another dog digging may look for a bone) in which "communication" of the actor's intentions to the observer is a mere side effect of an action intended for a practical end to (2) explicitly communicative actions that are directed at the observer rather than acting upon objects in the physical world. Thus, the duality between language and praxis can be extended to include a third component of communicative gestures for bodily communication generally and manual gesture more specifically that has an important but relatively small overlap with language and praxis.

We have seen one form of this in the great apes (Chapter 3), but with the restriction that any one group in the wild has a very limited set of gestures—there seems to be no conscious realization that one can create new gestures as needed. There are certainly unlearned gestures for great apes, suggesting that the production of at least some species-typical gestures is due to genetic predisposition, triggered by commonly available individual learning conditions, while the occasions for use have to be learned, as is the case for vocal development in monkeys (Seyfarth & Cheney, 1997). However, there is good evidence that great apes can also invent or individually learn new gestures. Building on this, let me suggest three types of bodily communication:

> *Body mirroring* establishes (unconsciously) a shared communicative space that has no meaning in itself but in which turn taking can be situated (e.g., Oberzaucher & Grammer, 2008). This is like echolalia/echopraxia (recall pathway (e) of Fig. 5-8 in Chapter 5) but is nonpathological if restricted to "basic body mirroring" that does not transgress social conventions (which can inhibit a subordinate from mirroring a superior, while allowing it for a close acquaintance).
>
> *Emotional communication:* We have evolved facial gestures for the expression of emotions (Darwin, 1872/1965), and it has been argued that a mirror system for such expressions could account for empathy when pathway (e) of Figure 5-8 (in Chapter 5) induces in us the motor state for the emotion.

However, in line with the discussion in Chapter 5, "emotion recognition" is not the sole province of a set of mirror systems. If I were to see someone advancing toward me with a knife, I would recognize his anger yet feel fear; I would not empathize as I struggled to protect myself. And, indeed, much of the literature on mirror neurons does distinguish between low-level visuomotor reaction and a more comprehensive understanding of the other's emotions.

Intentional communication: In most cases, body mirroring proceeds spontaneously, as does emotional interaction. By contrast, gestures—like language—
may be used as part of intentional communication, where the actions of the
"communicator" are more or less chosen for their effect on the "commu-
nicatee." In the cases of the apes or the cats discussed in Chapter 3, such
intended communication seems primarily instrumental, trying to elicit
some immediate action located in the here and now. By contrast, humans
can employ intentional communication for a vast range of speech (and gesture and sign) acts—sharing interests, telling stories, registering degrees
of politeness, asking questions, and so on. Among the most challenging
questions for the evolution of language is its ability to support "mental time
travel" (Suddendorf & Corballis, 1997, 2007), the ability to recall the past
and to plan and discuss possible outcomes for the future. Certainly, this
must involve integration of the human language system with the systems
"beyond the here and now" for episodic memory and the planning of future
courses of action that we met in property 6 — but this topic takes us beyond
what we can handle here and now in the present volume.

We have seen that what turns a movement into an action is that it is associated with a goal, so that initiation of the movement is accompanied by the
creation of an expectation that the goal will be met. For example, brushing
a fly off one's jacket and smoothing the jacket might employ the same hand
motion yet, having different goals, be quite different actions. Macaques
use hand movements primarily for praxis. The mirror system allows other
macaques to recognize these actions and, it is speculated, act on the basis of
this understanding. Similarly, the macaque's orofacial gestures register emotional state, and primate vocalizations can also communicate something of
the current situation of the macaque. We also saw that the mirror system in
macaque is the homolog of Broca's area in humans, and that there is a mirror
system for grasping in or near Broca's area in the human brain. Our aim is to
trace the path whereby the mirror system's involvement in both carrying out
and observing grasping evolved across 25 million years to provide the basis for
the shared meaning of language, what we call language parity, whereby an
utterance means roughly the same for both speaker and hearer. Rizzolatti and
Arbib[9] developed the Mirror System Hypothesis (which we "previewed" at the
end of Chapter 1).

The Mirror System Hypothesis: The mechanisms that support language in the human brain *evolved atop* a basic mechanism not originally related to communication. Instead, the mirror system for grasping with its capacity to generate and recognize a set of actions provides the evolutionary basis for *language parity*—the property that an utterance means roughly the same for both speaker and hearer. In particular, human Broca's area contains, but is not limited to, a mirror system for grasping that is homologous to the F5 mirror system of macaque.

The Mirror System Hypothesis roots speech in communication based on manual activity. Some critics have dismissed the Mirror System Hypothesis on the grounds that monkeys do not have language and so the mere possession of a mirror system for grasping cannot suffice for language. But the key phrase in the Mirror System Hypothesis is "evolved atop"—mirror systems expanded their roles in concert with other brain regions as the human brain evolved. The Mirror System Hypothesis provides a neurological basis for the oft-repeated claim that hominids had a (proto)language based primarily on manual gestures before they had a spoken language.[10]

In the section "Auditory Systems and Vocalization" of Chapter 4, we saw (see Fig. 4-8 for the anatomy) that the neural mechanisms involved in voluntary control over the initiation and suppression of monkey vocalizations rely on the mediofrontal cortex, including anterior cingulate cortex (ACC) but not on area F5, which includes the mirror system of the frontal lobe, which has been of such interest to us. Our Mirror System Hypothesis explains why it is F5, rather than the cingulate area involved in macaque vocalization, that is homologous to the human's frontal substrate for language by asserting that a *specific* mirror system—the primate mirror system for grasping—evolved into a key component of the mechanisms that render the human brain language-ready. It is this specificity that allows us to explain in this book why language is multimodal, its evolution being rooted in the execution and observation of hand movements and extended into speech. But we also saw that the region of F5 containing mirror neurons for grasping overlaps a region in F5 of "mouth mirror neurons," some of which discharge during the execution of ingestive actions yet are triggered by observation of communicative mouth gestures. The latter include lip smacking, lip protrusion, tongue protrusion, teeth chatter, and lips/tongue protrusion (Ferrari, Gallese, Rizzolatti, & Fogassi, 2003). In this way ingestive actions are the basis on which communication about feeding is built. This complements but does not replace communication about manual skills in the macaque.

An apparent "paradox," easily resolved, is that actions are typically expressed in languages as verbs, but most words are not verbs. However, the Mirror System Hypothesis does not claim that language evolved by the

Table 6-1   Some crucial stages postulated in the Mirror System Hypothesis

Pre-Hominid

1. **A mirror system for grasping:** matching action observation and execution for grasping. Shared with common ancestor of human and monkey
2. **A simple imitation system for grasping**. Shared with common ancestor of human and great apes

Hominid Evolution

3. **A complex imitation system:** *complex imitation* combines the ability to recognize another's performance as a set of familiar movements with the ability to use this recognition to repeat the performance, and (more generally) to recognize that another's performance combines actions that can be imitated at least crudely by variants of actions already in the repertoire, with increasing practice yielding increasing skill

4. **Protosign:** a manual-based communication system, breaking through the fixed repertoire of primate vocalizations to yield an open repertoire
5. **Protospeech and multimodal protolanguage:** This rests on the "invasion" of the vocal apparatus by collaterals from communication system based on F5/Broca's area

Cultural Evolution in Homo Sapiens

6. **Language:** The transition from action-object frames to verb-argument structures which express them; syntax and a compositional semantics: Co-evolution of cognitive & linguistic complexity

immediate conversion of neural mechanisms for performing actions into neural mechanisms for symbolizing those actions. Instead, it posits a crucial evolutionary transition in the way in which pantomime (Chapter 8) can express the identity of an object by indicating its outline, or by miming a characteristic action or use involving this type of object. This makes possible the later transition from pantomime to conventional signs as the beginning of a long road of abstraction. In due course, a mirror system emerges that is not tied to praxic actions, but rather relates to the actions of speaking or signing words and larger utterances.

The "openness" or "generativity" that some see as the hallmark of language (i.e., its openness to new constructions, as distinct from having a fixed repertoire like that of monkey vocalizations) is present in manual behavior. The issue, then, is to understand the evolutionary changes that lifted this capability from praxic action to communicative action.

The original Mirror System Hypothesis (Arbib & Rizzolatti, 1997; Rizzolatti & Arbib, 1998) is simply the assertion that the mechanisms that get us to the role of Broca's area in language depend in a crucial way on the mechanisms established to support a mirror system for grasping. Table 6–1 summarizes the stages that I now hypothesize in offering one strategy for refining this hypothesis, and it is based on more than 12 years of research published since the original papers with Rizzolatti. I believe that the overall framework is robust, but there are many details to be worked out, and a continuing stream of new and relevant data and modeling will guide future research. Chapters 7 through 10 will spell out the details, and the last three chapters will show how the mechanisms of the language-ready brain that made it possible for languages to get started still operate in how the child acquires language, the recent emergence of new sign languages, and the historical processes of language change. We close this chapter with a brief foretaste of the arguments that those chapters will develop.

Simple and Complex Imitation

Chapter 7: Merlin Donald's (1991, 1998, 1999) theory of the evolution of culture and cognition posits three stages that separate the modern human mind from that of our common ancestor with the chimpanzees:

1) The introduction of a supramodal, motor-modeling capacity, which he calls *mimesis*, and the exploitation of this capability to create representations with the critical property of voluntary retrievability.
2) The addition of a capacity for lexical invention, and a high-speed phonological apparatus, the latter being a specialized mimetic subsystem.
3) The introduction of *external memory* storage and retrieval, and a new working memory architecture.

The Mirror System Hypothesis is broadly consistent with this general framework, but it places special emphasis on the form of mimesis related to the visual control of hand movements as providing the basis for the evolutionary path that led to the emergence of the language-ready brain.

Chapter 7 discusses the crucial early evolutionary stages extending the mirror system for grasping to support imitation (Stages 2 and 3 in Table 6–1). I will argue that complex imitation is a key capability in distinguishing humans from other primates. It is one thing to acquire an observed plan of action by a long process of observation accompanied by trial and error, as the great apes seem able to do—this is what I call *simple imitation*—and quite another to just observe a behavior and acquire the plan, that is, to be capable of *complex imitation*. This combines the ability to recognize another's performance as a set of familiar movements with the ability to use this recognition to repeat the performance. This presupposes a capacity for *complex action analysis*, the ability to recognize that another's performance combines actions that can be more or less crudely imitated by variants of actions already in the repertoire and attempt to approximate the performance on this basis, with increasing practice yielding increasing skill.

Complex imitation was of great advantage for sharing acquired praxic skills. It was thus adaptive for protohumans independently of any implications for communication. However, in modern humans it undergirds the child's ability to acquire language, while complex action analysis is essential for the adult's ability to comprehend the novel compounds of "articulatory gestures." As we shall see in Chapter 7, monkeys have little or no capacity for imitation, whereas apes have a capacity for what I call simple imitation. But when it comes to complex imitation, apes pale in comparison to humans. Apes learn to imitate simple behaviors by using a mechanism called behavior parsing. Even using this method, it still takes an ape several months to master the structure of, for example, feeding on a novel type of food like nettles that requires some special strategy. Humans need just a few trials to make sense of a relatively complex behavior in terms of its constituent actions, and the various intermediate goals these actions must achieve on the way to ultimate success. Interestingly, even newborn infants can perform certain acts of imitation, but this capacity for neonatal imitation—such as poking out the tongue on seeing an adult poke out his tongue—is quantitatively different from that for complex imitation.

To imitate a novel behavior, one must attend to what is being imitated. Joint attention is even more important for the evolutionary development of imitation: Recognizing the object of another's attention and sharing that recognition may provide crucial information about the intricacies of the imitated behavior. The dramatic contrast in monkey, ape, and human imitation ability indicates that something important must have occurred to expand upon the mirror system for grasping found in monkeys to support apes' ability for simple imitation, and then further expand its interactions with various brain regions to go beyond a basic mirror system to support the human ability for more complex imitation. The notion of over-imitation will play a crucial role in the discussion, as will the cooperation between a direct and indirect path for imitation.

Via Pantomime to Protosign

Chapter 8: As we saw in Chapter 3, discussing "Vocalization and Gestures in Monkey and Ape," the call repertoires of nonhuman primates are both small and closed and specified by the genome, whereas the gestural repertoires of apes are still small but are open in that new gestures can be learned and adopted by a community. This suggests that the path to human language might need to progress through manual gesture. But how? Chapter 8 will argue that the crucial breakthrough came with the development of pantomime. The great apes may have discovered by chance that certain of their gestures were instrumentally effective in communicating to others, but new gestures were rarely adopted by a whole group.

By pantomime, I mean here the ability to use reduced forms of actions to convey aspects of other actions, objects, emotions, or feelings—the *artless* sketching of an action to indicate either the action itself or something associated with it. I do not mean the highly skilled art of a Marcel Marceau nor the type of entertainment, the Christmas panto, enjoyed each year by the English. Nor do I mean the highly structured form of communication involved in playing a game of charades, where meaning may be conveyed by varied well-rehearsed strategies such as using a conventional sign to indicate "sounds like," followed by an artful attempt to convey the sound of a word (again, a conventionalized symbol) rather than its meaning.

In pouring water from a bottle, I must grasp the bottle, then position and rotate it so that water flows into my glass. In pantomiming this action by holding my hand as if it were holding an upright cylinder and then moving it and turning it above my glass, the action becomes intransitive and sketchy in that it no longer acts on an object, the bottle, and so the action is no longer constrained to match the object's affordance. The observer, recognizing the action from which the sketch is derived, might then respond by passing a bottle of water or by pouring water in my glass. Flapping one's arms in a "wing-like" manner could indicate an object (a bird), an action (flying), or both (a flying bird). Examples linked to feelings or emotions could include a downturning of the lips or miming the brushing away of tears to feign sadness.

Pantomime, then, allows the transfer of a wide range of action behaviors to communication about action and much more—whereby, for example, an absent object is indicated by outlining its shape or miming its use. The power of pantomime—once the brain mechanisms and social understanding for it are in place—is that it allows a group to consciously communicate information about novel requests and situations that could not otherwise have been indicated.

The downside to pantomime is that it can often be ambiguous—for example, a certain movement could suggest myriad things: "bird," "flying," "bird flying," and so on. If pantomime engendered an explosion of semantics for gestural communication, then the high probability for ambiguity would seem to require the development of conventionalized gestures to disambiguate the pantomimes, as well as the conventionalization of certain pantomimes. This suggests that the emergence of symbols occurred when the ambiguity or "cost" of pantomiming proved limiting. The result is a system of protosign that can only be fully comprehended only by initiates but gains in both breadth and economy of expression.

Protosign and Protospeech: An Expanding Spiral

Chapter 9: Protosign provides the scaffolding for the emergence of protospeech, with protosign and protospeech then developing in an expanding spiral (shown to the left of Stages 4 and 5 in the table). Here, I am using "protosign" and "protospeech" for the manual and vocal components of a protolanguage, in the sense of an open system of communication that has not yet attained the power of human language. The claim here is that hominids had at least some aspects of protosign—a (proto)language based primarily on manual gestures—before they had a language based primarily on vocal gestures. This remains controversial and one may contrast two extreme views on the matter:

1. Language evolved directly from vocalizations as speech (MacNeilage, 1998).
2. Language first evolved as signed language (i.e., as a full language, not protolanguage), and then speech emerged from this basis in manual communication (Stokoe, 2001).

My approach is closer to (2) than to (1), but I shall argue for the *Doctrine of the Expanding Spiral:*

(a) that our distant ancestors (e.g., *Homo habilis* through to early *Homo sapiens*) first had a (possibly quite limited) protolanguage based primarily on manual gestures ("protosign") that—contra (1)—provided essential scaffolding for the emergence of a protolanguage based primarily on vocal gestures ("protospeech"), but that
(b) the hominid line saw advances in both protosign and protospeech feeding off each other in an expanding spiral so that—contra (2)—protosign did not attain the status of a full language prior to the emergence of early forms of protospeech.

My view is that the "language-ready brain" of the first *Homo sapiens* supported basic forms of gestural and vocal communication (protosign and protospeech) but not the rich syntax and compositional semantics and accompanying conceptual structures that underlie modern human languages.

I want to stress here, further, the essential plasticity of the mirror system. It does not come prewired with a specific set of grasps but rather (recall the MNS models of Chapter 5) expands its repertoire to adaptively encode the experience of the agent. This is an important aspect of the emergence of increasing manual dexterity; and it becomes crucial for the role of a mirror system for phonological articulation at the heart of the brain's readiness for language.

Ascribing a crucial role to protosign as a step in human language evolution thus goes against the hypothesis that evolution went from monkey vocalizations to human speech purely in the vocal-auditory domain, without any role for gesture. The "speech-only" view, if true, would make it harder to explain the signed languages of the deaf or the use of gestures by blind speakers. But if we reject the "speech-only" view, we must explain why speech arose and became dominant for most humans. We will argue that once protosign had established that conventionalized gestures could augment or even displace pantomime in providing a highly flexible semantics, then protospeech could "take off" as conventionalized vocalizations began to contribute increasingly to the mix. Finally, we take a brief look at how the demands of an increasingly spoken protovocabulary might have provided the evolutionary pressure that yielded a vocal apparatus and corresponding neural control to support the human ability for rapid production and coarticulation of phonemes that underpins speech as we know it today.

How Languages Got Started

Chapter 10: We turn to the issue of how languages emerged from protolanguages. The chapter will start by framing the debate between Derek Bickerton and a view I share with the linguist Alison Wray. For Bickerton (1995), a *protolanguage* is a communication system made up of utterances comprising a few words much like the more basic content words—like nouns and verbs—of a modern language, with these words put together without syntactic structure. For example, we need no grammar to interpret "apple boy eat" correctly, but we do need rudimentary grammar (even if only an agreed convention about word order) to tell who hit whom in the sentence "John Bill hit." Moreover, Bickerton asserts that the notion of protolanguage is far broader than being a precursor of true languages. For him, infant communication, pidgins, and the "language" taught to apes are all protolanguages in this sense. Bickerton hypothesizes that *Homo erectus* (the hominid species that preceded *Homo* *sapiens*) communicated by a protolanguage in his sense and that language just "added syntax."[11]

Alison Wray's (1998, 2000) counterproposal is that in much of protolanguage a complete communicative act involved a *unitary utterance* or *holophrase*, the use of a single symbol, formed as a sequence of gestures, whose component gestures—whether manual or vocal—have no independent meaning. A Just So story[12] may help to clarify the argument. Unitary utterances such as "grooflook" or "koomzash" might have encoded quite complex descriptions such as "The alpha male has killed a meat animal and now the tribe has a chance to feast together. Yum, yum!" or commands such as "Take your spear and go around the other side of that animal, and we will have a better chance together of being able to kill it." The important point is that the holophrases get invented and spread because *they signal an event that is either frequent and somewhat important, or very important even if it is rare*. In the same spirit, I will argue that the "language-readiness" possessed by the first *Homo sapiens* did include the ability to communicate both manually and vocally—*protosign* and *protospeech*, with the prefix "proto" here having no Bickertonian implication—but that such protolanguages were at first composed mainly of "unitary utterances."

I also argue that words coevolved culturally with syntax through *fractionation*. The following, overly simple, example may clarify what I have in mind.[13] Imagine that a tribe has two unitary utterances concerning fire—packing into different "protowords" the equivalent, say, of the English sentences "The fire burns" and "The fire cooks the meat"—which, by chance, contain similar substrings that become regularized so that for the first time there is a sign for "fire." Perhaps the original utterances were "reboofalik" and "balikiwert," and "falik" becomes the agreed-on term for fire, so the utterances become "reboofalik" and "falikiwert." Eventually, some tribe members regularize the complementary gestures in the first string to get a sign "reboo" for "burns." Later, others regularize the complementary gestures in the second string to get a sign for "cooks meat." However, because of the arbitrary origin of the sign for "fire," the placement of the gestures that have come to denote "burns" relative to "fire" differs greatly from those for "cooks meat." It thus requires a further invention to regularize the placement of the gestures in both utterances, and so the utterances make the transition to nonunitary utterances or protosentences—say "reboo falik" and "iwert falik." Thus, as words fractionate from longer strings of gestures, at the same time the protosyntax emerges that combines them. Of course, as we shall see in Chapter 10, this is only one of the mechanisms whereby language begins to emerge from protolanguage.

How the Child Acquires Language

Chapter 11: An influential (though not the latest) version of Chomsky's theory suggests that we can describe principles that govern the syntax of all human languages with a few parameters capturing key differences between the way those principles apply in different languages. The result is a Universal Grammar, which frames a basic description of the syntax of any language by simply setting parameters appropriately. However, I disagree with those who, like Chomsky himself, assert that Universal Grammar is genetically specified in the brain of each normal human child and that—in this version of his theory, the principles and parameters approach—learning the syntax of a language amounts simply to the "throwing of switches" in the child's brain to set parameters to match the structure of the sentences the child hears around her.

Rather than develop my argument contra an innate Universal Grammar in these pages I will instead introduce Jane Hill's specific computational model of language acquisition in the 2-year-old child, a model we may now recognize as a forerunner of the comprehensive approach to child language later developed by Michael Tomasello and his colleagues within the general framework of construction grammar. The model shows how the child repeating larger and larger fragments of the speech she hears comes, week by week, to extend the number and generality of the constructions (Hill called them templates) that put words together. The key point is that a holophrase like *want-milk* (where the child has not yet come to treat *want* and *milk* as separate words) can in time yield a very specific construction *want X*, where the "slot" X can be filled by any word that describes something the child wants. The slot fillers form a very specific *semantic* category. But as the child develops more general constructions such as *X did A to Y*, each slot filler comes to define a category that has lost much of its semantic mooring and so can be seen as being a more purely *syntactic* category.

How Languages Emerge

Chapter 12: We will study Nicaraguan Sign Language (NSL) and Al-Sayyid Bedouin Sign Language (ABSL), two new sign languages that emerged in groups of deaf people without being variations on already existing sign languages. Emerging patterns of motion description in NSL exemplify the processes of fractionation and consequent formation of new constructions that we saw as being a key to how languages got started. We will also look at the crucial role of social interaction in the emergence of NSL and the crucial role of NSL in the emergence of the Nicaraguan Deaf community. The word order of ABSL differs from that of Arabic, the spoken language of the Al-Sayyid Bedouin. Probing that word order offers general notions relevant to our study of how the brain got language, suggesting how the original syntax of languages may have been rooted in the structure of action. ABSL also gives us a window into the emergence of phonology.

Finally, Chapter 12 addresses the daunting question: If NSL and ABSL each emerged in the course of a few decades, is it really plausible to claim that early *Homo sapiens* had only protolanguages, with the first true languages being invented only in the past 100,000 years?

How Languages Keep Changing

Chapter 13: The final chapter achieves two goals. The first is to suggest a time line for the changes posited by the Mirror System Hypothesis to occur before there were languages. This is done by relating stages posited in Table 6-1 to the archeological record on stone tools produced by putative prede- cessors of *Homo sapiens*. The earliest known stone tools are assigned to the Oldowan Industry (ca. 2.6–1.4 million years ago), and we argue that they exhibit a complexity akin to the tool making of present-day chimpanzees in the wild. The Early Acheulean (ca. 1.6–0.9 million years ago) can be char- acterized by elaborate flake production and by the emergence of large cut- ting tools, but it would seem that at this time *Homo* still possessed only simple imitation, suggesting that they communicated with a limited repertoire of vocal and manual gestures akin to those of a group of modern great apes. The Late Acheulean (ca. 0.7–0.25 million years ago) saw production of blanks as the basis of more sophisticated shaping to achieve different tool forms. We argue that this was the period in which complex imitation emerged, and com- munication gained an open-ended semantics through the conscious use of pantomime. *Homo sapiens* was then the first species of *Homo* to have complex imitation and a language-ready brain.

The second goal is to suggest how mechanisms operative in the original transition from protolanguages to languages are still operative in the pro- cesses whereby languages change. Note the crucial distinction. In Chapters 10 and 12 we studied how languages emerge from something like protolan- guage, whereas in historical linguistics, we study how people who already have language develop new ones. The discussion focuses on two themes: (1) the way in which pidgins develop into creoles, incorporating elements of vocabulary from one language and some grammar from another as the basis for a multigeneration process of grammatical enrichment; and (2) the process of grammaticalization whereby over time information expressed in a string of words or a supplementary sentence becomes transformed into part of the grammar—a crucial engine for language change. And finally, we see that language keeps evolving.

7

Simple and Complex Imitation

In its broadest sense, *imitation* involves acting in a way that follows the example of the behavior of another. As such, it can involve immediate repetition of an observed action already in the observer's repertoire, or it can involve learning a new skill based on observation of the actions of others. Again, it may involve copying a limited set of properties of the observed action, or it may involve reproduction of both the subgoals of the observed behavior and (in more or less detail) the movements involved in achieving them. In the sense of most importance to our discussion, addressing the major role that imitation plays in learning by human children, imitation includes copying a novel, otherwise improbable action or some act that is outside the imitator's prior repertoire in such a way that the imitator, on the basis of (possibly repeated) observation, comes to add that action to his or her repertoire.

In this chapter, we will get a sense of the different forms of imitation exhibited by primates, but especially apes and humans. There is little evidence for vocal imitation in monkeys or apes,[1] whether in imitating a known vocalization or acquiring a novel one, and so we will focus on imitation of praxic actions that act upon objects in the physical world, seeing which types are exhibited by monkeys, which by apes, and which by humans. I will use the term "complex imitation" for the range of imitation of which humans are capable, and I will use "simple imitation" for imitation in apes. However, the terminology must not blind us to the very real skills in imitation that apes possess.

Our understanding of complex imitation will set the stage for our analysis in the next chapter of how praxic skills in imitation may underwrite development of communicative skills in the manual domain, leading to a limited repertoire of shared gestures in a group of apes, and to protosign, a manual form of protolanguage in early humans.

Imitation in Apes and Monkeys

There is a large literature on imitation, and different authors include different behaviors under this inclusive umbrella. Judy Cameron (personal communication) offered the following observation from the Oregon Regional Primate Research Center: "Researchers at the Center had laboriously taught monkeys to run on a treadmill as a basis for tests they wished to conduct. It took 5 months to train the first batch of monkeys in this task. But they then found that if they allowed other monkeys to observe the trained monkeys running on a treadmill, then the naïve monkeys would run successfully the first time they were placed on a treadmill." Is this imitation, or is it just that the monkey comes to associate running with the treadmill as a result of this observation?

Voelkl and Huber (2000) had marmoset monkeys observe a demonstrator removing the lids from a series of plastic canisters to obtain a mealworm. When subsequently allowed access to the canisters, a marmoset that observed a demonstrator using its mouth also used its mouth to remove the lids, whereas marmosets that had not seen use of the mouth demonstrated prior to testing were almost certain to use their hands. Voelkl and Huber (2000) suggest that this may be a case of *true* imitation in marmosets, but I would argue that it is a case of *effector enhancement*, directing attention of the observer to a particular object or part of the body or environment. This is to be distinguished from *emulation* (observing and attempting to reproduce results of another's actions without paying attention to details of the other's behavior). As Byrne and Russon (1998) note, in such cases the way the observer responds to the enhanced stimulus or reaches that goal is a matter of individual learning or prior knowledge, and it is not directly influenced by the observed techniques. They unify these and related phenomena as instances of *observational priming*. Visalberghi and Fragaszy (2001) reviewed data on attempts to observe imitation in monkeys, including their own studies of capuchin monkeys. They conclude that there is a huge difference between the major role that imitation plays in learning by human children and the very limited role, if any, that imitation plays in social learning in monkeys.

Observational priming can increase the chance that a known behavior is used in a new context but without satisfying our earlier criteria for imitation in its fullest sense in which the imitated act should not already be part of the animal's repertoire and that the success of the act depends on the specifics of the act as performed by the observed other(s). Such imitation can only be tested in situations requiring the observer to act in some way toward a goal using actions we would not expect the observer would/could normally deploy beforehand, but this is not the only type of imitation we will consider even as we move beyond observational priming.

What about apes? Myowa-Yamakoshi and Matsuzawa (1999) observed chimpanzees in a laboratory setting. The chimpanzees typically took 12 trials to learn to "imitate" a behavior but in doing so paid more attention to where the manipulated object was being directed than to the actual movements of the demonstrator. The chimpanzees focused on using one or both hands to bring two objects into relationship, or to bring an object into relationship with the body, rather than the actual movements involved in doing this. For example, seeing the human demonstrator pick up a pan with one hand and move it to cover a ball on the floor, the chimpanzee eventually "imitated" this by picking up the pan in one hand and the ball in the other, inserting the ball in the pan in midair. In other words, the chimpanzee observed the relation between the objects (but not between the objects and the floor), but it could not separate out the actual movements that were used to secure the observed goal.

Chimpanzees do use and make tools in the wild, with different tool traditions found in geographically separated groups of chimpanzees. Boesch and Boesch (1982) have observed chimpanzees in Taï National Park, Ivory Coast, using stone tools to crack nuts open, although Jane Goodall has never seen chimpanzees do this in the Gombe in Tanzania. The Taï chimpanzees crack harder shelled nuts with stone hammers and stone anvils. They live in a dense forest where suitable stones are hard to find. The stone anvils are stored in particular locations to which the chimpanzees continually return. To open soft-shelled nuts, chimpanzees use thick sticks as hand hammers, with wood anvils. The nut-cracking technique is not mastered until adulthood. Young chimpanzees first attempt to crack nuts at age 3 years and require at least 4 years of practice before any benefits are obtained.

Teaching is virtually never observed in the great apes (Caro & Hauser, 1992). Chimpanzee mothers seldom if ever correct and instruct their young. Tomasello (1999) comments that, over many years of observation, Boesch observed only two possible instances in which the mother *appeared* to be actively attempting to instruct her child, and that even in these cases it is unclear whether the mother had the goal of helping the young chimpanzee learn to use the tool. We may contrast the long and laborious process of acquiring the nut-cracking technique with the crucial role of caregivers in assisting a child's growing skill at imitation (at least in certain societies).

Imitation by apes can extend to other complex behaviors. For example, gorillas learn complex strategies to gather nettle leaves, which are high in protein but can be painful to gather without an appropriate strategy (Byrne & Byrne, 1993). Skilled gorillas grasp the stem firmly, strip off leaves, remove petioles bimanually, fold leaves over the thumb, pop the bundle into the mouth, and eat. But complex feeding skills such as this are not acquired by obvious look-hard-so-you-can-learn—the young seem to look at the food, not at the movements involved in food processing (Corp & Byrne, 2002).

The final skill has two components—learning a new set of basic actions such as bimanual removal of petioles, and learning how to assemble these actions. The challenge for learning how to assemble actions is that the sequence of basic actions varies greatly from trial to trial (recall our example of opening a childproof aspirin bottle in Fig. 2-8 in Chapter 2). Byrne (2003) implicates what he calls *imitation by behavior parsing*, a form of statistical learning whereby certain states of the feeding process become evident from repeated observation as being common to most performances (e.g., having nettles folded over the thumb); these then become *subgoals* that can anchor trial-and-error learning of movement patterns that can achieve them, thus breaking down the complexity of the overall task. Apparently, the young ape, over many months, may acquire the skill by coming to recognize the relevant subgoals and derive action strategies for achieving subgoals by trial and error—each animal was found to have a different preferred set of functionally equivalent variants. However, once low-level elements that achieve the same overall function are lumped into classes, the evidence suggests that gorillas can effectively copy the hierarchy of goals and subgoals. These provide the means to organize actions in terms of their relation to such subgoals. Information on such states is further given by the distribution of pauses, optional omission of parts of sequences, and smooth recovery from interruptions. As Byrne and Russon (1998) observe, short-term memory capacity might set a limit on how deep a hierarchy the mind of a gorilla or a human could expand "without getting in a muddle." Gorilla food preparation appears organized into shallow hierarchies, and perhaps gorillas can only keep track of two embedded goals even with the aid of the "external memory" present in physical tasks.

In such feeding strategies as studied by Byrne and Byrne (1993), the basic actions seem to be learned by trial and error rather than imitation, that is, they do not attend to the details of the actions that they observe. Each animal was found to have a different preferred set of functionally equivalent variants. Byrne and Russon (1998) thus contrast *imitation by behavior parsing* with *action-level imitation.* The latter involves reproduction of the details, more or less precisely, of the manual actions another individual uses; that is, in the latter case the observer can attend to details of an observed movement to more quickly learn how to achieve a subgoal.

Complex Imitation: Mirror Neurons Are Not Enough

Many people writing about mirror neurons seem to embrace the "myth" that having mirror neurons is sufficient for imitation. But it is one thing to recognize an action you yourself can perform; it is another thing to see someone perform a *novel* action and add it to your repertoire. A popular headline for articles about mirror neurons is "Monkey See, Monkey Do." However, this is not true. The neurophysiological data on the F5 mirror neurons in the macaque brain tell us this: "If an action is in the monkey's repertoire, then observation of that action when executed by another will activate the appropriate mirror neurons." But imitation goes beyond observation of an action to execution of that action. The MNS model (recall Fig. 5-3 in Chapter 5) showed how potential mirror neurons could become mirror neurons if the activity of the canonical F5 neurons for a particular grasp was used as a training signal to enable these particular mirror-neurons-in-the-making to learn what trajectories of the hand approaching an object were examples of this particular grasp. Imitation involves the *reverse* process of adding a new action to one's own repertoire as a result of observing how others employ that action to achieve some goal.

Our earlier discussion suggests that imitation in monkeys is limited to observational priming, and so we must conclude that having a monkey-like mirror system for grasping is *not* sufficient for imitation. I hypothesize that getting beyond this limitation was one of the crucial evolutionary changes in the "extended" mirror system that in concert with other brain regions yielded a specifically human brain. A further hypothesis is that humans have what I call *complex imitation*, whereas other primates do not (Arbib, 2002). In many cases of praxis (i.e., skilled interaction with objects), humans need just a few trials to make sense of a relatively complex behavior if the constituent actions are familiar and the subgoals these actions must achieve are readily discernible, and they can use this perception to repeat the behavior under changing circumstances.

Complex imitation is defined as combining three abilities:

(1) *Complex action recognition*, the perceptual ability to recognize another's performance as resembling an assemblage of familiar actions.
(2) *The actual imitation*, grounded in complex action recognition, to repeat the assembled actions.[2]
(3) More subtly, the recognition of another's performance as *resembling* an assemblage of familiar actions enables the imitator to further attend to how novel actions differ from the ones they resemble, providing the basis for acquiring the ability to perform these variant actions.

The latter process may yield fast comprehension of (much of) the overall structure of the observed behavior. However, this new motor schema may require a great deal of learning and practice to get tuned to yield truly skillful behavior.

On this basis, *complex imitation* is akin to *action-level imitation*. However, the aforementioned formulation makes explicit the underlying ability for complex action recognition with the implication that recognition of the form of an assemblage of actions may be used for cognitive processes other than those of imitation. It also offers a strategy for "reproduction of the details, more or less precisely, of the manual actions another individual uses" by recognizing ways in which a novel action or movement may be seen as a variant of one already known to the observer.

By contrast, then, I will use the term *simple imitation* for the capacity of apes, even though it is not all that simple—we have seen that it includes imitation by behavior parsing, and in a few pages will see that it avoids the pitfalls (but also misses the advantages) of over-imitation.

Jeannerod (1994) has noted the role of mental rehearsal and "motor imagery" in humans improving their skills, whether in sport or piano playing. Here, the "parsing of action" proceeds internally, without the overt action that constitutes imitation. Instead, what is tuned is (1) the expectation of the action, so that one comes better and better to "understand" (not necessarily consciously), (2) what variants of one's actions would match those of the master, and (3) what cues must be taken into account to effect a smooth transition from one subaction to another.

In Figure 2-8 in Chapter 2, we saw how an action such as opening a child-proof aspirin bottle is analogous to (but is not) a "sentence" made up of "words," where these "words" are basic actions akin in complexity to "reach and grasp": a hierarchical sequence whose subsequences are not fixed in length but instead are conditioned on the achievement of goals and subgoals. Depending on the actual bottle cap,

(grasp press_down_&_turn) (regrasp pull_up_&_turn) (remove lid)

or

(grasp press_down_&_turn) (regrasp pull_up_&_turn) (regrasp pull_ up_&_turn) (remove lid)

could be equally appropriate "action sentences." Just imitating one of these sequences on every occasion would not count as learning how to open the bottle. Thus, the ability to imitate *single* actions is just the first step toward complex imitation. The full ability involves not only (1) parsing a complex movement into more or less familiar pieces and then performing the corresponding composite of (variations on) familiar actions but also (2) expanding the repertoire of basic actions as well as (3) the flexible re-assembly of actions in terms of affordances and subgoals.

Our notion of complex imitation incorporates the *goal-directed imitation* of Wohlschläger, Gattis, and Bekkering (2003). Based on their findings of systematic errors in human imitation, they posited that the imitator does not imitate the observed movement as a whole, but rather decomposes it into its separate aspects. These aspects are hierarchically ordered, and the highest aspect becomes the imitator's main goal. This hierarchical structuring of subgoals is possibly incomplete, possibly erroneous. But, through increased attention being paid to its subgoals, the imitator may achieve a finer-scaled decomposition of the observed movement, resulting through successive approximation in execution of a more congruent behavior. As in the program-level imitation of apes, successful imitation here requires learning not only what subgoals must be achieved to obtain the overall goal but also the ability to discriminate which subgoal is currently most important, and which specific actions (some of them novel) must be deployed to achieve each subgoal. Thus, when I speak of imitation here, I do not speak only of the imitation of a movement but also of the linkage of that movement to the goals it is meant to achieve. The action may thus vary from occasion to occasion depending on parametric variations in the goal. We may contrast the full notion of complex imitation here with the notion of *emulation*, which we saw involved observing the goal of another's action and attempting to reach it without paying attention to details of the other's movements.

We see that a brain that supports complex imitation must include more than mirror neurons:

1) To imitate an action already in the repertoire, we need a link from the mirror neurons that recognize the action to the canonical neurons that will then support performance of the observed action.

2) A greater challenge is for the imitator to use observation to acquire an action not already in the repertoire. This involves recognizing the goal of the action and the means used to achieve that goal, but it may also be achieved by recognizing the goal and using trial and error to find a means for achieving it.

This distinction may be illustrated by considering the task of assembling a piece of furniture purchased from IKEA. In many cases, we look at the picture of a subassembly and proceed to put pieces together without inspecting the detailed instructions. If we succeed in reaching the goal of matching the picture, all well and good. But if we fail, we have two choices—to disassemble the structure and try different strategies until, by chance, we succeed. Or we may actually read the instructions and, if they are well presented, follow them step by step to reach our goal.

The implication is that, to the extent that the mirror system is part of an imitation system, it must be augmented by other subsystems. Moreover, different systems may be brought into play to yield the different strategies that together constitute the overall human capacity for imitation. For example, Tessari and Rumiati (2004) discuss the "switching" between strategies as a function of cognitive burden and task demands. The aim of their study was to bring to the surface the strategic use of imitative processes in the context of a two-route model: (a) direct imitation, used in reproducing new, meaningless actions, and (b) imitation based on stored semantic knowledge of familiar meaningful actions. The issue of "direct" versus "indirect" imitation will be taken up when we consider the cognitive neuropsychological model of limb praxis due to Rothi et al. (1991) in the section "The Direct and Indirect Path in Imitation" later in this chapter. There we will suggest an important variation of the model—showing how the two paths may work together to tweak the observer's recognition of an action.

To summarize: Monkeys have little or no capacity for imitation beyond observational priming and macaques had their common ancestor with humans some 25 million years ago. Apes have an ability for imitation by behavior parsing and had their last common ancestor with humans some 5 to 7 million years ago. These facts make it plausible that our evolutionary path took us through the emergence of imitation by behavior parsing before 7 million years ago, with complex imitation being an emergent of hominid evolution.

Evolution is not directed toward some distant end. If a change in the genome is passed on through many generations, then—barring some catastrophe that accidentally wiped out those with more advantageous genetic endowments—the change must be either neutral or offer some selective advantage. It is highly implausible that the genetic changes underlying complex imitation were selected because they would *eventually* prove useful for language. Instead, my hypothesis is that complex imitation for hand movements evolved because of its adaptive value in supporting the increased transfer of manual skills and thus preceded the emergence of protolanguage in whatever modality. This is a case of *exaptation*, the process whereby a biological adaptation originally selected for one function is later appropriated for another.[3] Exaptation provides a mechanism to explain how complex structures could evolve over time. For example, how could a bird's wing evolve if there were no adaptive value in having a forelimb that was "somewhat wing-like" but could not support flight? One answer is that a forelimb covered in air-trapping feathers might be an efficient insulator. This would provide a selective advantage for wing-like forelimbs that could *later* be exapted for flight.

In short, the claim here is that in human evolution the emergence of brain mechanisms that support imitation by behavior parsing and complex imitation was adaptive because of its utility in the social sharing of practical skills, long before there was language. This is a claim about *human* evolution and the importance of our increasing skill at manipulation. This is clearly different from an evolutionary path that would support the evolution of *vocal* learning in various species of birds and in whales and dolphins. It seems reasonable to suspect (though no data are available except for songbirds) that dolphins and parrots and certain other bird species do have mirror neurons, and that these had to be augmented to form neural systems that support imitation. Some critics of the Mirror System Hypothesis suggest that this would bring into question the importance of mirror neurons in the development of humans. But I see no force in this "criticism." Our hypothesis is neither (1) that having mirror neurons gives you language nor (2) that having a capacity for imitation is based only on mirror neurons for grasping. Neither dolphins nor birds have hands and thus they lack manual dexterity. Our concern is to trace the evolution of humans from our common ancestors with extant nonhuman primates. The Mirror System Hypothesis seeks to explain what is unique about the evolution of the human language-ready brain, and it provides support for the view that this passed through a capacity for complex imitation of manual actions as the basis for pantomime (Chapter 8) to support in turn the emergence of protosign to serve as the scaffolding for the emergence of protospeech (Chapter 9).

In summary, human imitation differs from the capability of the great apes in three ways:

(1) We can learn by program-level imitation more quickly than apes can. We can perceive—more or less immediately and with more or less accuracy—that a novel action may be approximated by a composite of known actions associated with appropriate subgoals.

(2) We can learn deeper hierarchies than apes can.

(3) We have a greater capacity for action-level imitation—depending on circumstances, we may develop our own way of reaching a subgoal or, failing to do so, we may pay more attention to the details of the demonstrator's actions and modify our actions accordingly.

In any case, note that these ape studies are based on *manual* imitation. Apes have neither a vocal tract with the right morphology, nor adequate neural control, to produce the range of syllables that humans deploy when speaking. Moreover, when the young ape imitates some aspects of the adult's feeding, the adult's behavior is not aimed at communicating the means or the practical goal of the imitated action (the communicative possibility of these being recognized is an unintended "side effect"). However, as we saw in Chapter 4, apes can deploy these skills for a limited form of gestural communication. In his book *The Ape and the Sushi Master*, Frans de Waal (2001) argued that Westerners emphasize imitation and teaching as the basis of human culture and too readily deny shared characteristics between human and animals. As a counterexample to this Western view, de Waal suggested that the Japanese sushi master neither teaches nor instructs his apprentice. The apprentice watches his master at work for several years without ever being allowed to practice. After this, he will successfully prepare his first sushi with considerable skill. However, when I talked to the Japanese owner of my local sushi bar, he denied de Waal's account. His sushi master had provided constant and rigorous training, hitting him vigorously whenever he made a mistake! The point is not to deny de Waal's point that we share much with our ape cousins, but it is necessary to resist his attempts to dissolve all differences in a thorough-going anthropomorphism. All humans certainly learn by observation, but this can lead to complex imitation, not only simple imitation, and humans can benefit from the explicit instruction that only humans can provide.

Neonatal Imitation

Let us now add human development to comparative primatology in our discussion of imitation. Meltzoff and Moore (1977) found that 12-to-21-day-old infants could "imitate" four different adult gestures: lip protrusion, mouth opening, tongue protrusion, and finger movement (Fig. 7-1). (Later studies showed facial "imitation" in an infant only 42 minutes old.) What is worth stressing is that the newborns' first response to seeing a facial gesture is activation of

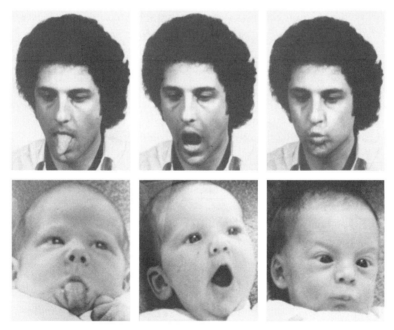

FIGURE 7-1.   Photographs of 12- to 21-day-old infants imitating facial expressions demonstrated by an adult. Imitation is innate in human beings, which allows them to share behavioral states with other "like-me" agents. (From Meltzoff & Moore, 1977. Reprinted with permission from AAAS.)

the corresponding body part. Seeing tongue protrusion, the infant might not protrude the tongue at first but might simply move the tongue—but not some other body part. Meltzoff and Moore call this *organ identification*—recall the earlier mention of "effector enhancement." Thus, "organ identification" may be present at birth and serve as a foundation for *neonatal "imitation."*[4] In this regard, it is worth recalling that in the MNS model, the transfer from recognition of a grasp in one's own repertoire to its recognition as a grasp in another's repertoire comes because the mirror neuron system treats the hand of the other equivalently to a hand of the self. The issue of whose hand is doing the grasping is no concern of the mirror system—but certainly important to parts of the brain that separate *self* from *other*.

But why did I place "imitation" in quotes in the previous paragraph? It is because there is good evidence that neonatal imitation is very different from the imitation of novel performances or of actions that the child has learned. The necessary abilities for this seem only to emerge when the child is 9 to 12 months old. Moreover, neonatal imitation is based on moving single organs and thus differs from complex, goal-directed imitation.[5]

Bodily correspondence in neonatal imitation may be a necessary precursor for complex imitation, but biological evolution may have selected for neonatal "imitation" quite independently from imitation more generally. Monkey neurophysiology shows that the recognition of faces and hands is supported neurally; otherwise we would not have the mirror neurons that can respond specifically to manual actions and others that respond to orofacial actions, as documented in Chapter 5. Intriguingly, there is now evidence for neonatal imitation in very young monkeys (Ferrari et al., 2006) but not for imitation in older monkeys. Moreover, Myowa-Yamakoshi et al. (2004) observed two chimpanzees that, at less than 7 days of age, could discriminate between, and imitate, human tongue protrusion and mouth opening. Yet by the age of 2 months, they no longer imitated the gestures. Instead, they would frequently open the mouth in response to any facial gesture they observed. This suggests that the brain mechanisms exploiting neonatal organ identification may have expanded as hominids evolved. For example, humans have speech, whereas chimpanzees do not, but Studdert-Kennedy (2002) discusses data consistent with the view that the human infant at first "imitates" sounds by moving one articulator (e.g., tongue, jaw, or lips) at a time and only later coordinates articulators. Neonatal imitation resembles effector matching and the "contagion" in yawning or smiling, which extends to emotional contagion in which people automatically mirror the postures and moods of others. Since emotional states are closely linked to certain facial expressions, observation of a facial expression often results in mirrored (but mainly inhibited) premotor activation in the observer and a corresponding "retrodicted" emotional state.

But this is a long way from both imitation by behavior parsing and complex imitation.

Over-imitation

Another contrast between humans and chimpanzees is provided by the study of *over-imitation*. In contrast to nonhuman primates, when young children learn by imitating they focus more on reproducing the specific actions used than the actual outcomes achieved. Here we are looking at immediate imitation, but the presumption is that the strategy for immediate imitation of a novel behavior is a crucial precursor for addition of the skill to the observer's long-term repertoire.

In a study by Horner and Whiten (2005), young wild-born chimpanzees and 3- to 4-year-old children observed a human demonstrator use a tool to retrieve a reward from a puzzle box. The demonstration involved both causally relevant and irrelevant actions, and the box was presented in each of two conditions: opaque and clear.

When chimpanzees were presented with the opaque box, they reproduced both the relevant and irrelevant actions, thus imitating the overall structure of the task. When the box was presented in the clear condition, they instead ignored the irrelevant actions in favor of a more efficient technique in which they only carried out those actions that they saw achieving a clear subgoal of changing the mechanism toward the state in which it released the reward. These results suggest that the favored strategy of chimpanzees is *emulation*, observing and attempting to reproduce results (subgoals) of another's actions without paying attention to the other's actual behavior, when sufficient causal information is available. However, if such information is not available, chimpanzees are prone to employ a more comprehensive copy of an observed action.

In contrast to the chimpanzees, children imitated all the demonstrated actions to solve the task in both conditions, at the expense of efficiency. Indeed, from about 18 months of age, children over-imitate in that what they copy and may include arbitrary and unnecessary actions. And chimpanzees do not. Are chimpanzees smarter than humans in this regard?

Horner and Whiten suggest that the difference in performance of chimpanzees and children may be due to a greater susceptibility of children to cultural conventions, perhaps combined with a differential focus on the results, actions, and goals of the demonstrator.

Nielsen and Tomaselli (2009) documented similarities exhibited by children from Brisbane, a city in Australia, and children from remote Bushman communities in southern Africa. They suggest that over-imitation is a universal human trait, rather than being a culture-specific consequence of the pedagogical approach adopted by parents in Westernized cultures. The Bushman children are recent ancestors of true hunter-gatherers living in communities where many aspects of traditional culture are maintained, whereas the Brisbane children are typical of those living in large, Westernized, industrialized cities. They argue that, although seemingly maladaptive, over-imitation reflects an evolutionary adaptation fundamental to the development and transmission of human culture. Directly replicating others affords the rapid acquisition of novel behaviors while at the same time avoiding the potential pitfalls and false end-points that can come from trial-and-error learning. Even when children aged 3 to 5 years were trained to identify the causally irrelevant parts of novel action sequences performed by an adult on familiar household objects, such as retrieving a toy from a plastic jar after first stroking the side of the jar with a feather (Lyons, Young, & Keil, 2007), they still reproduced causally irrelevant actions—despite being specifically instructed to copy only the necessary actions. In other words, children who observe an adult intentionally manipulating a novel object have a strong tendency to encode all of the adult's actions as causally meaningful. This allows children to rapidly calibrate their causal beliefs about even the most opaque physical systems, but it also carries a cost. Despite countervailing task demands, time pressure, and even direct warnings, children are frequently unable to avoid reproducing the adult's irrelevant actions because they have already incorporated them into their representation of the target object's causal structure.

Could it be that young children's propensity for over-imitation is that they lack the maturity to discern the causal relations between the model's actions and the outcome of those actions? No. Older children tested by Nielsen and Tomaselli were even more inclined than the younger children to copy the model. Also, children who were first given the opportunity to discover the affordances of the test apparatus still reproduced the model's actions and did so at similar rates to children who were not given such an opportunity. Even when children discovered on their own how to open by hand all three apparatuses used in the study, each of these children persisted in copying an adult's subsequent demonstration of a more complicated method incorporating irrelevant actions. It is thus unlikely that children's high-fidelity imitation is solely attributable to their capacity for causal understanding. Instead, young children are drawn toward copying the actions they see adults perform, so much so that children will persistently replicate the actions of an adult even if such actions interfere with production of the desired outcome.

Although at first glance such behavior seems maladaptive, we view it as quintessential to the development and transmission of human culture. Consider the multitude of complex social activities humans engage in. We make tools together, court each other, develop political institutions, construct dwellings, and prepare meals. But precisely *how* we engage in these activities differs, often strikingly, from one community to another: Human behavior varies profoundly across cultures. Nielsen and Tomaselli (2009) argue that, in understanding aspects of human behavior that are culturally instantiated, it is knowing the *way* things are done that is important, not *what gets done*. For them, over-imitation provides a glimpse into the origins of our human propensity to follow those around us and to do as others do, irrespective of the logic underpinning such behavior. I think this is mistaken, and that what I call the IKEA effect is more relevant; that is, over-imitation evolved to support complex imitation. Social discriminability is a consequence, not a cause, of this ability.

Nonetheless, children do not blindly copy everything they see adults do. Children will make judgments about what actions to copy based on a host of variables, including the apparent intentions of the person they observe and the situational constraints confronting both this "model" and child. For example, Carpenter et al. (1998) explored infants' ability to discriminate between, and their tendency to reproduce, the accidental and intentional actions of others. Infants aged 14 through 18 months watched an adult perform a series of two-step actions on objects that made interesting results occur. Some of the modeled actions were marked vocally as intentional ("There!"), and some were marked vocally as accidental ("Woops!"). Following each demonstration, infants were given a chance to make the result occur themselves. Overall, infants imitated almost twice as many of the adult's intentional actions as her accidental ones. Infants before age 18 months thus may understand something about the intentions of other persons. This understanding represents the human infants' first step toward adult-like social cognition and underlies their acquisition of language and other cultural skills.

In any case, let us return to the notion that *complex imitation* (our extension of *action-level imitation*) involves reproduction of the details, more or less precisely, of the manual actions another individual uses; that is, in the latter case the observer can attend to details of an observed movement to more quickly learn how to achieve a subgoal. We earlier (Chapter 5) saw the equation action = movement + goal, but the point is that the over-imitating child may reproduce an action in which certain subcomponents are not associated with a discernible goal. The only function of such a movement Y is that "it's what you do before you do action X" so that the composite Y;X appears to be the action one must take to reach whatever goal is achieved upon completion of X.

A Cooperative Framework

In defining complex imitation, we contrasted the long and laborious process of acquiring the nut-cracking technique studied by Boesch and Boesch (1990) with the comparative rapidity with which human adults can acquire at least the rudiments of (some) diverse novel skills. This may well reflect not only changes in the brain that affect the child's learning skills but also those affecting the way in which others interact with the child. In the next section, we will discuss the crucial role of caregivers in assisting complex imitation in young children. By contrast, Michael Tomasello[6] has stressed that chimpanzee mothers seldom if ever help their offspring to learn. He (2008, 2009) sees the patterns of cooperation exhibited by humans but not by apes as providing the "stage zero" on which the evolution of language is based:

T0. Collaborative activities
T1. Pragmatic infrastructure for natural gesture
T2. Communicative conventions
T3. Grammaticalization of constructions

What is crucial for Tomasello for Stage T1 is that (a) chimpanzees can imitate the praxis of another chimpanzee, but the imitated chimpanzee seldom if ever modifies its behavior to assist the imitator; and (b) the gestures developed by chimps (see Chapter 3) are *instrumental* in that they serve to get another to do something the gesturer wants, whereas even a young child may gesture *declaratively* to direct another's attention to (aspects of) an item of interest. *Instrumental gesture* is firmly rooted in the here and now (with a little assist from working memory of recent events relevant to the current situation), whereas the declarative mode opens the way to what Suddendorf and Corballis (1997) call mental time travel. I will not seek to explain the "declarative opening" in this volume but will indeed build on it in the next chapter by exploring how pantomime provides the bridge from praxis to protosign, corresponding to the transition from Tomasello's T1 to T2. We will then be in a position to address the issue of "grammaticalization of constructions" both within the cultural evolution of the earliest protolanguages and recent languages (Chapter 10) as well as in the rapid emergence over a few decades of new sign languages (Chapter 11).

In view of this, let's consider the role of the human caregiver in helping the child learn about her world by focusing on studies by Pat Zukow-Goldring (1996, 2001), which involved both Anglo and Latino children in Los Angeles. While child-rearing practices certainly differ greatly from culture to culture— recall our earlier discussion of Bushman communities in southern Africa— they do establish a baseline for cross-cultural comparison (elsewhere). The

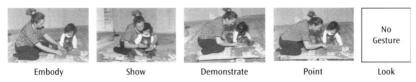

| Embody | Show | Demonstrate | Point | Look |

FIGURE 7-2.   Attention-directing gestures: Caregivers act on the infant during an *embody*, display an action to a watchful infant during a *show*, and act first and then invite the infant to join in during a *demonstration*. No action is displayed during *points* and *looks*. (From Zukow-Goldring & Arbib, 2007.)

initial aim of the research was to study what caregivers do when infants initially misunderstand messages directed to them. At a stage when the child has little or no command of language, more explicit verbal messages do not assist the infant in understanding the caregiver message. However, providing perceptual information that makes the message transparent does reduce misunderstanding. In later research, Zukow-Goldring came to realize that in many of those interactions the caregivers were inviting the infants to imitate using various strategies for *assisted imitation* (Zukow-Goldring & Arbib, 2007). These studies demonstrated that in acquiring a new practical skill, the child must learn not only to recognize *affordances* (perceptual cues as to aspects of the environment that can support various kinds of interaction—we saw affordances for manual action in Chapter 4) but also learn to mobilize *effectivities* (different ways of coordinating parts of the body to achieve some desired effect upon the environment). However, the caregiver–child relation is not merely a matter of transferring praxic skills but also initiates the social process of understanding the relation between perceiving and acting as shared between first person (the child) and third person (the caregiver, and others).

Caregivers often *embody* infants in the sense that they provide effects on the infant's body that help the infant pay attention to experiences relevant to acquiring new affordances and effectivities, or caregivers act in tandem with them as the two go through the motions of some activity together (Fig. 7-2). The caregiver can help the infant learn how to do what the other does to achieve similar benefits or avoid risks, by noticing and linking the effectivities of her own body with affordances for action. Many authors have suggested that the infant comes to recognize that others are like her, but Zukow-Goldring (2006) has stressed the converse: The child has the chance to see and feel that her own movements are "like the other's." This is crucial; the child's cognitive growth rests on expanding her repertoire to include skills exhibited by those around her, rather than shrinking her observation of others to actions already in her repertoire. The infant's fragmentary, flawed attempts to imitate actions elicited very careful and elaborate tutoring on the part of the caregivers studied here, directing attention to relevant affordances and effectivities, nudging the infant toward a culturally relevant approach to activities and the use of artifacts. Thus, the perceiving and acting of infant and caregiver continuously affect the perceiving of the other. The caregiver directs infants to notice the content of messages, such as specific elements, relations, or events over the myriad other possibilities available. The collection of attention-directing interactions in these studies included instances of perceptual impera-tives expressed by caregivers (both English- and Spanish-speaking Americans), such as look!/¡mira! (important evidence for the role of the "*mira system*" in child development?), listen!/¡oye!, touch!/¡toca!, and so on, as well as the accompa-nying gestures, the gestures alone, and the infants' subsequent actions.

Caregivers may also display how to do something to an observing infant without giving the infant a chance to act. However, in assisted imitation, after displaying the activity caregivers invite the infant to join in by orienting or offering the object to the infant and/or saying, e.g., "Now, you do it!" "Let's do it," or "Do you want to do X?" In demonstrations, the infant must pick up or detect a familiar or somewhat novel coupling of affordance and effectivity in order to imitate successfully. As the child becomes more experienced, pointing to some affording part of an object, or even just looking at it may suffice. For points, the infant must detect affordances for action by noticing where a ges-ture's trajectory through space converges with some target of attention. For looks, no gestures accompany the caregiver's speech. Instead, only the care-giver's words and gaze direct the infant to discover the affordances for action (Fig. 7-2).

To develop these ideas, we focus on just one later naturalistic study of the role of the caregiver in infant development through this process of assisted imitation (Zukow-Goldring, 2006; Zukow-Goldring & Arbib, 2007). In this example a child aged 14.5 months plays with a vibrating toy that has a hid-den affordance, a spring inside the toy to which a string is attached. When the mother pulls the ring that unwinds the string and then releases the string so it will snap back in, the toy will start to vibrate. Then the mother places the vibrating toy on the infant's tummy, yielding an enjoyable sensation for the infant. Once the child is motivated to elicit this sensation, assisted imitation can begin. The caregiver invites the infant to imitate by orienting the ring on the back of the toy toward the infant, making the affordance for pulling promi-nent, and saying, "You do it!" As a result, the infant grasps the ring (grasping is already within her repertoire). The caregiver embodies the necessary action for the infant by holding the infant's hand and toy steady as she pulls the toy away from her. The infant can feel the effectivity of the body's work of holding steady against the tension as well as the string on the spring's affordance as the string unwinds. As a result of this, the infant will then pull the string out slowly and hold on tightly as the string pulls her hand back toward the toy. The toy vibrates weakly at most because little tension is left. After a while, success comes by accident. The infant pulls forcefully. The string snaps from her fingers. The hand and string move as one; the end effector "migrates" from the hand to the leading edge of the string attached to the spring. The forceful pulling and quick release lead to a vigorously vibrating toy and many repetitions of the act. Although the infant knew that the toy afforded vibrating, she did not know how to use her body to elicit this, until both caregiver and toy educated her attention. Overall, the resulting dynamic coupling of effectivities and affordances leads to more adept behavior. Furthermore, extending the end effector from the hand to some part of a tool or object (Arbib, Bonaiuto, Jacobs, & Frey, 2009) increases the detection of new effectivities as well as new affordances as the coupling continues to unfold.

One challenge posed by this work is to understand how "programs" like that for the vibrating toy are learned in such a way that a single experience can reconfigure what the infant knows into a successful form that can be acted upon thereafter. In much skill learning, many trials may be required to tune the parameters of the system (encoded in patterns of synaptic weights) to yield consistently successful behavior. Here, by contrast, we have moved "up the hierarchy" so that a single restructuring of the program may yield success that will thereafter be acted upon—one-shot learning. Our brief discussion of augmented competitive queuing (chapter 5) offers a step in this direction. Of course, much practice and tuning may be required to hone a behavior that is awkwardly performed into a form where the behavior is executed with skill and grace.

The Direct and Indirect Path in Imitation

We have emphasized various forms of imitation of behaviors that reach some praxic goal. In addition, humans have the ability to imitate complex "meaningless" movements that are not directed toward objects. This ability becomes important for communication, as these intransitive actions can effect communicative goals. The subtleties in going from "recognizing a familiar action" to "imitating a complex behavior based on an interweaving of variations on familiar actions" was illustrated in the following description of a dance class[7]:

> The percussion is insistent. Dancers move in rows from the back of the hall toward the drummers at the front. From time to time, the mistress of the dance breaks the flow and twice repeats a sequence of energetic dance moves. The dancers then move forward again, repeating her moves, more or less. Some do it well, others not so well.

Imitation involves, in part, seeing the instructor's dance as a set of familiar movements of shoulders, arms, hands, belly, and legs. Many constituents are variants of familiar actions, rather than familiar actions themselves. Thus, one must not only observe actions and their composition but also novelties in the constituents and their variations. One must also perceive the overlapping and sequencing of all these moves and then remember the "coordinated control program" so constructed. Memory and perception are intertwined.

As the dancers perform, they both act out the recalled coordinated control program and tune it. By observing other dancers and synchronizing with their neighbors and the insistent percussion of the drummers, they achieve a collective representation that tunes their own, possibly departing from the instructor's original. At the same time, some dancers seem more or less skilled—some will omit a movement, or simplify it, and others may replace it with their imagined equivalent. (One example: the instructor alternates touching her breast and moving her arm outward. Most dancers move their arms in and out with no particular target.) Other changes are matters of motor rather than perceptual or mnemonic skill—not everyone can lean back as far as the instructor without losing balance.

These are the ingredients of imitation.

To address such behaviors, we now offer an analysis of praxic actions that gives a deeper significance to this apparent departure from goal-directed behavior, going beyond the "IKEA effect" and the observation that the overimitating child may reproduce an action in which certain subcomponents are not associated with a discernible goal. To this end, we will look at a classical conceptual model of apraxia, and then reframe it to gain new insights into the building up of a motoric repertoire.

People with *apraxia* ("without praxis") have brain damage that impairs their ability to carry out learned purposeful movements, despite having the physical ability to move the appropriate limbs or other effectors. De Renzi (1989) reports that some apraxics exhibit a *semantic deficit*—having difficulty both in classifying gestures and in performing familiar gestures on command—yet may be able to copy the pattern of a movement of such a gesture without "getting the meaning" of the action of which it is part. I call this residual ability *movement imitation* to distinguish it from imitation based on recognition and "replay" of a goal-directed action. I have elsewhere called this *low-level* imitation, but I now reject this because I want to see it as part and parcel of the transition from *imitation by behavior parsing* to *complex imitation*. We saw that in the latter case the observer can attend to details of an observed movement, but now we ponder how this ability can be divorced from the context provided by a praxic subgoal.

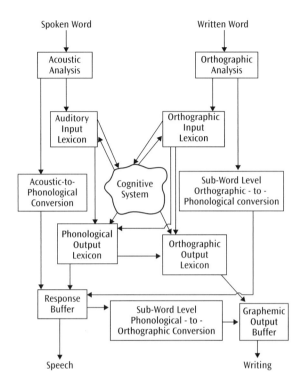

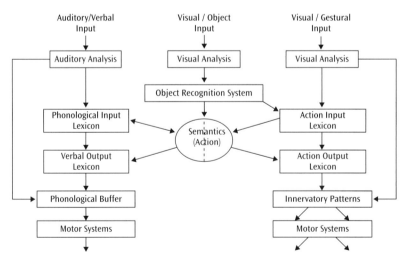

FIGURE 7-3.   (*Top*) A process model for the recognition, comprehension, and production of spoken and written words and nonwords (Patterson & Shewell, 1987). (*Bottom*) A model of praxis and its relation to semantics, naming, and word and object recognition based on the Patterson-Shewell model (Rothi et al., 1991).

To address De Renzi's data, Rothi, Ochipa, and Heilman (1991) proposed a dual-route imitation model to serve as a platform for studying apraxia (Fig. 7-3 bottom). Since our task in this book is to trace an evolutionary progression from praxis to language, it is intriguing to note that Rothi et al.'s model was inspired by a model for the recognition, comprehension, and production of spoken and written words and nonwords (Patterson & Shewell, 1987). At the left of Patterson and Shewell's figure (Fig. 7-3 top), we see that repeating a spoken word may proceed in one of two ways—we may recognize the word as an entry in the "auditory input lexicon" and use this to retrieve the motor plan for speaking the word from the "phonological output lexicon" (the *indirect* route), or we may simply repeat the sequence of phonemes we have heard, invoking "acoustic-to-phonological conversion" (the *direct route*). This is the duality of patterning of Chapter 2, but with a new twist—when we are used to speaking a word, we do not string together the motor plans for each meaningless sound that underlies it; instead, we invoke a "motor program" that yields smooth pronunciation of the word as a whole. However, if what we hear is a nonsense word, or a word that is new to us, we must break it down into its constituent phonemes and reassemble them to pronounce the novel "word" as best we can. The right-hand side of Patterson and Shewell's figure offers a similar analysis for writing, though, strangely enough, it omits the direct route of letter-by-letter copying of a nonword or novel word. Finally, the model offers somewhat different paths for linking speaking and writing. To go from a spoken word to a written form for it, one may either go from the phonological output lexicon directly to the orthographic output lexicon to drive the graphemic output buffer, or one may employ acoustic-phonological conversion to load the response buffer but, rather than speaking the result, use subword-level phonological-to-output orthographic conversion to spell out the response buffer's contents via the graphemic output buffer. Conversely, reading a word may employ subword-level orthographic-to-phonological conversion to drive speech via the response buffer. Unspecified cognitive processes drive further links between the systems for speech and writing.

Now let's see how Rothi, Ochipa, and Heilman (1991) transformed this into a dual-route imitation model for praxis (Fig. 7-3 bottom). Essentially, they have taken the Patterson-Shewell model and replaced the writing system by a more general action system. As we can see, the left-hand sides of both diagrams (for speech) differ only in relabeling of the components. On the right of Rothi et al.'s diagram, the *direct route* for imitation of meaningless and intransitive gestures converts a visual representation of limb motion into a set of intermediate limb postures or motions for subsequent execution. The *indirect route* for imitation of known gestures recognizes and then reconstructs known actions regardless of whether they are object-directed. (Note: For some apraxics, performance of an action upon an object may be far better when the object is present than when pantomime of the action must be performed in the absence of the object.) Let us consider the parallels between language and praxis illustrated here. The *lexicon* is the collection of words in a language or the repertoire of a speaker or signer. The *phonological input lexicon* contains the perceptual schemas for recognizing each spoken word in the lexicon on hearing it, while the *phonological output lexicon* contains the motor schemas for pronouncing each spoken word in the lexicon. Note that one might be able to recognize a word when pronounced in diverse accents yet repeat it in one's own accent. This contrasts with the direct path in which one tries to imitate how a word is pronounced, a strategy that can also work for nonwords or words that one does not know. If a word is in the lexicon, then its recognition and production (in the *phonological* lexicon) are to be distinguished from what the word actually means, given in the model by the link between the lexicon and the box for *semantics*.

To proceed, we replace the term "action lexicon" used in the figure by the term *praxicon* to denote the collection of praxic actions (practical actions upon objects; the type of action impaired in apraxia) within the repertoire of a human (or animal or robot). Thus, the *input praxicon* corresponds, approximately, to the mirror neurons that recognize actions, while the *output praxicon* adds the canonical neurons involved in the performance of actions—but probably augmented by the systems for understanding and planning shown in Figure 5-7 (in Chapter 5), with the degree of involvement varying from occasion to occasion. These form the indirect pathway. The direct pathway is based on the fact that we can also imitate certain novel behaviors that are not in the praxicon and cannot be linked initially to an underlying semantics.

For Rothi et al. (1991), the language system at the left of Figure 7-3 simply serves as a model for their conceptual model of the praxis system at right, with semantics playing a bridging role. For us, the challenge is to better understand the right-hand side as a sketch of praxic abilities that could have served as the basis for the evolution of protolanguage as a core competence of the language-ready brain, a topic that we take up in the next chapter. To start this process, let's note that, strangely enough, Rothi et al. seem to focus only on single actions, thus omitting an "action buffer" in which various actions are combined. To move forward, we consider a variant of their model (Fig. 7-4) in which an action buffer is included (building on comments by Arbib & Bonaiuto, 2008).

The new model has no language component—our concern is to understand praxis and imitation as they may have existed in a prehuman brain that could support complex imitation but not language. Nonetheless, there is a crucial lesson we can learn from Patterson and Shewell (1987, Fig. 7-3 top), namely, that that their direct paths for speech and writing may be meaningless but

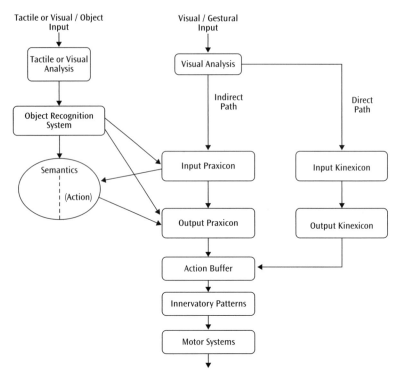

FIGURE 7-4.   A variant of the Rothi et al. dual-route model of praxis. We remove the language component since our concern is to understand praxis and imitation as they may have existed in a prehuman brain that could support complex imitation but not language. The key novelty of this model is that actions specified by both the direct and indirect routes (the latter via the praxicons) may be combined in the action buffer.

they are not arbitrary—they yield "gestures" that are composites of phonemes and letters, respectively. The key here is the duality of patterning of language. A key innovation of our model (though not made explicit in Fig. 7-4) is that now *we postulate duality of patterning for actions as the key to complex imitation.* However, unlike a particular language where the phonology establishes a relatively small set of meaningless units from which to compose words (from which we compose larger utterances), the world of action imposes no such limits. We have already been at pains to distinguish actions from movements. I suggest that our vocabulary of movements can be increased in two ways:

(1) Abstracting away from goals: A movement originally acquired as a means to achieve a goal becomes available as a separate resource. Where the original action may have been parameterized by the need to match the affordances of an object, the abstracted movement can be parameterized to match

other types of context. For example, in the MNS model (Chapter 4) we saw how a trajectory of hand and arm could be generated to match the affordances and location of an object. But our earlier discussion of Chapter 3 introduced the notion of ontogenetic ritualization. Here a praxic trajectory became truncated by criteria based on communicative success which no longer required an end-state matching the affordances of an object. We will return to this concept in our discussion of pantomime in the next chapter.

(2) "Tweaking" actions: Until now, when we have spoken of combining movements or actions, our emphasis has been on putting them together in sequences (which may or may not express an underlying hierarchy). But we may also combine them by executing them together in a coordinated way—our prime example of this being the simultaneous execution of reach and grasp. What I want to emphasize here, however, is that—unlike the reach and grasp example—there are actions (I call them tweaks) that we have acquired not as goal-directed in themselves but because they allow us to modify an action to make it more successful. Thus, in assembling a piece of furniture, we may insert a table leg into a hole in the table only to have it fall out once we let go. However, we may discover that if we tweak the original action by giving the leg a simple twist as the leg enters the hole, we will secure the leg in place.

The point, then, is that our prior motor experience equips us with a rich set of tweaks that are meaningless in themselves but allow us to modify an action to form another that is more effective. In the original motivation for the two models of Figure 7-3, the direct and indirect paths were considered as *alternatives*—one either employed the indirect path to execute a known action stored in the praxicons (or produced a word already in the lexicons) or one employed the direct path to execute a meaningless action (or produce a non-word or unknown word).

However, proceeding from an evolutionary basis in which praxis precedes gestural communication and (proto)language, our hypothesis is as follows:

(1) The indirect path is the basic pathway, supporting the acquisition of actions that can achieve a specific goal. This pathway is supported by trial-and-error learning in which supervised learning (e.g., mediated by cerebellum) and reinforcement learning (e.g., mediated by the basal ganglia) can adjust the synapses in a variety of neural circuits to tune the action to become more successful over repeated trials.

(2) The direct pathway evolved to enable the observed difference between an observed action and one's unsuccessful attempt to emulate it to be used on future trials to elicit a tweak to be combined with the original action to yield a more successful action. The collection of such tweaks could be added both as

movements abstracted away from the goals of the actions that employed them or by trial-and-error learning of ways to adjust actions in varied circumstances.

Our variation of the Rothi et al. model provides the key mechanism for the third component of our definition of complex imitation: recognizing ways in which a novel action or movement may be seen as a variant of one already known to the observer. We thus obtain duality of patterning for actions but with important differences from language:

- Tweaks are parameterizable to yield varied movement patterns.
- Many actions can be acquired through trial and error without being reduced to tweaks.
- Even if an action was originally built up through tweaks, the result may become optimized through learning into an integrated whole that becomes added to the praxicon,

A corollary of this analysis is that the direct path is not so direct. It too involves a mirror system–like structure. If there is room for yet more terminology, we might speak of an input and an output *kinexicon* containing those movements already in the "vocabulary" of tweaks and of movements abstracted away from praxic goals.

With this, we come to the third evolutionary stage of the scheme shown in Figure 7-4:

(3) The direct pathway became available for production of movements decoupled from the indirect path.

This sets the stage for our discussion of pantomime and protosign in the next chapter.

Human Imitation Is Complex

In Chapter 6, I singled out complex imitation as a key component of language readiness, but I also emphasized that the extension of childhood and the participation of caregivers in the cognitive development of the child were also crucial characteristics. Thus, the first and seventh properties listed in the section "Protolanguage Versus Language" were as follows:

Complex action recognition and complex imitation: *Complex action recognition* is the ability to recognize another's performance as a set of familiar movements designed to achieve specific subgoals. *Complex imitation* is the ability to use this as the basis for flexible imitation of the observed behavior. This extends to the ability to recognize that such a performance combines novel actions that can be approximated by (i.e., more or less crudely be imitated by) variants of actions already in the repertoire.

Paedomorphy and sociality: Paedomorphy is the prolonged period of infant dependency that is especially pronounced in humans. This combines with the willingness of adults to act as caregivers and the consequent development of social structures to provide the conditions for complex social learning.

In this chapter, we have defined complex imitation as being akin to what Byrne and Russon (1998) call *action-level imitation* in contrast to *imitation by behavior parsing.* In either case, the imitator will learn to recognize key points that define subgoals for the observed behavior, but we used the IKEA effect to distinguish between using any means at hand to achieve a subgoal, and careful attention to the movements used as a basis for either employing the observed action, or seeking to approximate the movement that has been observed. In other words, the human ability for complex imitation does not preclude frequent recourse to imitation by behavior parsing. However, our discussion of over-imitation reinforced this distinction, emphasizing that children may repeat actions even if their relevance to a goal is not apparent. We saw that even though there are cases in which such over-imitation may seem counterproductive, overall it makes cultural evolution possible on a scale denied to nonhumans. Nonetheless, we cautioned that children will not blindly imitate movements if they can understand, for example, why their performance depends on some limitation of the performer that does not apply to them.

If the action is familiar, then recognition of a movement can yield its successful performance. But if the action is not familiar, one may only capture certain of its elements in first trying to perform it. The result may be twofold: Errors in achieving the subgoal may provide learning feedback that can adjust the motor schema to yield greater success across multiple attempts, but, perhaps more important, it may direct attention, on the next trial, to features of the movement that were not noticed previously. Our discussion of our version of the dual-route model (Fig. 7-4) showed how a direct route structured to provide tweaks (already in the kinexicon) to build new motor schemas from those already in the praxicon could markedly speed the process of finding a successful movement over blind trial and error. Nonetheless, as any athlete or instrument player or other skilled performer knows, much practice may be required to assure the synaptic tuning that maintains an action at its peak effectiveness—mere tweaking using the kinexicon is not enough.

Since complex imitation involves parsing a complex movement into a composite of (variations on) familiar actions, this must be grounded in the prior development of a basic set of actions and a basic set of composition techniques (of which forming a two-element sequence is perhaps the simplest). I do *not* posit a fixed set of "primitive actions" that is innate or acquired early in life. Rather, I suggest that at any stage of life there is a (increasing) repertoire of overlearned actions (which may themselves have hierarchical structure whose execution has become automatized) that provide the basis for learning new skills. As such, actions that are "basic" at one stage of life may disappear as they become subsumed in skills that see more frequent use at a later stage. I should add that when I speak of a "stage" in ontogeny, I do not have in mind some fixed time period that is preset by the genes, but rather a typical pattern that emerges in normal development through the coalescence of a multitude of maturational and experiential changes. This process yields both the mastery of ever finer details and the increasing grace and accuracy of the overall performance.

The property of *paedomorphy and sociality* takes us beyond complex imitation to address ways in which the initial population of the praxicon and kinexicon is built up, while providing the young child with a basic set of affordances and effectivities. Here we emphasize that human evolution has endowed humans with the social substrate for child–caregiver interactions that supports the ability to learn by *assisted imitation* as one means for building up the capability for complex imitation. The key here is that we posit that evolution has not only modified the learning abilities of children and adults but has also endowed adults with skills that make the sharing of experiences a key aspect of social cognition, with a resultant amplification of the child's learning through the repeated education of attention to salient aspects of the physical and social world.

In other words, while I select complex imitation as a vital preadaptation within praxis for the later emergence of language readiness, I am in no way restricting the complexity of human imitation to complex imitation alone.

Notes Toward Related Modeling

Let's close by relating all this to some of our earlier analysis of the control of hand movements. Our MNS models of the mirror system for grasping in the monkey (Chapter 5) demonstrate how the mirror system may come to detect grasps that are already in the (monkey or human) infant's repertoire. But this raises the question of how grasps entered the repertoire. To simplify somewhat, there are two answers:

(1) Infants explore their environment and as their initially inept arm and hand movements successfully contact objects, they learn to reliably reproduce the successful grasps, with the repertoire being tuned through further experience.

(2) With more or less help from caregivers, infants come to notice certain novel actions in terms of similarities and differences from movements already in their repertoires, and on this basis they learn to produce some version of these novel actions for themselves. The second approach takes us into the realm of assisted imitation.

My group already has an interesting model relevant to the first approach in the Infant Learning to Grasp Model (ILGM; Oztop, Arbib, & Bradley, 2006; Oztop, Bradley, & Arbib, 2004). This study shows that the young infants may at first come to grab objects, with varying success, solely as a result of the innate grasp reflex—this exists only in young infants, and it is the reflex whereby the hand instinctively closes around an object that contacts the palm. ILGM then offered a computationally implemented model whereby neural networks could learn which of the resulting handshapes were successful in achieving a secure grasp of an object. The model employs reinforcement learning based on a "joy of grasping" signal whereby positive reinforcement of a grasp increased with increasing stability of the grasp. A complementary model developed a learning network that could come to recognize the affordances of an object (Oztop, Imamizu, Cheng, & Kawato, 2006). Current work is developing ILGA (Integrated Learning of Grasps and Affordances), a model of infant learning of grasps and affordances, in which the learning of affordances and the learning of grasps is intertwined—the vocabulary of affordances is built up as the set of visual indicators that a successful grasp will ensue on a certain part of an object; the affordances are learned simultaneously with the transformation that links the perceived affordance to grasps (effectivities) appropriate to it.

The models specify that if the infant pays attention to an object or to his hand and an object, he will be able to extend his repertoire of executed and identifiable grasps—extending his stock of affordances and effectivities in the process. However, the modeling does not address how the infant comes to attend to these visual stimuli. Clearly, models that address the naturalistic experiments like the vibrating toy study must encompass a wider range of sensory data concerning a range of objects and information about the body of the infant, the behavior of the caregiver, and interactions between infant and caregiver. We must then model how the caregiver directs the attention of the infant to get the infant to notice the coupling of effectivities and affordances as they dynamically unfold. Successful focusing of attention by the caregiver means that the infant's "search space" is limited to the neighborhood of successful grasps and manipulations, rather than involving a time-consuming trial-and-error process that includes many configurations far removed from those required for successful completion of the task. In any case, our example makes clear that the affordances to be learned go well beyond affordances for a stable grasp.

All this suggests that detailed modeling of the phenomena described in this chapter involves, at least, the following: The MNS models exploit connectivity from canonical neurons (those that encode a grasp already in the system's repertoire) to the mirror neurons to provide the training signal to neurons that are to learn to become mirror neurons for similar grasps by detecting the visual signals for the trajectories of hand–object relationships related to that grasp. New modeling will explore ways to build an "evolved" imitation ability exploiting capacities like those of the ILGA model by augmenting MNS capabilities with the reverse connection. In this way, the detecting of trajectories performed by another (e.g., the caregiver) can provide the training signal for recruiting new canonical neurons to develop a controller for a grasp describable by similar external patterns of goals and affordances.

The notion that mirror neurons may come to detect actions frequently performed by others even though canonical neurons do not exist to control that action raises the further possibility that the infant may come to detect movements that not only are *not* within the repertoire but that never come to be within his repertoire. In this case, the cumulative development of action detection may proceed to increase the breadth and subtlety of the range of actions that are detectable but cannot be performed by infants. Recalling the earlier discussion of complex and goal-directed imitation, we see that the emphasis must shift from single actions to sequences of actions, where the refining of individual actions and the transition from one action to the next depends crucially on ceaseless cycles of action-coupled perception of actions by the infant in a particular environment. Moreover, since the caregiver will modify her actions in response to the child, our future modeling will extend to the dyad of caregiver-child interaction, setting the stage for the evolution of brain mechanisms that can support the cooperative phenomena of conversation as biological and cultural evolution build language atop praxis.

8

Via Pantomime to Protosign

From Praxis to Intended Communication

In Chapter 3, "Vocalization and Gesture in Monkey and Ape," we saw that the motor schemas for monkey vocalizations were almost entirely innate, though young monkeys could learn to be more specific in the conditions under which they released these innate motor schemas. For example, a young monkey might at first initiate the eagle call in response to any creature flying overhead, but it would eventually learn—on the basis of the presence or absence of calls by those around it—to release it only in the presence of predatory eagles or in response to the eagle calls of others. Such calls also showed an audience effect: The call was more likely to be made when others were present. By contrast, whatever the innate components of ape gesture, it became clear that, perhaps by a combination of ontogenetic ritualization and social learning, a group of apes could add new gestures to their repertoire. Moreover, ape gestures can be adapted to the attentional state of specific individuals, with the gesture used more likely to make a distinctive sound or include a component of touching the other if the signaler was not in the other's field of visual attention. It thus seems that ape gestures satisfy at least three of the properties reviewed in the section "Protolanguage Versus Language" in Chapter 6:

> **Property 2: Intended communication:** Communication is intended by the utterer to have a particular effect on the recipient, rather than being involuntary or a side effect of praxis.
> **Property 3: Symbolization:** The ability to associate symbols with an open class of events, objects, or actions—though the "openness" of ape gestures is limited indeed.
> **Property 4: Parity:** What counts for the producer must count as approximately the same for the receiver.

Although the novel gestures used by an ape group provide an "open" set of symbols that is not confined to a fixed, innate repertoire like most monkey vocalizations, they are nonetheless "not very open"—a group might have 10 or so gestures in its novel repertoire. I will argue that pantomime provided the bridge to a "very open" set of gestures, and that this paved the way for proto-sign (this chapter) and protospeech (the next chapter).

Building on our Chapter 5 discussion, I suggest that our last common ancestor with monkeys had (1) F5 mirror systems for both manual and inges-tion-related orofacial actions, and (2) a mirror system for the control and rec-ognition of facial expressions of emotion by systems that exclude F5. There are few data on imitation of facial expression by apes (but see the discussion of "Facial Expressions" in Chapter 3 and of neonatal imitation in Chapter 7), though we saw in Chapter 7 that apes do have "simple imitation" for manual actions of some complexity. The data on ape gesture suggest that this capacity for simple imitation of hand movements extended to communicative gestures as well as praxic actions. We have seen that ontogenetic ritualization may have been crucial here, converting a praxic action to change the behavior of a conspecific into a communicative gesture that would have the same effect. With this, the transition to "Intentionality" has been achieved, along with "Symbolization." Nonetheless, the fact remains that the number of gestures used by any ape, even that star turn Kanzi, is far less than the number of words that are mastered by a typical 3-year-old human child, and that the child has syntactic abilities that seem to elude the ape. I think the key difference *can be traced back to* the following:

Complex action recognition and imitation: *The ability to recognize another's performance as a set of familiar movements designed to achieve specific sub-goals and to use this as the basis for flexible imitation of the observed behavior. This extends to the ability to recognize that another's performance combines novel actions that can be approximated by (i.e., more or less crudely be imitated by) variants of actions already in the repertoire.*

But note the key qualification "can be traced back to." In this chapter we delin-eate the evolutionary changes that built on this foundation to yield capacities for pantomime and protosign, and then in Chapter 9 we suggest how protospeech then develops with protosign to yield protolanguages far richer than the ges-tural repertoire of apes. Chapter 11 will show how complex action recognition and imitation can operate on protolanguages to yield the first constructions that eventually yielded a critical mass of grammatical structures—driving a histor-ical process spanning across a spectrum of protolanguages to yield languages. Chapter 11 will then show the continuing relevance of the mechanisms neces-sary for language to get started in our distant ancestry. It will link construction grammar to both the way in which children now acquire the language of the communityaround.

Symbolization becomes immensely enriched with the extension of imi-tation from the imitation of hand movements to the ability to in some sense

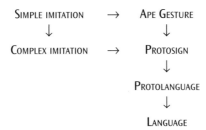

FIGURE 8-1.   A sketch of key elements of the Mirror System Hypothesis. The left-hand column suggests that the capability for simple imitation allows apes (and, presumably, the common ancestor of apes and humans) to acquire a small repertoire of communicative manual gestures, but it required the evolution of mechanisms for complex imitation (in the hominid line) to support the open-ended symbol creation of pantomime and, through extensive conventionalization, protosign and then (adding protospeech to expand upon protosign) protolanguage. It is argued (Chapter 11) that the transition from protolanguage to language was then a matter of cultural rather than biological evolution.

project the degrees of freedom of movements involving other effectors (and even, say, of the passage of the wind through the trees) to create hand movements that could evoke something of the original in the brain of the observer. This involves not merely changes internal to the mirror system but its integration with a wide range of brain regions involved in the elaboration and linkage of perceptual and motor schemas. We then add that this was limited in the case of ape gestures by the restriction to simple imitation, and it was "unleashed" for protohumans by the emergence of complex imitation (Fig. 8-1).

A key point about the success of gesture is that the observer can distinguish the gesture from the praxic action on which it is based. One way to do this is by a separate facial gesture. A young chimpanzee may make a "play face" as it hits another to signal that it wants to engage in rough-and-tumble play, rather than in outright aggression.

Recall (Chapter 3) the notion of *ontogenetic ritualization*:

- Individual A performs behavior X.
- Individual B reacts consistently with behavior Y.
- Subsequently B anticipates A's performance of the complete behavior X by performing Y after observing only some initial segment X' of X.
- Subsequently, A anticipates B's anticipation and produces the initial step in a ritualized form X^R (waiting for a response) *in order to* elicit Y.

To link this to evolution of, and beyond, a monkey-like mirror system for grasping (assumed to be a property of the brain of the last common ancestor of macaque, chimpanzee, and human), recall that Umiltà et al. (2001) observed mirror neuron activity in macaque F5 in response to the sight of someone grasping an object, and reported that it required congruence between the motion of the hand with the observed location and affordance of the object, or the encoding in working memory of the data for that object, now behind a screen to activate mirror neurons related to the kind of grasp linked to that relationship. In other words, the mirror neuron was activated for observation of the *transitive* action (the motion of the hand to act upon the object) but not for the *intransitive action* (the identical motion of the hand in the absence of a target object).

In the original interaction, A acts upon B to elicit behavior Y. The process of ontogenetic ritualization transforms what may have been a transitive action X into (if you will pardon the neologism) a *semi-transitive* action X^R, which is a ritualized form of X but which still succeeds in eliciting behavior Y. A's original behavior X, if carried to completion, would have acted upon some affordance of an object or (possibly) the observer B. The ritualized behavior X^R is still stimulated by the sight of that affordance, but since it does not go to the completion of X, it becomes less constrained by that affordance and does not involve action upon it.

To carry this forward to the transition from pantomime to protosign, let us recall that an ape usually draws attention to an object as a means to act with or upon it—we say the attention is *instrumental*—whereas humans may share attention for *declarative* purposes, simply out of shared interest.[1]

Apes mainly use their gestures imperatively (Pika, Liebal, Call, & Tomasello, 2005), whereas human children gesture for declarative purposes as well to direct the attention of others to an outside object or event (Bates, Camaioni, & Volterra, 1975; Liszkowski, Carpenter, Henning, Striano, & Tomasello, 2004). I do not know whether the emergence of pantomime preceded the rise of declarative (i.e., noninstrumental) attention, or whether it was the other way round. More likely, the two capabilities evolved in tandem as increasing capability in the one opened new capabilities for the other. In any case, communication about outside entities might have triggered the expanded use of pantomime to share these experiences. Conversely, the emergence of a basic ability to communicate many imperatives symbolically might have created the need to communicate more about objects to which the desired actions should be directed.

In Chapter 3, we distinguished *dyadic* gestures, which refer only to the direct interaction between the communicating agents (the dyad) from *triadic* gestures that relate the dyad to some external object or agent, thus forming a triad. We agreed to call triadic gestures *referential*, with that third object or agent being the reference of the gesture (though the gesture may be freighted with meaning relevant to action, rather than a labeling of the referent). Thus, the need noted previously to communicate more about objects to which the desired actions should be directed would encourage triadic, referential, communication, which could then be expanded for purely declarative purposes when no instrumental purpose was served. This propensity might also express the need to create a medium for the evaluation of social bonds in humans, to test and strengthen social relationships, and thus to share experiences as part of a social relationship. In our closest relatives, bonobos and chimpanzees, social grooming permeates virtually every aspect of social life. It might therefore represent their medium to evaluate and invest in social relationships (Dunbar, 1996).

Pantomime

Pantomime (or, simply, mime) involves expressing a situation, object, action, character, or emotion without words, and using only gestures, especially imitative gestures, and other movements. In Chapter 6, I took pains to distinguish pantomime from the art of Marcel Marceau, or the highly convention-laden productions of a game of charades. Instead, I stressed the *artless* sketching of an action to indicate either the action itself or something associated with it. A charade is parasitic on language, so that we may convey a word by breaking it into pieces and miming each of them—we might mime "today" first by holding up two fingers and enduring some ribaldry until someone says "two," at which we nod assent, and then mime the sun rising in the hope that someone will yell out "day" and someone else will then say "today." Or we can have a conventionalized gesture for "sounds like" and then pantomime a word that rhymes with the intended word, hoping that the audience will get the mimed word and then find the rhyme that fits the context of the previous words. In what follows, I will be using pantomime in the "pure" sense of a performance that resembles an action of some kind and can thus evoke ideas of the action itself, an associated action, object, or event, or a combination thereof. For example, in Chapter 6 we discussed examples of miming pouring water from a bottle, miming a flying bird. and miming the brushing away of tears to feign sadness. Our headache is to imagine the meaning of such pantomimes to humans who do not yet have protolanguage, let alone language, noting that our use of words and phrases to define these mimes may clarify distinctions that might be inaccessible to thought at this early stage.

Let's battle on. I want to argue now that, building on the skill for complex imitation, pantomime provided the breakthrough from having just a few gestures to the ability to communicate freely about a *huge variety* of situations, actions, and objects. Where imitation is the generic attempt to reproduce movements performed by another, whether to master a skill or simply as part of a social interaction, pantomime is performed with the intention of getting the observer to think of a specific action or event. It is essentially communicative in its nature. The imitator observes; the pantomimic *intends* to be observed.

Again in Chapter 3, we went beyond ontogenetic ritualization to discuss the development of pointing by chimpanzees who could count on a human response of a kind they would not elicit from chimpanzees in the wild. This led us from ontogenetic ritualization to the idea of *human-supported ritualization*:

- Individual A *attempts* to perform behavior X to achieve goal G, but fails—achieving only a prefix X'.
- Individual B, a human, infers goal G from this behavior and performs an action that achieves the goal G for A.
- In due course, A produces X' in a ritualized form X^R to get B to perform an action that achieves G for A.

Though I introduced this notion to account for why it may be that chimps in captivity point while those in the wild do not, I noted that this ability on the part of A was far more widespread than the primate line, certainly being possessed by domesticated cats. Recall the example where a tentative motion down the hall toward the room with the food dishes means "feed me." The cat's performance of the prefix of the action of walking down the hall is intended not simply to enable the action itself to proceed to completion, but rather to initiate a human behavior pattern which will finally lead to the cat achieving its goal of eating. And note that this is a cooperative behavior involving cat and human, not a behavior in which the actions are those of the cat alone. Thus the cat's behavior seems to take us beyond quasi-transitive actions in an important way. Here, a fragment of an action directed toward some sub-goal of an overall behavior comes to signal the instrumental request to the observer to assist the cat in achieving the overall goal of that behavior, and so that action is no longer constrained to approximate an action directed toward that goal.

We may see here a precursor of metonymy—using something as a substitute for or symbol of something else with which it has a semantic association.[2] The suggestion, then, is that pantomime rests on three abilities:

i) Recognition that a partial action serves to achieve the overall goal of the behavior of which it is part. As we have seen, this ability may be quite widespread, and it is not confined to primates.
ii) The recognition that a fragmentary action is part of a behavior that could achieve a goal G as a basis for assisting the other in the achievement of goal G. This seems to be part of the cooperative framework for human action that may be missing in many of the animals with which humans interact.

iii) The reversal of that recognition to consciously create actions that will stand in metonymic relationship to some overall goal, whether praxic or communicative. This appears to be uniquely human.

In trying to communicate using pantomime (as we might do when traveling in a foreign land), we may act out some situation, or we may indicate an object by outlining its shape or miming an action that is typically associated with the use of such an object. As such, the pantomime taps directly into our praxic system, providing a behavior in the absence of the situation or object that it is based on. The pantomimed action cannot take advantage of the affordances of a visible object to constrain its metrics; but it has the advantage that, in the absence of an object, less precision is required in shaping the hand than is needed to match the affordances of a specific object.

Where both ontogenetic ritualization and human-assisted ritualization are happenstance, pantomime allows the envisioning of a goal to initiate a process of creating a gesture, or sequence of gestures, that will remind the observer of an overall behavior that will achieve that goal as a means of instilling recognition in the observer. It thus creates an ad hoc but open semantics for communicating about a wide range of objects, actions, and events.

As Stokoe (2001) and others emphasize, the power of pantomime is the ability to create an open-ended set of complex messages exploiting the primates' open-ended manual dexterity. It provides open-ended possibilities for communication that work without prior instruction or convention. *But not all concepts are readily pantomimed—the concepts available to our ancestors who had pantomime but neither protolanguage nor language may have been no more than a fragment of those we have today.* In what follows I will make clear that pantomime is very different from protosign, which is itself very limited with respect to modern signed languages, which are fully expressive languages in the manual modality, not protolanguages or crude systems of supplementary gestures.

From Pantomime to Protosign

Pantomime has *limitations*: It's hard to pantomime blue. And even when a pantomime may be feasible, it may be too "costly" in that it can take time to decide what pantomime to produce for a given situation, and even longer to act it out. Moreover, the result may be confusing to the observer. Imagine trying to pantomime the concept of "a wedding" both concisely and without ambiguity. The process of ritualization—but without being ontogenetic—may come to the rescue.

A further critical change en route to language emerges from the fact that in pantomime it might be hard, for example, to distinguish a movement signifying "bird" from one meaning "flying." This inability to adequately convey shades of meaning using "natural" pantomime provides an "incentive" for the invention of conventionalized gestures, which could in some way combine with or modify the original pantomime to disambiguate which of its associated meanings was intended. This in turn gives an opening for abstract gestures to be created as elements for the formation of compounds that can be paired with meanings in more or less arbitrary fashion. Note that whereas a pantomime can freely use any movement that might evoke the intended observation in the mind of the observer, a disambiguating gesture must be conventionalized.[3] However, to say that it is conventionalized does not require that it bear no resemblance to the original form. As we saw in looking at signs of sign language—and as we stressed in adjusting Peirce's trichotomy to extend the notion of symbol to include signs that were iconic or indexical—once a group agrees on which performance is the agreed-upon convention, it is irrelevant whether it might appear iconic, in whole or in part.

Supalla and Newport (1978) observe that AIRPLANE is signed in American Sign Language (ASL) with tiny repeated movements of a specific handshape, while FLY is signed by moving the same handshape along an extended trajectory. These signs are part of a modern human language rather than holdovers from protosign. Nonetheless, they exemplify the mixture of iconicity and convention that, I claim, distinguishes protosign from pantomime. It also makes the point that our notion of *conventionalization of pantomime* needs to be extended—conventionalization may come about not only by truncating or in some other way simplifying a pantomime but also by willfully finding some arbitrary change in a gesture to make it carry a distinctive burden of meaning—as in arbitrarily adding a small back-and-forth movement to the airplane-like handshape to distinguish the sign for AIRPLANE from that for FLY. Again, I cannot emphasize too strongly that ASL is a fully expressive modern language, not a protosign system. However, it seems fair to suggest that protohumans must have invented distinctions like that exemplified in Figure 8-2 to enable protosign to have made necessary distinctions that pantomime could not convey readily.

As our ancestors moved to an expanded repertoire of declarative communication, the measure of success may not have been the elicitation of some instrumental behavior Y so much as the elicitation of shared attention and some further declaration that suggests that the original pantomime has been understood. On this basis, we replace the notion of ontogenetic and human-assisted ritualization by the notion of *conventionalization of pantomime* as follows:

Part 1: A Dyadic Core: Two individuals come to share a conventionalized form of a pantomime.

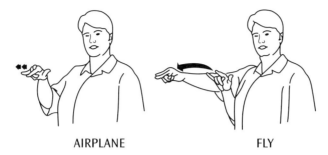

AIRPLANE   FLY

FIGURE 8-2.   In ASL, the signs for AIRPLANE and FLY use the same airplane-like handshape, but the choice of hand movement to distinguish them—a small movement back and forth for AIRPLANE, a single long movement for FLY—is purely conventional. (From Stokoe, 2001; following Supalla & Newport, 1978.)

- Individual A performs pantomime X with the intention of drawing individual B's attention to situation Z.
- Individual B reacts with behavior Y that involves paying attention to Z, and possibly performing another pantomime appropriate to sharing interest in Z.
- Subsequently B anticipates A's performance of a (possibly simplified, possibly modified) version X' of X by attending to Z.
- Subsequently, A produces X' without trying to produce all of X when wishing to get B to attend to Z.
- Moreover, B too adopts this convention, and instead of attempting an ad hoc pantomime, instead uses X' to draw A's attention to situation Z.

This process may then be iterated, until the use of the original pantomime X is replaced by a comparatively short conventionalized sign X§, which henceforth is used by A and B to communicate about Z.

Part 2: Adoption by the Community. Meanwhile, as A and B establish such a conventionalized sign, they can convey it to others of their group by performing both the sign and an appropriate pantomime together. If others find this conventionalization worth *imitating*, understanding that the conventionalized sign X§ can be used to communicate about Z may become established. Note that we see the two faces of imitation here, but in the communicative domain: (a) the goal of communicating about Z; and (b) the movement pattern required to produce a recognizable version of X§.

With this, a system of protosign is established. Note that three stages were involved:

1   The group had to have the ability to "get the idea" of pantomime, so that the strange antics of another group member could be understood, making

it possible to convey a huge range of novel meanings—but at the price of considerable effort both to generate a pantomime that was likely to be understood and to understand which of the possible interpretations was intended.

2 The development of *conventionalization of pantomime* as a means of replacing pantomimes with protosigns that required reduced effort both to generate and to interpret.

3 The shared understanding of the *idea* of conventionalization of pantomime. Earlier, I said that as A and B establish a conventionalized sign, they can convey it to others by performing both the sign and an appropriate pantomime. However, there is a big difference between doing this on a case-by-case basis where there may be a low probability that others will "make the connection," and "getting the general idea" so that the pairing of a novel sign with a pantomime can be recognized immediately as the attempt to teach a new protosign. (Recall our earlier discussion of the role of the caregiver—and note that caregivers and teachers do not restrict their care to infants but may assist others of all ages to learn new skills, both praxic and communicative.)

The Swiss linguist Ferdinand de Saussure (Saussure, 1916) stressed the difference between the *signifier* (e.g., a word) and the *signified* (e.g., the concept that the word denotes). Irrespective of whether we are talking about the words of a language or the "protowords" of a protolanguage, we must (in the spirit of Saussure) distinguish the "signifier" from the "signified." In Figure 8-3, we distinguish the "neural representation of the signifier" (top row) from the "neural representation of the signified" (bottom row).[4] We distinguish

- the mirror system—by which I mean both the appropriate mirror and canonical neurons—for the articulatory action which expresses the signifier (recognizing and producing the shape of a gesture, the sound of a spoken word), from
- the linkage of the sign to the neural schema for the signified (the concepts, situations, actions, or objects to which the signifier refers).

These distinctions may be illuminated by briefly examining the semantic somatotopy model of action-word processing (see, e.g., Pulvermüller, 2005, for a review). Most readers will recall seeing pictures of a distorted homunculus stretched across the primary motor and sensory cortices of the human brain. This is a somatotopic representation in that place (topos) on the body (soma) is related to place on the cortical surface. In particular, the motor cortex and premotor cortex exhibit a somatotopic arrangement of the face, arm/hand, and foot/leg representations. Moreover, the language and action systems in the human brain appear to be linked by cortico-cortical connections, according to inferences from the connections of homologous regions of the monkey brain

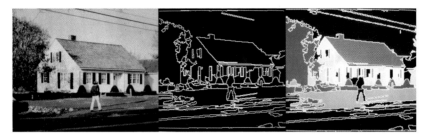

FIGURE 1-3. Segmentation of a scene into candidate regions provides the bridge between the original image and the interpretation of a scene in VISIONS by associating regions of the image with schema instances. In this example, VISIONS classifies regions of the scene as sky, roof, wall, shutter, foliage, and grass, but it leaves other areas uninterpreted. (Figures supplied by kind courtesy of Allen Hanson.)

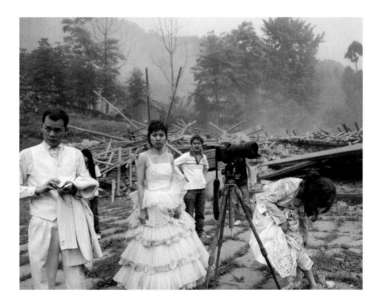

FIGURE 2-1. An unusual wedding scene described by one viewer as follows: "uh … it looks like it was supposed to be a wedding shoot … but … um … there appears to be some sort of natural disaster … probably an earthquake of some sort um … buildings collapsed around them … they're dusty uh … the bride looks kind of shell-shocked … and … all their clothes are … ruined [laugh] … more or less … (Photo available at: http://cache.boston.com/universal/site_graphics/blogs/bigpicture/sichuan_05_29/sichuan3.jpg)"

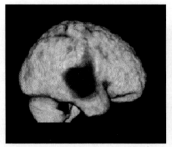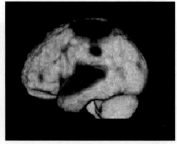

FIGURE 2-3. This figure is based on brain imaging of people who have mastered both English and ASL. It shows in purple those parts of the brain that are more active for speaking than for signing, and in red those areas that are more active for signing. Much of the purple area is related to hearing, while much of the red area is related to the spatial structuring of action. By contrast, areas like Broca's area implicated in less peripheral aspects of language processing are used equally in both spoken and sign language, and thus they do not show up in the comparison. (Adapted, with permission, from a slide prepared by Karen Emmorey. See Emmorey et al., 2002; Emmorey, McCullough, Mehta, Ponto, & Grabowski, 2011, for related data.)

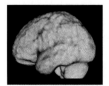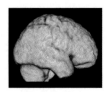

BRUSH-HAIR   READ

FIGURE 2-4. Whereas pantomime and signing dissociate with left hemisphere damage, there is no difference in brain activation between "pantomimic" and nonpantomimic *signs*. (Adapted, with permission, from a slide prepared by Karen Emmorey.)

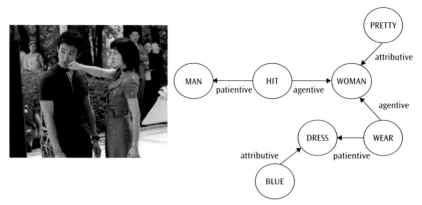

FIGURE 2-10.   (*Left*) A picture of a woman hitting a man (original image from "Invisible Man Jangsu Choi," Korean Broadcasting System). (*Right*) A SemRep graph that could be generated for the picture. Arbib and Lee (2007, 2008) describe how Template Construction Grammar may operate on this to yield the sentence "A pretty woman in blue hits a man."

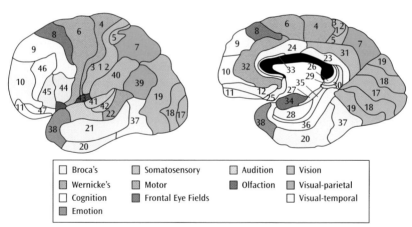

FIGURE 4-5.   Brodmann's areas in the human brain. These are all areas of cerebral cortex. There are many other regions of importance to us, including cerebellum, basal ganglia, and hippocampus.

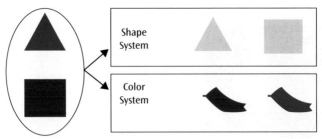

FIGURE 5-8. The classic binding problem for vision: Which color should be bound to which shape?

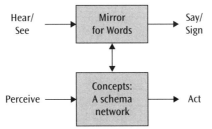

FIGURE 8-3.   The bidirectional Saussurean sign relation links (neural codes for) words (signifiers) and concepts (signifieds). For us, the signifier is the phonological form of the word, the neural code for which is linked to the neural schema for the concepts (note the plural) that the word may be used to express. On our account, it is not necessary that the relation between signifier and signified be arbitrary, only that it be conventionalized.

(though, of course, the monkey does not have language). Pulvermüller and his colleagues studied action words that relate to different body parts (such as "lick"/face, "pick"/hand, and "kick"/foot). For example, Hauk, Johnsrude, and Pulvermüller (2004) used functional magnetic resonance imaging of human subjects to compare cortical activation during movement and during passive reading of action words. Leg-related words activated areas that overlap or are adjacent to areas involved in foot movements, and there were similar relationships between arm-related words and finger movements. (The pattern of adjacency seemed weaker for face-related words and tongue movements.) Pulvermüller argued for a common neural substrate involved in the processing of actions and the meaning of action words. Three observations: (1) In our terminology, we would say that the signified for such an action word may be encoded in the brain regions that provide the motor schemas for the corresponding action. (2) However, the neurons encoding the signifier (the word as articulatory action) are encoded in a different region of the brain, and they do not inherit somatotopy from these actions. (3) Relatively few words are verbs encoding actions associated with the use of a specific body part, and we use many verbs (e.g., *fly*) for actions we do not perform (at least not, in this case, without the help of an airplane). Thus, we would agree with Papeo et al. (2010) that action performance and action-word understanding can be dissociated, as they demonstrate with studies of patients with left-brain damage, while further emphasizing that most words are not action words and have no natural somatotopy for their signification.

Another important caveat: It is often seen as intrinsic to Saussure's approach that the linguistic sign in his sense must be intrinsically arbitrary. However, it is irrelevant to our use of this terminology whether or not an account can be given of the relation of the signifier to the signified through, e.g., pantomime or onomatopoeia or etymology or any other history that precedes the conventional adoption of the signifier with this particular signification. Moreover, the relation between signifier and signified is by no means one to one—we can say "dress" or "frock" or "garment" to express the mental schema for the clothes someone is wearing and, as made especially clear by the notion of metaphor, the intended meaning (conceptual elaboration) of a word may be inferred only by careful consideration of context. Thus, we may think we know what the concepts are that link to the words "sky" and "cry" but in the sentence "The sky is crying" we must give up at least one of those concepts, perhaps to interpret the sentence to mean "It is raining, and the situation is tinged with sadness." Arbib and Hesse (1986) explored at some length this process of meaning inference within a network of schemas, working out from schemas most often activated by the words of a sentence while constrained by the constructions that combine them.

When a conventionalized gesture is not iconic, it can only be used within a community that has negotiated or learned how it is to be interpreted. *This use of noniconic gestures requires extending the use of the mirror system to attend to a whole new class of hand movements, those with conventional meanings agreed upon by the protosign community to reduce ambiguity and extend semantic range.* But something more is at work. Even if a gesture is iconic, the broader brain mechanisms it engages when it is being used within the context of (protosign) communication will be different from those when it is engaged as an action or pantomime. This makes sense if we recall the equation *action = movement + goal*. The same movement is part of a different action when the goal is part of communication rather than part of praxis.[5,6]

Pantomime is not itself part of protosign but rather a scaffolding for creating it. Pantomime involves the production of a motoric representation through the transformation of a recalled exemplar of some activity. As such, it can vary from actor to actor, and from occasion to occasion. The pantomime succeeds to the extent that it evokes within the observer the neural representation of something akin to what the pantomimic sought to communicate. By contrast, the meaning of conventional gestures must be agreed upon by a community. With time and within a community these gestures become increasingly stylized and their resemblance to the original pantomime may (but need not) be lost. But this loss would be balanced by the *discovery* that when an important distinction cannot be conveniently pantomimed an arbitrary gesture may be invented to express the distinction. Deixis (e.g., pointing at an object or an ongoing event) presumably plays a crucial role here—what cannot be pantomimed may be shown when it is present so that the associated symbol may be of use when it is absent.

Protosign, then, emerges as a manual-based communication system rooted originally in pantomime but open to the addition of novel communicative gestures as the life of the community comes to define the underlying concepts and makes it important to communicate about them. Once a group has acquired the understanding that new symbols can provide noniconic messages, the difficulty of separating certain meanings by pantomime encourages creation of further new signs. We thus distinguish two roles for imitation in the transition from complex imitation through pantomime to protosign in the evolution of manual-based communication:

1) The transition from *praxic action* directed toward a goal object to *pantomime* in which similar actions are produced away from the goal object. In pantomime, imitation is extended from imitation of hand movements to mapping of other degrees of freedom onto arm and hand movements.

2) The emergence of conventionalized gestures to ritualize or disambiguate pantomimes. In these gestures, imitation must turn to the imitation of intransitive hand movements as protosigners master the specific manual signs of their protosign community.

With this, the parity/mirror property from Chapter 6 follows automatically—what counts for the signer must count (approximately) for the observer. Or does it? The situation is subtle, and to appreciate this subtlety we must reconsider the path from pantomime to conventional communicative gestures.

1) When pantomime is of praxic hand actions, then the pantomime directly taps into the mirror system for these actions.

2) However, as the pantomime begins to use hand movements to mime different degrees of freedom (as in miming the flying of a bird), a dissociation begins to emerge. The mirror system for the pantomime (based on movements of face, hand, etc.) is now different from the recognition system for the action that is pantomimed, and—as in the case of flying —the action may not even be in the human action repertoire.

3) Moreover, we have seen that the pantomime is not restricted to actions. Indeed, we saw that a pantomime may encompass a whole Action-Object frame, such as "bird flying." However, the system is still able to exploit the praxic recognition system because an animal or hominid must observe much about the environment that is relevant to its actions but is not in its own action repertoire.

4) Nonetheless, this dissociation now underwrites the emergence of actions that are defined only by their communicative impact, not by their praxic goals. What the Mirror System Hypothesis adds is that there is a neural mechanism that supports this parity, and it is grounded in the mirror system being extended to support not only complex imitation of praxic skills but also complex imitation of communicative gestures.

5) Nonetheless, these communicative actions no longer find their meaning by direct linkage into action systems, and instead succeed by their linkage into broader brain systems whose activation can provide the

necessary signifieds, providing the neurological realization of the scheme of Figure 8-3.

6) And this says nothing of interacting contexts, as the neural patterns of such communicative actions interact not only with each other, but also with patterns in working memory, long-term memory and goal systems, and so on, in affecting both the mental state and ongoing action of the hearer.

Chapter 2 reviewed neurological evidence that signed languages consist of linguistic gestures and not simply elaborate pantomimes. As illustrated by Figure 2-4 in Chapter 2, even signs that resemble pantomimes in a modern sign language are conventionalized and are thus distinct from pantomimes. My hypothesis is that the mechanisms that distinguish sign language from pantomime also distinguished protosign from pantomime. Elsewhere (Arbib, 2005a), I stated that the transition from pantomime to protosign does not seem to require a biological change. However, the evidence marshaled here has caused me to change this view.

The transition from slow and sporadic use of ad hoc pantomime to fast and frequent habitual use with increasing mastery of conventionalization of pantomime might have been both the drive for as well as the fruit of the development of the ability to segregate (whether structurally or just functionally) the neural code for the symbols from the neural code for the actions or objects they represent. In pantomime mode, one's brain seeks to relate the observed performance directly to one's stock of representations of actions and objects, whereas in protosign mode, the representation of the protosign symbol stock provides a necessary bridge between observation and interpretation.

With this, we have established a progression of mirror systems and the broader systems of which they are part for the following:

1) Grasping and manual praxic actions
2) Imitation of grasping and manual praxic actions
3) Pantomime of grasping and manual praxic actions
4) Pantomime of actions outside the pantomimic's own behavioral repertoire (e.g., flapping the arms to mime a flying bird)
5) Conventional gestures used to formalize and disambiguate pantomime (e.g., to distinguish "bird" from "flying")
6) Conventionalized manual, facial, and vocal communicative gestures ("protowords") separate from pantomime

All this was done without appeal to the mechanisms involved in the vocalization of calls as used by nonhuman primates. In the next chapter, we will see how vocalization reenters the picture, with protospeech building upon protosign in an expanding spiral.

Getting the Idea of (Proto)Language

Helen Keller's *Story of My Life* (1903/1954) provides a dramatic example of these various capabilities at work in a modern child (she lived from 1880 to 1968) struggling to communicate despite being deaf and blind. She developed normally and was already saying a few words at the age of 19 months when she had a high fever which left her deaf and blind. But still she struggled to learn and to communicate. She would hang on to her mother's skirt to get around, and would feel people's hands to try to find out what they were doing—learning many skills in this way, such as milking a cow and kneading bread dough. She could recognize people by feeling of their faces or their clothes. She made up 60 signs, conventionalized pantomimes, to communicate with her family—if she wanted bread, she pretended to be cutting a loaf; if she wanted ice cream, she would hug her shoulders and shiver. But she became very frustrated because she couldn't talk. Her family found a teacher named Anne Sullivan who taught Helen the signs for the letters of the alphabet. Then she would "spell" the words in Helen's hand to communicate with her. One day Anne led Helen to the water pump and pumped water on her hand. She spelled the letters W-A-T-E-R as the water ran over Helen's hand. She did this over and over again. At last it dawned on Helen that the word "water" meant the water which she felt pouring over her hand. This opened up a whole new world for her. She ran everywhere asking Anne the name of different things and Anne would spell the words in her hand.

The story of Helen Keller is well known, but others preceded her. In *American Notes*, the book recounting his visit to the United States in 1842, Charles Dickens tells of Laura Bridgman, a deaf, blind girl at the Perkins Institution for the Blind in Watertown near Boston, and recounts a similar story of how she came to learn English. He quotes the account of her tutor on how he instructed her.[7] Let me just offer a short extract:

> . . . on the 4th of October, 1837, [her parents] brought her to the Institution.
>
> For a while, she was much bewildered; and after waiting about two weeks, until she became acquainted with her new locality, and somewhat familiar with the inmates, the attempt was made to give her knowledge of arbitrary signs, by which she could interchange thoughts with others.
>
> There was one of two ways to be adopted: either to go on to build up a language of signs on the basis of the [home sign] which she had already commenced herself, or to teach her the purely arbitrary language in common use: that is, to give her a sign for every individual thing, or to give her a knowledge of letters by combination of which she might express her idea of the existence, and the mode and condition of existence, of any thing. The former

would have been easy, but very ineffectual; the latter seemed very difficult, but, if accomplished, very effectual. I determined therefore to try the latter.

The first experiments were made by taking articles in common use, such as knives, forks, spoons, keys, &c., and pasting upon them labels with their names printed in raised letters. These she felt very carefully, and soon, of course, distinguished that the crooked lines spoon, differed as much from the crooked lines key, as the spoon differed from the key in form.

Then small detached labels, with the same words printed upon them, were put into her hands; and she soon observed that they were similar to the ones pasted on the articles. She showed her perception of this similarity by laying the label *key* upon the key, and the label *spoon* upon the spoon. She was encouraged here by the natural sign of approbation, patting on the head.

Learning to spell is immensely harder than learning to recognize the sound pattern of a spoken word (if one can hear) or the visual pattern of a signed word (if one can see), but these dramatic stories of the keys that unlocked the world of words for Laura Bridgman and Helen Keller help us appreciate how amazing is the transition into protolanguage made by our distant ancestors and the process whereby modern children make this incredible transition from learning the instrumental meaning of a few words to finally "getting the idea of language," usually around the age of 2 or so, with a consequent explosion in acquiring many new words and putting them together in increasingly sophisticated ways. However, the story of Helen Keller tells us even more: Helen was able to develop a "home sign" of 60 signs, but her breakthrough came because in Anne Sullivan she had a caregiver who could provide the support Helen needed to get the idea first of words themselves and then of how to combine them in novel ways. And similarly for Laura Bridgman. This emphasizes again the importance of property 7 (Chapter 6) of the language-ready brain:

Paedomorphy and sociality: *Paedomorphy is the prolonged period of infant dependency, which is especially pronounced in humans. This combines with the willingness of adults to act as caregivers and the consequent development of social structures to provide the conditions for complex social learning.*

I shall have much more to say about "getting the idea of language" in Chapter 12 when we discuss "How Languages Emerge."

9

Protosign and Protospeech:
An Expanding Spiral

As we saw in the last chapter, the Mirror System Hypothesis suggests that the path to language went through protosign, rather than building speech directly from vocalizations. It shows how praxic hand movements could have evolved into the communicative gestures of apes and then, along the hominid line, via pantomime to protosign. And yet speech is now the predominant partner for most human use of language, even though embedded in the multimodal mix of hand, face, and voice. How did protosign lead on to protospeech, and why did speech become dominant? This chapter will offer some answers.

Building Protospeech on the Scaffolding of Protospeech

Nonhuman primates certainly have a rich auditory system (Chapter 4) that contributes to species survival in many ways, of which communication is just one. As a result, the protolanguage system did not have to create the appropriate auditory system "from scratch." However, since apes seem unable to produce human-like vocalizations, changes in the vocal apparatus as well as its neural control were required from those of our common ancestors with the chimpanzees to support spoken language as we know it today. Clearly, some level of language-readiness and some intermediate form of *vocal* communication preceded this—a core of *protospeech* was needed to provide pressures for evolution of the vocal apparatus of modern humans. Thus, it is quite possible that early humans—as well as Neanderthals and their *Homo erectus* precursors—may have had protospeech without having languages with syntax and semantics akin to that of modern languages.

The preview of this chapter in Chapter 6 contrasted two extreme views on the role of protosign in relation to protospeech:

(1) Language evolved directly as speech.
(2) Language evolved first as signed language (i.e., as a full language, not protolanguage) and then speech emerged from this basis in manual communication.

I offer an intermediate approach, the *Doctrine of the Expanding Spiral*, namely that our distant ancestors initially had protolanguages based primarily on protosign that (thanks to the open-ended semantics inherited from pantomime) provided essential scaffolding for the emergence of protospeech, and that the hominid line saw advances in both protosign and protospeech feeding off each other in an expanding spiral (Arbib, 2005b). On this view, protosign did not attain the status of a full language prior to the emergence of early forms of protospeech. My view is that the "language-ready brain" of the first *Homo sapiens* supported basic forms of gestural and vocal communication (protosign and protospeech) but not the rich syntax and compositional semantics and accompanying conceptual structures that underlie modern human languages.

It might be possible to develop a variant of the Mirror System Hypothesis that emphasizes speech rather than gesture, downplaying the evidence on the flexibility of ape gesture cited earlier. We saw in Chapter 4 that some mirror neurons for manual action in the macaque are *audiovisual* in that if the action has a distinctive sound—such as that for breaking a peanut or tearing paper—the neuron could be activated either by hearing or seeing the action, or both (Kohler et al., 2002). We also saw that the orofacial area of F5 (adjacent to the hand area) contains a small number of *mouth mirror neurons* related to communicative gestures as well as ingestive actions (lip smacking, etc.) (Ferrari, Gallese, Rizzolatti, & Fogassi, 2003). This suggests that macaque F5 is also involved in nonmanual communicative functions (Fogassi & Ferrari, 2007). Some people argue that these results let us apply the Mirror System Hypothesis to vocalization directly, "cutting out the middleman" of protosign. But the sounds studied by Kohler et al.—breaking peanuts, ripping paper—cannot be created in the absence of the object, and there is no evidence that monkeys can use their vocal apparatus to mimic the sounds they have heard. Moreover, the lip smacking, teeth chatter, and so on associated with "mouth mirror neurons" are a long way from the sort of vocalizations that occur in speech. This weakens any case that these neurons might serve vocal communication, but it does demonstrate that mirror neurons do receive auditory input that could be relevant to the protosign-protospeech transition. Ferrari et al. (2003) state that "the knowledge common to the communicator and the recipient of communication *about food and ingestive action* became the common ground for social communication. Ingestive actions are the basis on which communication is built" (my italics). However, their strong claim that "Ingestive actions are the basis on which communication is built" might better be reduced to "Ingestive actions are the basis on which communication about feeding is built," which complements but does not replace communication based on manual skills. Our hypothesis, instead, is that the evolution of a system for voluntary control of intended *gestural* communication based in part on F5/Broca's area provided the basis for the evolution of creatures with more and more prominent connections from F5/Broca's area to the vocal apparatus. This in turn could provide conditions that led to a period of coevolution of the vocal apparatus and its integration with the neural circuitry for control of gesture and protosign.

All this provides the basis for the following hypothesis:

Protospeech builds on protosign in an expanding spiral: Neural mechanisms that evolved for the control of protosign production came to also control the vocal apparatus with increasing flexibility, yielding protospeech as, initially, an adjunct to protosign.

The argument in support of this is that protosign built on pantomime to provide the key ability for the free creation of novel gestures to support an open-ended semantics and then refined the semantic range of its symbols by adding conventionalized gestures. Once established, the open-ended use of communicative gestures could be exploited in providing adaptive pressures for evolving the vocal apparatus (including its neural control) in a way that made protospeech possible. The capacity to use conventionalized manual communicative gestures (*protosign*) and the capacity to use vocal communicative gestures (*protospeech*) evolved together in an expanding spiral to support *protolanguage* as a multimodal communicative system.

It must be confessed that the *Doctrine of the Expanding Spiral* remains controversial. The present chapter is based in part on a paper (Arbib, 2005b) that includes a critique of MacNeilage's (1998) argument that the speech system evolved without the support of protosign. MacNeilage and Davis (2005) offer a spirited argument against my critique. The crux of our disagreement is that I say that they provide too little insight into how sounds came to convey complex meanings, and they note that they offer a rich account of the development of speech in present-day children. The task of this chapter, then, is to examine some of the controversies and show why the *Doctrine of the Expanding Spiral* remains a convincing view of the available data.

As we have seen, monkeys already have orofacial communicative gestures, and these may certainly support a limited communicative role. However, they lack fine vocal control and the ability to develop a rich and varied repertoire of novel meanings. Apes can create gestures with novel meanings, but only in a very limited way. The main argument of Chapter 8 was that the use of pantomime (which apes lack) made it possible to acquire a burgeoning vocabulary, while the discovery of a growing stock of conventional signs (or sign modifiers) to mark important distinctions then created a culture in which the use of arbitrary gestures would increasingly augment and ritualize (without entirely supplanting) the use of pantomime. Our task now is to show how this use of arbitrary gestures could provide the scaffolding for the development of protospeech.

Once an organism has an iconic gesture, it can both modulate that gesture and/or symbolize it (noniconically) by "simply" associating a vocalization with it. Once the association had been learned, the "scaffolding" gesture (like the pantomime that supported its conventionalization, or the caricature that supports the initial understanding of some Chinese ideograms[1]) could be dropped to leave a symbol that need have no remaining iconic relation to its referent, even if the indirect associative relationship can be recalled on some occasions. One open question is the extent to which protosign must be in place before this scaffolding can effectively support the development of protospeech. Since there is no direct mapping of sign (with its use of concurrency and signing space) to phoneme sequences, I think that this development is far more of a breakthrough than it may appear at first sight. The next section offers some relevant data supporting the hypothesis that the human brain system involved in observation and preparation of grasp movements has strong links with cortical areas now involved in speech production.

Linking Manual Actions and Speech Production

Consider the plausibility of a hand-mouth linkage in nonhuman primates, even though these creatures lack speech or even protospeech. One of the most important uses of the hand is to bring food or drink to the mouth. Thus, the shape of the hand and the nature of what it is carrying will lead to anticipatory shaping of the mouth to drink or to eat, to take food whole or to bite off a piece, and so on. This may provide the link between hand and voice in humans.

Massimo Gentilucci and his colleagues in Parma[2] have investigated the tight link between manual actions and speech production, showing that manual gestures relevant to communication can have natural vocal concomitants that may have helped the further development of intentional vocal communication. Before describing their work, we need a little background on how speech can be visualized. Basically, a speech signal can be converted into a picture called a spectrogram that shows—with time running along the horizontal axis and frequency defining the vertical axis—how much energy is contained in each frequency band. This will hold relatively constant over time during the maintained sounding of a vowel, but it will change over the pronunciation of each word or the singing of a melody. In vowels, we look for frequency bands of higher energy than adjacent bands. Starting from the lowest frequency, the

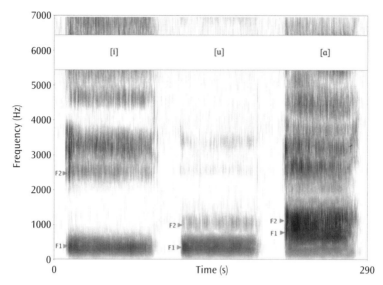

Figure 9-1.   Spectrogram showing the frequencies of first and second formants (F1 and F2) of three vowels as pronounced by a Louisiana native. For each of the three vowels, time runs along the horizontal axis and frequency defines the vertical axis. (From the Wikipedia entry for "Formant." This file is licensed under the Creative Commons Attribution 2.0 generic license.)

center frequencies of these bands are called the *first formant, second formant*, and so on (Fig. 9-1). Usually, the first two formants, *F1* and *F2*, are enough to disambiguate the vowel.

In one study, the Gentilucci group asked each subject to bring fruits of varying size (a cherry or an apple) to the mouth and pronounce a syllable instead of biting the fruit. The fruit size affected both the kinematic pattern of the mouth aperture and the vocal emission of the subjects. Formant 2 (F2) was higher when bringing the large fruit rather than the small one to the mouth. Fruit size influenced the vocal tract configuration, which in turn modified the frequency of F2.

In another study, subjects observed two types of manual action, a bringing to the mouth action and a grasping action, presumably implicating the mirror system for manual actions. In each case, the action was performed with a small or a large fruit and the subjects had to pronounce a syllable at the end of the movement. The second formant varied during the bringing to the mouth task, whereas the first formant varied during the grasping task.

These studies highlight the potential role of upper limb action in the shaping of vocal signs. They suggest that the emergence of voice modulation and thus of an articulatory movement repertoire could have been associated with, or even prompted by, the preexisting manual action repertoire. In light of these and other data, Gentilucci and Corballis (2006) argue for a double hand/mouth command system that may have evolved initially in the context of ingestion and later formed a platform for combined manual and vocal communication.

Such linkages may be quite ancient in the primate line, as shown by a study that found spontaneous vocal differentiation of coo-calls for tools and food in Japanese monkeys. Iriki et al. (1996) trained two Japanese monkeys to use a rake-shaped tool to retrieve distant food. There were intriguing changes in bimodal neurons of parietal cortex, but our concern for now is with the monkeys' vocalizations. In a subsequent study from Iriki's group, Hihara et al. (2003) observed that, after training, the monkeys spontaneously began vocalizing coo-calls in the tool-using context. They then trained one of the monkeys to vocalize to request food or the tool:

> **Condition 1:** When there was no food on the table, the monkey produced a coo-call (call A), in response to which the experimenter put a food reward on the table, but out of the monkey's reach. When the monkey again vocalized a coo-call (call B), the experimenter presented the rake within its reach. The monkey was then able to retrieve the food.
> **Condition 2:** In this condition, there was no food on the table, but the experimenter placed the tool on the table within the monkey's reach. When the monkey vocalized a coo-call (call C), the experimenter set a food reward that was within reach for use of the rake.

The monkey spontaneously differentiated its coo-calls to ask for either food or tool during the course of this training—in other words, call A and call C were similar, and both differed from call B. Hihara et al. speculate that this process might involve a change from emotional vocalizations into intentionally controlled ones by associating them with consciously planned tool use. However—noting the work of Gentilucci's group—I would instead attribute this to unconscious manual-vocal interaction, though here the modulation of vocalization depends on "intention to act" rather than execution of the action itself.[3]

Together, the human and macaque data suggest that the emergence of voice modulation and thus of an articulatory movement repertoire could have been associated with, or even prompted by, the preexisting manual action repertoire. I thus argue that such modulation could provide a powerful means for building toward protospeech once a protosign repertoire began to develop. Note, though, that these modulations might have been quite subtle and hard to perceive. Animals that could exaggerate the modulations would have the selective advantage that their gestures could be understood through the accompanying vocalization even by conspecifics who were not paying visual attention to the gesturer. Thus, over many generations, more and more of the population would have the ability to vocalize information in a way that allowed the vocalizations to be used even in the absence of the accompanying gesture. This would accelerate selection as more and more creatures would omit or truncate manual gestures to the point of unintelligibility, putting those who could not join in vocally at a competitive disadvantage.

This scenario addresses a common question for models of language evolution: How can it be of advantage for an exceptional individual to gain the ability to produce novel signals unless others have evolved the ability to detect those signals? Both the pantomime-to-protosign transition posited in Chapter 8, and the amplify-vocal-correlates hypotheses given here, obviate this problem. In each case, the better producer of communicative gestures is more likely to succeed in his or her acts of communication even with the previously existing receptive capabilities of the group or tribe.

There is always a temptation to find one key mechanism and think that it is the only one that is important. However, the increased vocal control that emerged according to the aforementioned scenario could also allow protohumans to exploit other resources—not just manual-vocal interactions—to expand their protospeech repertoire. To see this, consider another Just So story: Imagine a protohuman tribe that used a limited form of protosign to communicate about the world around, with particular signs for several different kinds of fruit. When someone bit into a piece of sour fruit by mistake, he or she would make a characteristic face and intake of breath at the bitter taste. This orofacial gesture would become part of protospeech when, first, someone came up with the innovation of mimicking this sound to warn others not to eat a sour fruit and, secondly, the idea caught on and a number of tribe members came to adopt this warning. This would lead the way to a conventionalized variant of this reaction as the symbol for "sour" in a tribe. This symbol for "sour" is a vocal-facial gesture, not a manual gesture. It exemplifies a mechanism that would lead to protospeech symbols that are not generated from protosign.

The suggestion, then, is that whatever processes of brain evolution that built atop manual mirror neurons to make pantomime of manual actions possible also would have made facial expressions possible. But note that the original base that we may postulate for the last common ancestor of the human-chimpanzee's expressive repertoire of manual actions is vastly greater than the expressive repertoire of their orofacial actions. However, the ability to create novel sounds to match degrees of freedom of manual gestures (for example, rising pitch might represent an upward movement of the hand, as well as the other examples we have just discussed) might coevolve with the ability to imitate novel sound patterns for onomatopoeia to yield other vocal gestures not linked to manual gestures. Over time, an increasing number of symbols would have become vocalized, freeing the hands to engage in both praxis and communication as desired by the "speaker." Corballis (2002) offers cogent reasons like these for the selective advantage of incorporating vocalization in an originally hand-based communicative repertoire. Unlike speech, signing is not omni-directional, does not work in the dark, and does not leave the hands free. However, the fact that modern humans can learn sign language as readily as spoken language shows that the central mechanisms of the language-ready brain are multimodal rather than specific to speech.

The human vocal tract with all its necessary adaptations (including the maladaptation that involves the risk of choking, the price we pay for speech) suggests that it took a cumulative process of natural selection and, moreover, that the selection was related to increasing sophistication of vocal communi-cation. However, a discussion of the relevant paleoanthropological evidence for evolution of the vocal system is outside the scope of this volume. What is in its scope is to argue that it was protosign that created a rich enough communi-cative ability to create the adaptive pressure for this evolution.

If protosign was so successful, why did spoken languages come to predomi-nate over signed languages? As in much of evolutionary discussion, the answer must be post hoc. One can certainly imagine a mutation that led to a race of deaf humans who nonetheless prospered mightily as they built cultures and societies on the rich adaptive basis of signed languages. So the argument is not that speech *must* triumph, any more than that having a mirror system *must* lead to (proto)language. However, signers can still sign while showing some-one how to use a tool, and sign might actually be better than speech when the tool is not present. Emmorey (2005, p. 114) thus argues against the expand-ing spiral on the grounds that "If communicative pantomime and protosign preceded protospeech, it is not clear why protosign simply did not evolve into sign language" and preempt the evolution of spoken language. However, I do not claim that the evolution of protosign (both biological and cultural) was "completed" before protospeech was initiated, nor that protosign attained the status of a full language prior to the emergence of early forms of protospeech. Rather, once hominids had come to employ pantomime and discovered how to use conventional gestures to increasingly augment, ritualize, and in some part replace the use of pantomime, then protospeech followed naturally as vocal gestures entered the mix. Indeed, if hominid protolanguage combined protosign and protospeech, we need not worry about how a fully successful system of signed language could become displaced by speech.

But Did Speech Evolve Directly From Vocalization?

Seyfarth et al. (2005) assert that brain mechanisms for language evolved from the call systems of nonhuman primates without involvement of manual gesture. Stressing the parallels between social structure and language structure, they suggested that language evolved through the increasingly flexible use of vocalizations to signal such relations. For example, they have demonstrated that there are some calls that a baboon will only make to another who is subordinate on the social hierarchy, while others are only made to a dominant other. Different call types are given in different social contexts, and listeners respond appropriately (Cheney & Seyfarth, 2007). I agree that social structure ensures "having plenty to talk/sign about" but do not believe that it provides the means per se to develop (proto)language.

Seyfarth et al. also observe that primate vocal repertoires contain several different call types that grade acoustically into one another, yet primates produce and perceive their calls as more or less discretely different signals. Moreover, the grunts used by baboons (and probably many other primates) differ according to the placement of vowel-like formants. Thus, a number of the properties of speech are already present in the vocalizations of nonhuman primates. A problem here is that the term "speech" is ambiguous; it can mean "spoken language," but it can also refer just to the sounds from which language could be composed. I would view these data as relevant more to the latter sense of "speech"—to evolution of the articulatory apparatus rather than language. We do indeed need to explain evolution of the speech apparatus, even if we espouse a form of "gestural origins."

With this, let me focus on Peter MacNeilage's (1998) theory of the evolution of speech production. He distinguishes three levels of mammalian vocal production:

- *Respiration:* the basic cycle is the inspiration-expiration alternation with the expiratory phase modulated to produce vocalizations.
- *Phonation:* the basic cycle is the alternation of the vocal folds between an open and closed position ("voicing" in humans). This cycle is modulated by changes in vocal fold tension and subglottal pressure level, producing variations in pitch.
- *Articulation:* In his view, articulation is based on the syllable, defined in terms of a nucleus with a relatively open vocal tract, and margins with a relatively closed vocal tract. Modulation of this open-close cycle in humans takes the form of typically producing different phonemes, consonants (C), and vowels (V), respectively, in successive closing and opening phases.

Each spoken language (or, more precisely, each accent for a given language) has a relatively small fixed set of phonological units that have no independent meaning but can be combined and organized in the construction of word forms (the *duality of patterning* of Chapter 2). These units vary from language to language, but in each spoken language these units involve the choreographed activity of the *vocal articulators*, the lips, tongue, vocal folds, velum (the port to the nasal passages), as well as respiration.[4] But what are these units? Different authors have argued for features, gestures, phonemes (roughly, segments), moras (each mora consists of a consonant followed by a vowel; the mora is the basic unit for word formation in Japanese), syllables, gestural structures, and so on.

MacNeilage (1998) views the CV syllable—such as *da* or *gu*—as the basic unit of articulation and argues that language evolved directly as speech, rejecting any role for manual gesture in language evolution. However, in evaluating his theory, we must revisit the two senses of "speech" and distinguish *syllabic vocalization* from *spoken language*. The first is simply the uttering of sounds; the latter uses those sounds to convey meaning, and—as we have seen—spoken language must provide an open-ended set of sound combinations *linked to* an open-ended set of meanings. Thus, my main critique of MacNeilage's evolutionary theory is that his original theory gives no insight into the evolution of speech in the sense of spoken language as distinct from speech as the ability to articulate syllables. We shall see that the updated version of the theory (MacNeilage & Davis, 2005) goes part way, but only a very small part of the way, to meeting this objection. But first, a brief rhetorical jeu d'esprit (certainly not a reasoned scientific criticism since it applies to English, not to languages generally) of the claim that the basic syllable is CV. MacNeilage and Davis (2001) assert that:

(i)   Words typically begin with a consonant and end with a vowel.
(ii) The dominant syllable type within words is considered to be consonant-vowel (CV).

However, neither sentence supports its own claim, at least as far as English is concerned. In (i), only 1 of the 11 words conforms to the claim it makes; while in (ii), less than half of the 22 syllables conform! Indeed, the CVC syllable is basic in English, whereas the CV mora is basic in Japanese, but each allows variation from this norm. And note, too, the importance of tones in Chinese and clicks in certain African languages. However, jeu d'esprit aside, Jusczyk et al. (1999) found that 9-month-old English learners are sensitive to shared features that occur at the beginnings, but not at the ends of syllables. Specifically, the infants had significant listening preferences for lists in which the items shared either initial CV's, initial C's, or the same manner of articulation at syllable onsets. This suggests that infants may only later develop sensitivity to features that occur late in complex syllables. This certainly accords with the argument (MacNeilage & Davis, 2001) for the developmental priority of the CV syllable, and it may be true that the CV form is the only universal syllable form in languages (Maddieson, 1999). What then explains the evolution of the wide range of other "syllable-level" units used across the world's languages? Derek Bickerton (personal communication) sees a mix of drift and culture, specifically a trade-off between word length and syllabic complexity, as providing the answer. A language that has only CV syllables soon has to start lengthening words, so you get things like *humuhumunukunukuapua'a* (a Hawaiian fish—the word means "triggerfish with a snout like a pig") with 12 syllables. A language that allows high syllabic complexity has words like *strength* with six consonants to one vowel.

A more general concern is with the tendency to equate what is seen in the human infant with what must have developed in human evolution. At a trivial level, we know that hominids could make tools and hunt animals, and we know that modern human infants cannot, and so it is dangerous to equate "early in ontogeny" with "early in phylogeny." Closer to the language issue, recall from the section "Teaching 'Language' to Apes" of Chapter 3 that the bonobo Kanzi and a 2.5-year-old girl were comparable in their comprehension of 660 sentences phrased as simple requests (72% correct for Kanzi, 66% for the girl) but that this seemed to mark the limits of Kanzi's abilities. This suggests that the brain mechanisms that support the full richness of human language may not be fully expressed in the first 2 years of life yet, given the appropriate developmental grounding, eventually prove crucial in enabling the human child to acquire language.

But let us return to MacNeilage's Frame/Content (F/C) theory. The central notion is that there is a CV syllable structure frame, into which "content" is inserted prior to output. He argues that the speech frame may have been exapted from the combination of the mandibular cycle originally evolved for chewing, sucking, and licking with laryngeal sounds. However, I would claim that the mandibular cycle is too far back to serve as an interesting way station on the path toward syllabic vocalization. To illustrate this point, consider the evolution from rhythmic movements in our fish-like ancestors to the human capability for discrete goal-seeking movements of the hands. Among the stages we might discriminate are the following: swimming; visual control of trajectory; locomotion on land; adaptation to uneven terrain (so that two modes of locomotion emerge: modulation of rhythmic leg movements and discrete steps, e.g., from rock to rock); brachiation; bipedalism; and finally dexterity encompassing, for example, grooming (note the jaw/hand tradeoff), tool use, and gesture. It seems to me no more illuminating to root syllable production in mandibular oscillation than to root dexterity in swimming.

Schaal et al. (2004) report results from human functional neuroimaging that show significantly different brain activity in discrete and rhythmic movements, although both movement conditions were confined to the same single wrist joint. Rhythmic movements merely activated unilateral primary motor areas, while discrete movements elicited additional activity in premotor, parietal, and cingulate cortex, as well as significant bilateral activation. They suggest that rhythmic and discrete movement may be two basic movement categories in human arm control that require separate neurophysiological and theoretical treatment. The relevance for the present discussion is to suggest that human speech is best viewed as an assemblage of discrete movements even if it has a rhythmic component, and thus it may have required major cortical innovations in evolution for its support.

An account of speech evolution needs to shift emphasis from ancient functions to the changes of the last 5 million years that set humans off from other primates, with the transition from a limited set of vocalizations to syllabification or other units of vocal articulation. Indeed, MacNeilage and Davis (2005) appear to be moving in this direction because they now note three further stages beyond evolution of the mouth close-open alternation (c. 200 million years ago) en route to spoken language:

- Visuofacial communication in the form of lip smacks, tongue smacks, and teeth chatters (established with the macaque-human common ancestor perhaps 25 million years ago)
- Pairing of the communicative close-open alternation with phonation to form protosyllabic "frames"
- The frame becoming programmable with individual consonants and vowels

The human transition to an omnivorous diet may well have been accompanied by what I would call the *oral dexterity* of an omnivore—the rapid adaptation of the coordination of chewing with lip, tongue, and swallowing movements to the contents of the mouth—to the evolution of the control of the articulators that make speech possible. These might be part of the evolutionary path from mandibular oscillations to a form of skilled motor control that has some possibility of evolving to provide articulators and neural control circuits suitable for voluntary vocal communication. The challenge is to fill in the aforementioned schematic to provide in detail the evolutionarily plausible stages that get us from chewing to deploying tongue, respiration, larynx, lips, and so on, in the service of spoken language—a challenge to be met whether one is for or against the vocal origins hypothesis.

With this it is time to note that whatever its merits as a theory of the evolution of syllabic vocalization, MacNeilage (1998) has little to say about the evolution of spoken language—the evolution of semantic form and phonological form and their linkage. I think it is only because MacNeilage ignores the distinction between the two senses of "evolution of speech" that he can argue as confidently as he does for the view that language evolved directly as speech, dismissing claims for the key role of manual gesture in the evolution of language. Unless one can give some account of how strings of syllables come to have meaning, it is hard to see what evolutionary pressure would have provided selective advantage for the transition from "oral dexterity" to skilled vocal articulation. Fortunately, MacNeilage (2008) has at last begun to address the question, giving two different answers: (a) that ingestive movements may form a basis for communication (we saw that orofacial mirror neurons in macaques seem to support the claim that ingestive actions are the basis on which communication about feeding is built, but this does not replace communication about manual skills); and (b) that words for "mother" and "father" might have emerged by conventionalization of the infant's first attempts at syllabification yielding *ma* and *da*. My response is not to deny these claims, but only to stress that neither seems to establish a rich semantics in the way that pantomime does.

Musical Origins

Darwin (1871) addressed the question of language evolution with the emphasis on song rather than gesture as the precursor. He laid out a three-stage theory of language evolution:

1) A greater development of protohuman cognition, driven by both social and technological factors.
2) The evolution of vocal imitation used largely "in producing true musical cadences, that is in singing." Darwin suggests that this evolved as a challenge to rivals as well as in the expression of emotions. The first protolanguage would have been musical, driven by sexual selection as was birdsong—so that this capacity evolved analogously in humans and songbirds.
3) Articulate language then owed its origins to the imitation and modification, aided by signs and gestures, of various natural sounds, the voices of other animals, and the human's own instinctive cries. This transition was again driven by increased intelligence. Once meaning was in place, actual words would have been coined from various sources, encompassing any of the then-current theories of word origins.

A key observation here is that language has "musicality"/prosody as well as semantic expression. The same words may convey not only information but also emotion, while increasing social bonding and engaging attention. The *musical protolanguage hypothesis* can be simply stated as "phonology first, semantics later." It emphasizes that song and spoken language both use the vocal/auditory channel to generate complex, hierarchically structured signals that are learned and culturally shared. Musical protolanguage provides hierarchically structured signals that include phrases but lack many other syntactic complexities. Music has a kind of free-floating "meaningfulness" that can attach itself to many types of group activity and can thus enrich events it accompanies with unifying, barrier-dissolving effects (Cross, 2003). Nonetheless, music lacks nouns, verbs, tense, negation, embedding of meanings—it lacks "propositional meaning." Moreover, just as protolanguage is not language, so is a musical protolanguage not music. For example, music in many cultures now uses a small number of discrete frequency units—*notes*—that together make up a *scale* (Nettl, 2000). A song in such a tradition allows only these units to be used. Similarly, time is typically evenly subdivided into discrete "beats" that occur at a relatively regular tempo, which are arranged according to a metrical structure of strong and weak events: the core ingredients of musical rhythm. Neither of these features is required in the model of protomusic we are discussing. Just like pantomime, neither protomusic nor, indeed, early protolanguages need have been built up from a small, discrete set of elements.

In elaborating the notion of musical protolanguage, Otto Jespersen (1921/1964) suggested that, initially, meanings were attached to vocal phrases in a holistic, all-or-none fashion with no articulated mapping between parts of the signal and parts of the meaning—this is the notion of a *holophrase* to be developed in the Chapter 10, but we will emphasize the way in which manual pantomime provided a natural and open-ended semantics as the basis for conventionalized protosigns. Jespersen went beyond Darwin's vague suggestions about "increasing intelligence," to offer a specific path from irregular phrase-meaning linkages to syntactic words and sentences. Pointing to the pervasiveness of both irregularities, and attempts (often by children) to analyze these into more regular, rule-governed processes ("over regularization"), Jespersen gave a detailed account for how such holophrases can gradually be analyzed into something more like words. The analysis of whole phrases into subcomponents occurs not just in language evolution and historical change, but in language acquisition as well. Children at first hear entire phrases as a whole, and then become increasingly capable at segmenting words out of a continuous speech stream. For modern children, though, the words are there to be analyzed out of the stream of speech. The task is harder by far if the words aren't already there, as I will argue (in Chapter 10) was the case as protolanguages—whether in the manual and vocal domains—gave way to words linked by constructions.

Mithen (2005) and Fitch (2010) have combined Darwin's model of "musical" or "prosodic" protolanguage and Jespersen's notion of holistic protolanguage to yield a multistage model that builds on Darwin's core hypothesis that protosong preceded language. The resulting model posits the following evolutionary steps and selective pressures, leading from the unlearned vocal communication system of the last common ancestor of chimpanzees and humans, to modern spoken language in all of its syntactic and semantic complexity:

1. *Phonology first:* The acquisition of complex vocal learning occurred during an initial song-like stage of communication (comparable to birdsong or whale song) that lacked propositional meaning. Darwin proposed a sexually selected function, whereas Dissanayake (2000) opts for a kin-selection model. The two suggestions are not mutually exclusive. On this view, vocal imitation—lacking in chimpanzees—was the crucial step toward language. Fitch notes the convergent evolution with that for "song" in songbirds, parrots, hummingbirds, whales, and seals.

2. *Meaning second:* The addition of meaning proceeded in two stages, perhaps driven by kin selection. First, holistic mappings between whole, complex phonological signals (phrases or "songs") and whole semantic complexes (context-bound entities: activities, repeated events, rituals, and individuals) were linked by simple association. Such a musical protolanguage was an emotionally grounded vocal communication system, not a vehicle for the unlimited expression of thought.

3. *Compositional meaning:* These linked wholes were gradually broken down into parts: Individual lexical items "coalesced" from the previous wholes.

4. *Modern language:* As the language of its community grew more compositional (i.e., with wholes replaced by composites of parts), pressure for children to rapidly learn words and constructions became strong. This drove the last spurt of biological evolution to our contemporary state. Fitch suggests that this last stage was driven by kin selection for the sharing of truthful information among close relatives.

The Mirror System Hypothesis differs from the aforementioned scenario by positing that rich meanings were scaffolded by pantomime and that the consequent emergence of protosign in turn scaffolded the emergence of protospeech. However, the notion of a holophrastic phase from which syntax emerges is one we share with Jespersen, Mithen, and Fitch. These processes that underwrite the transition from protolanguage to language will be our prime concern in Chapter 10. But on our account, the transition to compositional meaning is a general property that goes back to essentially human modes of praxis—complex action recognition and complex imitation—rather than being a specific sequel to the combination of vocal learning with increased cognitive ability.

Elsewhere (Arbib, 2012), a group of scholars report on their efforts to probe the mysterious relationships between music, language and brain. Their assessments are beyond the scope of this volume, but it may be helpful to round out this section with the efforts of Arbib and Iriki (2012) to tease apart the different social origins of language and music, without in any way precluding the finding that these two skills may share some neural resources while also exploiting mechanisms specific to one skill rather than the other: They argue that for an evolutionary perspective on language, the most basic situation is that of two people using words and sentences to develop a more or less shared understanding or course of action. Although there are diverse speech acts (Searle, 1979) it seems reasonable to ground dyadic communication at its most basic to states of the world and courses of action to change that state. However, the act of communication often augments the words with facial and bodily expressions which can inject emotion into the conversation. As for music, it is perhaps too easy from a modern, Western perspective to reduce it to the sound patterns that can be captured electronically, or to the asymmetrical relation between performers and audience. However, just as language involves hands and face as well as voice, it seems more appropriate to seek the roots of music in a triple integration of voice (song), body (dance), and instruments (with, perhaps, the rhythmic beat of the drum as the most basic form). And where the turn taking of a dyad sharing information may provide grounding for language, the grounding for music may be in a group immersed in music together, with joint activity building a social and emotional rapport.

Neurobiology of the Expanding Spiral

Pantomime allows a broad range of communication that does not require an agreed-on convention between sender and receiver, as noted by Stokoe (2001) and others. However, pantomime is limited, and we have seen that the range of communication can be greatly improved by the development of conventions on the use of gestures that may not directly pantomime anything but are developed by a community to refine and annotate the more obvious forms of pantomime—forms that themselves would become increasingly ritualized with use. The notion, then, is that the manual domain provided the initial support for the expression of meaning by sequences and interweavings of gestures, with a progression from "natural" to increasingly conventionalized gesture to speed and extend the range of communication within a community. Note, however, that the gestural system remains, in modern humans, an invaluable adjunct in the acquisition of new words—or in standing in for them when one travels outside one's language community.

I think it likely (though empirical data are sadly lacking) that anterior cingulate cortex contains a mirror system for primate vocal communications, and that a related mirror system persists in humans, but I suggest that it is a complement to, rather than an integral part of, the speech system that includes Broca's area in humans. We noted in Chapter 3 that the neural substrate for primate calls is in a region of cingulate cortex distinct from F5, which later is the monkey homolog of human Broca's area. We thus have sought to explain why F5, rather than the a priori more likely "primate call area," provided the evolutionary substrate for speech and language. Rizzolatti and Arbib (1998) answer this by suggesting three evolutionary stages:

1. A *distinct* manuobrachial (hand-arm) communication system evolved to complement the primate calls/orofacial communication system.
2. The "speech" area of early hominids (i.e., the area presumably homologous to monkey F5 and human Broca's area) mediated orofacial and manuobrachial communication but not speech.
3. The manual-orofacial symbolic system then "recruited" vocalization. Association of vocalization with manual gestures allowed them to assume a more open referential character and exploit the capacity for imitation of the underlying manuobrachial system.

It seems necessary to hypothesize that the expanding spiral of protosign and protospeech must have reached a critical level prior to the emergence of *Homo sapiens*, a level that provided and built upon the processes of natural selection that yielded a modern vocal apparatus and brain mechanisms to control it. My hypothesis is that these provided part of what constitutes the *language-ready brain* (and body)—but that these were established prior to the emergence of true languages, and that this latter emergence depended more on cultural than biological evolution, since otherwise it is hard to see what selective pressure could have brought about the further refinements in the vocal apparatus that made fluent (proto)speech possible.

The claim, then, is that the biological evolution of hominids yielded a mirror system embedded in a far larger system for execution, observation, and imitation of compound behaviors composed from orofacial, manual, and vocal gestures. I also accept that this system supported communication in *Homo erectus*—since otherwise it is hard to see what selective pressure could have brought about the lowering of the larynx, which, as Lieberman (1991) observes, makes humans able to articulate more precisely than other primates but afflicts them with an increased likelihood of choking. The Perth psychologist Colin McLeod (personal communication) quips that "The human vocal tract evolved so that we could cry out 'Help, I'm choking!' "—but the serious point is that an increased risk of choking must have been offset by a selective advantage of some kind, and advancing effectiveness of protospeech seems a likely candidate. Fitch and Reby (2001) showed that lowering of the larynx in the red deer may have been selected to deepen the animal's roar so that the animal would seem larger than it was. Thus, the lowering of the larynx in humans or prehuman hominids might have served a similar purpose—without denying that further selection could have exploited the resultant increase in degrees of freedom to increase the flexibility of speech production. Lieberman argues that the restructuring of the human supralaryngeal vocal tract to enhance the perceptibility of speech would not have contributed to biological fitness unless speech and language were already present in *Homo erectus* and in Neanderthals. I make the lesser claim that biological evolution equipped early humans with a set of brain mechanisms that made *proto*speech possible—and these brains proved to be language-ready, being rich enough to support the cultural evolution of human languages in all their commonalities and diversities.

Having argued why speech did not evolve "simply" by extending the classic primate vocalization system, I must note that the language and vocalization systems are nonetheless linked. Lesions centered in the anterior cingulate cortex and supplementary motor areas of the human brain—homologs of vocalization areas of monkey cerebral cortex—can cause mutism in humans, as they do in muting monkey vocalizations. Conversely, a patient with a Broca's area lesion may nonetheless swear when provoked. As Critchley and Critchley (1998) report, the 19th-century British neurologist Hughlings Jackson drew attention to the fact that many patients with extreme poverty of speech were nonetheless able to swear. His notion was that swearing is not, strictly speaking, a part of language but a practice that, like loudness of tone and violence of gesticulation, expresses the force of passing emotions. This leads to the hypothesis that the evolution of speech yielded the pathways for cooperative computation between cingulate cortex and Broca's area, with cingulate cortex involved in breath groups and prosodic shading, and Broca's area providing the motor control for rapid production and interweaving of elements of an utterance. The suggestion then is that *Homo habilis* and even more so *Homo erectus* had a "proto-Broca's area" based on an F5-like precursor mediating communication by manual and orofacial gesture. There are indeed endocasts of the skulls of early *Homo* that trace indentations in the inner skull that to some extent reflect the general shape of the surface of the cerebral cortex (see Wilkins & Wakefield, 1995, for a review), though they show nothing of the detailed parcellation of cortex akin to that studied by Brodmann. The issue is to hypothesize what apparent enlargements in an overall lobe of the brain might signify. Our development of the Mirror System Hypothesis driven by comparative neurobiology and primatology helps us begin to fill the gap.

The suggestion, then, is that a process of collateralization enabled this "proto" Broca's area to gain primitive control of the vocal machinery, thus yielding increased skill and openness in vocalization, moving from the fixed repertoire of primate vocalizations to the unlimited (open) range of vocalizations exploited in speech. Speech apparatus and brain regions could then coevolve to yield the configuration seen in modern *Homo sapiens*. Intriguingly (Jürgens, personal communication, 2006), squirrel monkey F5 does have connections to the vocal folds, but these are solely for closing them and are not involved in vocalization. I thus argue that the evolution of speech may have involved expansion of the F5 projection to the vocal folds to allow for vocalization to be controlled in coordination with the control of the use of tongue and lips as part of the ingestive system.

Building on our discussion in Chapter 4 of "Auditory Systems and Vocalization," note that although their vocalizations are controlled by brainstem mechanisms, monkeys can be conditioned to vary their rates of vocalization and that this ability relies on medial cortex, including the anterior cingulate cortex, rather than on lateral areas homologous to Broca's area (Jürgens, 2002). This supports initiation and suppression of a small repertoire of innate calls, not the dynamic assemblage and coarticulation of articulatory gestures that constitute speech. However, stimulation studies in macaque *have* demonstrated a larynx representation in ventral premotor cortex (Hast, Fischer, Wetzel, & Thompson, 1974), while anatomical studies showed connections of F5 with the anterior cingulate cortex (Simonyan & Jürgens, 2002). Preliminary data suggest that these connections may provide a weak pathway whose evolutionary expansion could support the linkage of the lateral and medial systems. Coudé et al. (2011) trained two monkeys to vocalize (coo-call) for a reward when a piece of food was placed on a table facing them. The monkeys' vocal production and neuronal activity were recorded simultaneously. In both monkeys Coudé et al. observed attempts to vocalize in which the orofacial gesture typical of vocalization was produced but no sound was emitted. This behavior occurred as often as actual vocalization, suggesting that voluntary control of vocalization may have been a poorly controlled side effect of orofacial control, akin to those discussed earlier for the studies from the Gentilucci and Iriki groups. However, the neurophysiology did find F5 neurons whose firing correlated with voluntary vocal production. Such results show that the debate is far from over concerning gestural versus vocal origins of the language-ready brain. My current position is that it was the demands of vocal expression of the open semantics opened up by protosign that provided the adaptive pressure for the evolutionary extension of manual and orofacial gestural control to the speech apparatus and its neural control.

Rather than supporting the move to eliminate protosign, then, the data on audiovisual and mouth mirror neurons are more consistent with the view that:

- manual gesture is primary in the early stages of the evolution of language-readiness, but that
- orofacial neurons lay the basis for later extension of protosign to protospeech, and that

- the protospeech neurons in the F5 precursor of Broca's area may be rooted in ingestive behaviors.

Here I need to make the usual evolutionary caveat: Macaques are not ancestral to humans. What is being said here is shorthand for the following: (a) There are ingestion-related mirror neurons observed in macaque. (b) I hypothesize that such neurons also existed in the common ancestor of human and macaque of 25 million years ago. (c) Noting (with Fogassi & Ferrari, 2004) that there is little evidence of voluntary control of vocal communication in nonhuman primates, I further hypothesize that evolution along the hominid line (after the split 5 to 7 million years ago between the ancestors of the chimpanzees and those of humans) expanded upon this circuitry to create the circuitry for protospeech.

Protosign Vindicated

In agreeing that the specific communication system based on primate calling was not the precursor of language, some people (e.g., Bickerton, 1995) have claimed that communication could not have been a causal factor in the evolution of language-readiness. They argue instead that it was the advantage of being able to represent and thus think about a complex world that favored language evolution, rather than communication about the physical and social world. However, we should not be constrained by such either/or thinking and in recent writing Bickerton (e.g., 2009) places the origin of language in communication and argues that the explosion in human cognition must have followed, not preceded, the emergence of language—virtually reversing his previous position. Indeed, the coevolution of communication and representation was essential for the emergence of human language. By representing more aspects of the world, we had more to talk about, but without communication those thoughts would remain inchoate. Both representation within the individual and communication between individuals could provide selection pressures for the biological evolution of language-readiness and the further cultural evolution of language and cognitive abilities, with advances in the one triggering advances in the other.

While many theories of language evolution have focused either on evolution of language as a separate faculty or as internal to systems of communication, the present theory emphasizes a capability that lies outside communication—namely the imitation of practical actions—and then suggests how it opened new possibilities that made language possible. In this respect, the theory has clear parallels with Merlin Donald's (1991, 1998, 1999) theory of *mimesis,* and the exploitation of this capability to create representations with the critical property of voluntary retrievability, as the key to the evolution of human intelligence. However, my core argument more specifically insists that complex imitation of *hand movements* was a crucial precursor to the development of an open system of communication because pantomime provided a rich semantic range that could ground the later emergence of conventionalized communicative utterances. The doctrine of the expanding spiral is that (1) protosign exploits the ability for complex imitation of hand movements to support an open system of communication; (2) the resulting protosign provides scaffolding for protospeech; but that (3) protosign and protospeech develop together thereafter. The strong hypothesis here is that protosign is essential to this process, so that the full development of protospeech was made possible by the protosign scaffolding.

As was clear from the example of sour fruit given earlier, I do not claim that meaning cannot evolve within the orofacial domain, but only that the range of such meanings is impoverished compared with those expressible by manual pantomime. Once a brain can support imitation in the manual domain, one must ask to what extent this would imply or be separate from imitation in the vocal domain, where imitation of familiar sounds from the calls of animals to the howling of the wind could also contribute core vocabulary, but from the vocal side. However, the crucial point here is that these are no part of the species-specific calls of nonhuman primates and that the available data on macaque F5 suggest a system very different from the "speech machine" that includes present-day Broca's area. A "speech-only" evolutionary hypothesis leaves mysterious the availability of this vocal-manual-facial complex, which not only supports a limited gestural accompaniment to speech but also the ease of acquisition of signed languages for those enveloped within it in infancy. However, the "protosign scaffolding" hypothesis has the problem of explaining why speech became favored over gestural communication, and we have offered some answers earlier in the chapter.

With this analysis of the Expanding Spiral of Protosign and Protospeech, we have basically completed the account of the processes posited by the extended Mirror System Hypothesis to underlie the biological evolution of the language-ready brain of modern humans. However, there are facets of language that would seem to be biologically grounded yet lie outside the main focus of our investigation. One is the linkage of the explicit syntax and semantics of language to emotional expression; the other, related aspect of language is its prosody and its linkage to music through song and dance. This book leaves these questions for investigation elsewhere (including Arbib, 2012), focusing primarily on delimiting a number of stages whereby our ancestors achieved—through biological and cultural evolution—the ability to develop and use an open-ended, and freely expandable, set of symbols for communication. With this, we will turn in Chapter 10 to the demonstration that the capabilities charted in Chapters 7 through 9 are indeed sufficient for languages, with their rich grammar as well as an open-ended lexicon, to emerge through a process of cultural, rather than biological evolution.

10

How Languages Got Started

The book is entitled *How the Brain Got Language*, while this chapter is called "How Languages Got Started." Why the switch from singular to plural? It has been the argument of this book that many different changes during *biological evolution* gave humans a *language-ready brain* but that it took *cultural evolution* to exploit the human brain's capabilities to the point where the potential for language (in the singular) became realized in the development of diverse languages (in the plural) as *Homo sapiens* developed different groupings in Africa and spread from there around the world. We have now established the core arguments of the Mirror System Hypothesis, which roots much of the evolution of the language-ready brain in praxis, but then shows how the resultant capabilities were exapted for communication so that the first *Homo sapiens*, according to this theory, already exploited protolanguage but did not yet speak or sign any languages in the sense of Chapter 6. It is time now to consider how cultural evolution, exploiting the adaptability of the brains of a community of humans whose brains were language-ready, achieved that final transition.

In the previous chapters we have charted an evolutionary sequence of brain mechanisms supporting a widening set of capabilities:

- Mirror system for grasping (shared with human-monkey common ancestor)
- "Simple" imitation (shared with ape-monkey common ancestor)
- Complex imitation, with related abilities for structuring behavior and for caregiving (unique to *Homo*)
- Pantomime
- Protosign and protospeech—multimodal protolanguage to yield a brain that is language-ready

Chapter 8 showed how pantomime provided an open-ended semantics, while protosign exploited pantomime but was differentiated from it by using ritualization and other means whereby a group can establish a set of shared conventional gestures. In this way, protosign provided the key ability for the free creation of arbitrary gestures to support an open-ended semantics.

Chapter 9 then showed how protospeech emerged as control mechanisms that had evolved for protosign came to also control the vocal apparatus with increasing flexibility, and then showed how protospeech and protosign evolved thereafter in an expanding spiral to support protolanguage as a multimodal communicative system. The efficacy of pantomime in creating an open-ended semantics was contrasted with the limited association of primordial sounds or facial gestures with meanings to argue against a "vocal-only" scheme in which a complex imitation system for vocalization led to protospeech directly, with no necessary involvement of manual gesture. However, Chapter 9 did touch briefly on the importance of understanding the evolution of a vocal apparatus (including its neural control) adequate to the demands of spoken language.

This chapter now takes on the challenge of explaining the *cultural* evolution of *languages* once the mechanisms supporting the earliest forms of protolanguage were all in place—going beyond the ability to perceive states of the world or social needs or situations, or to formulate courses of action, to provide a syntax and semantics with which to express explicitly the relations inherent in these prior capabilities. In Chapter 2 we presented *Construction Grammar* as providing a useful framework for the study of language, abandoning segregated rule systems for syntax, semantics, and phonology. Rather than limiting syntax to a few very general rules for combining elements of prespecified syntactic categories like noun and verb, we instead deploy a wide array of "constructions," which are either like elements of the lexicon or have slot fillers that may have to satisfy semantic as well as syntactic restrictions. It is only the merging of categories from different constructions that may blur the original semantic cues as to what entered into the earlier constructions, yielding more syntactic/less semantic categories. But such categories are often more language-specific than universal, and the number and variety of constructions in a language imply that speakers deploy a huge range of specialized knowledge to communicate successfully.

This chapter will offer a scenario for the invention of more and more constructions by humans who had begun to link a capacity for complex imitation to the demands of communication via protospeech and protosign.

From Holistic Protolanguages to Construction Grammar

We said that a protolanguage is an open system of communication used by a particular hominid grouping that was a possible precursor of "true" language—where a language is an open-ended system in which words and then phrases can be assembled according to some grammar that makes it possible to infer plausible meanings for novel utterances created "on the fly." Just as there are many different languages today, so there must have been diverse protolanguages in the distant past. And just as we can today chart the historical change of languages in recent millennia (to be sampled in How Languages Keep Changing in Chapter 13), so can we be rather confident that there was a spectrum of protolanguages across the time and space of "the dawn of humanity" from the truly primitive to those that had achieved a complexity little different in their properties from the simplest of "real" languages. Implicit in this statement, and consistent with a Construction Grammar approach, is that grammar is *not* all or none—so that it is not a matter of protolanguage + grammar = language but rather a continuum:

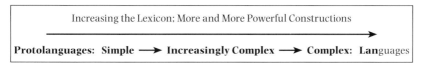

Even Alison Wray, who contributed to much of the theory (holophrasis) that I espouse below, has concerns about what use a partial grammar might be:

> [T]here is a critical level of complexity that must obtain for a creative grammar to be useful in expressing propositions. ... [I]t is difficult to imagine what advantage a primitive, half-way grammar would have for its users, over the highly successful interactional systems of other primates ... (Wray, 1998, p. 48)

Here I would disagree with Wray. The trouble comes, I think, from viewing a grammar as providing an all-or-none capacity to express propositions, or as comprising a rather small but exhaustive set of very general rules rather than as a set of independently useful constructions that have "stand-alone utility." My view is that language did not arise from protolanguage simply by "adding syntax" (including syntactic categories) in an all-or-none process. Rather, languages emerged from protolanguages through a process of *bricolage* (tinkering), which yielded many novelties to handle special problems of communication, with a variety of generalizations emerging both consciously and unconsciously to amplify the power of diverse inventions by unifying them to provide general "rules" that could be imposed on, or discerned in, a population of ad hoc mechanisms. Bricolage added "tools" to each protolanguage, such as that for counting up to larger and larger numbers. Many, but not all, of these became more or less regularized, with general "rules" emerging both consciously and unconsciously only as generalizations could be imposed on, or discerned in, a population of ad hoc tools. The result: a spiraling coevolution of communication and representation, extending the repertoire of achievable, recognizable, and describable actions, objects, and situations which could be thought and talked about.

To chart the transition from protolanguages to languages, we need first to better understand what form protolanguages might have taken as a basis for assessing the various mechanisms that may have led to more and more complex protolanguages until eventually some critical mass of features of modern language was achieved. Much of the debate over the notion of protolanguage focuses on whether it was compositional or holophrastic.[1]

The compositional view (Bickerton, 1995; Tallerman, 2007) hypothesizes that *Homo erectus* communicated by a protolanguage in which a communicative act comprises a few nouns and verbs strung together without syntactic structure. As noted in Chapter 6, Bickerton asserts that infant language, pidgins, and the "language" taught to apes are all protolanguages in this sense. On this view, the "protowords" (in the evolutionary sense) were so akin to the words of modern languages that these evolved from protolanguages simply by "adding syntax."

The holophrastic view (Arbib, 2005a; Wray, 1998, 2002) holds that in much of early protolanguage, a complete communicative act involved a "unitary utterance" or "holophrase" whose parts have no independent meaning yet whose overall meaning would be akin to that of a phrase or sentence of English, which is indeed composed of meaningful words. On this view, words coevolved culturally with syntax: As "protowords" were fractionated or elaborated to yield words for fragments of their original meaning, so were constructions developed to arrange the words to reconstitute those original meanings and (the advantage of this transition) many other meanings besides.[2]

If a vote were taken today among those who study language evolution, I suspect that a majority would favor the compositional view of protolanguage over the holophrastic view. Certainly, once you have discovered the combinatorial power of using syntax to combine words, then considering words as the building blocks of protolanguage, not just of language, does seem plausible. But if one has not yet discovered syntax, then labeling significant events or constructs seems the simpler strategy. And our earlier discussion of "partial grammar" suggests that a protolanguage might remain holophrastic in part even while other parts have become more compositional in their structure. Turning to writing systems, a much more recent invention than language itself, "phonetic writing systems are simpler than ideographic writing systems" is true if you start from sound patterns, but it is false if you start from pictures. There are many "self-evident truths" that were not always self-evident, and it is a feat of the imagination to think back to a possible past in which the culture had not yet made them self-evident.

In what follows, then, I will not only set forth the reasons that led me to favor the holophrastic view but will summarize some key objections from those who favor the compositional view—and do my best to answer them. The holophrastic view does *not* say, "Protolanguage was only and always a collection of holophrases." Rather, the crucial claim is that the earliest protolanguages were in great part holophrastic, and that as they developed through time, each protolanguage retained holophrastic strategies while making increasing use of constructions. Protolanguages formed a *spectrum:* (a) different groups of hominids would have adopted different protolanguage strategies at different times, and (b) a given group would have concurrently employed both holophrastic and compositional strategies, plus a range of distinct intermediates (perhaps for different semantic functions) with increasing use of compositional strategies. This is to be distinguished from positing a single evolutionary transition, or a series of transitions that led to an innate Universal Grammar (Pinker & Bloom, 1990).

I will argue for the general view that biological evolution contributed many changes that made the human use of language possible (i.e., created the genetic basis for a language-ready brain) but that the full exploitation of these changes rested on cumulative human inventions and, in turn, made possible new selective pressures based on the advantages of using increasingly expressive protolanguages.

Since the flexible use of language seems to us an inescapable part of the human condition, it is hard to imagine what it could have been like to be a protohuman who was more ape than human, and yet now had the capability to master the use of a protolanguage once the community of which he or she was a member began to invent (whether consciously or not) and exchange protowords. We know (see Chapter 3) that *biological* evolution yielded a repertoire of primate calls each of which describes a "situation," while apes were able to extend their range of innate communicative gestures through such mechanisms as ontogenetic ritualization and social learning. I have argued that protohumans and early *Homo sapiens* had gone further: (a) pantomime opened up the ability to communicate novel meanings; (b) conventionalization served to reduce ambiguities and speed communication, yielding a system of protosign; and (c) the mechanisms evolved to support protosign began to control vocalizations as well; thus (d) providing a selective benefit in subsequent refinements of the vocal apparatus and its control.

To get some feel for holophrases, recall from Chapter 3 the "leopard call" of the vervet monkey. It is emitted first by a monkey who has seen a leopard; the call triggers further calling by others and the leopard-appropriate escape behavior of running up a tree (Cheney & Seyfarth, 1990). The leopard call's meaning might be paraphrased by: "There is a leopard nearby. Danger! Danger! Run up a tree to escape—and spread the (proto)word." To this one might respond (Bridgeman, 2005), "It's only one word, because 'leopard' is enough to activate the whole thing." However, once one moves from species-specific calls to protolanguage, one might add new "protowords" to convey meanings like "There is a dead leopard. Let's feast upon it" or "There is a leopard. Let's hunt it so we can feast upon it"—and we clearly cannot use the leopard alarm call as the word for *leopard* in either of these utterances without triggering an innate and inappropriate response. Thus, on the *holophrastic view*, early protolanguage proceeded first by adding such holophrases.

At first, only a few protowords might have been added to the protovocabulary in each generation. (Even in modern society, "basic" words, e.g., "house" as distinct from "houseboat," are added only slowly—especially if we measure this in words per person per year that gain widespread currency.) Thus, adding new "protowords" would have been psychologically akin to adding a new primate alarm call to the repertoire, transcending the fixed biological inheritance by exploiting new neural pathways. We saw that different brain regions came to be responsible for the production of innate primate vocalizations and for the production of protowords. However, early humans would have no more perception of which brain regions produced observed behavior than modern humans normally do. As a result, addition of new protowords would be something that "just happened" in a community, rather than being the fruit of consciously directed invention. Early hominids just beginning to have protolanguage need have had no conception of language as we know it, any more than our ancestors of 10,000 years ago had any conception of reading or writing. Nonetheless, early protowords would differ *crucially* from primate calls in that new utterances could be *invented* (probably unconsciously, in the earlier generations) and then acquired through social learning within a community. Thus, the set of such protowords was open, whereas the set of calls was closed.

To place the holophrastic view within the context of the Mirror System Hypothesis, note that much of pantomime is holophrastic. I hypothesize that as protolanguage and protospeech evolved together (whether through biological or cultural innovations), many of the protowords shared this holophrastic feature—as a pantomime was reduced to a conventionalized protoword, whether in protosign, or in protospeech shaped in part by modulation of vocalizations by hand movements (Gentilucci, Santunione, Roy, & Stefanini, 2004). Protospeech could also build on protosign or be experienced psychologically as a variation on the theme of alarm calls but signaling more diverse situations, or be formed by tagging a snatch of song with some overall association (as in the Musical Origins model critiqued in Chapter 9). So, it becomes plausible, but not uncontroversial, to assert that many of the "protowords" of the earliest protolanguages were unitary utterances or *holophrases* more akin in their meaning to whole action-object frames than to the verbs or nouns that lie at the heart of languages like English.

More specifically, I hypothesize that—responding to "cultural selection" rather than "natural selection"—the users of the first protolanguages created novel protowords for *complex* situations that were *frequently important* to the tribe. Perhaps, at first, at most two or three such situations would be added to the "nameable" by an entire tribe in any one generation. Early protoconversations might then have been like interactions we now see in nonhuman primates, but with a few protowords interspersed. Following up on the variations on the leopard alarm mentioned earlier, we might suggest that as the leopard as predator became prey and as man the scavenger began to develop a protolanguage, he might have seen the carcass of a leopard and then emitted a new *socially defined* (rather than innate) holophrase meaning:

"There is a dead leopard. Let's feast upon it."

This might provide an early example of *displacement* (talking about things that are not present) if the one who had discovered the carcass was calling on members of the tribe to share his good fortune in scavenging the remains (Bickerton, 2009). The protoword might be accompanied by a pointing gesture to locate the (remains of the) leopard, or followed by beginning to run, signaling "the leopard is this way, follow me"—but again, the interpretation of the action was context dependent, with no correspondence between the parts of the action and the individual words of the English translation I have given. Furthermore, as man becomes a hunter he must add new protowords to his protovocabulary, such as one meaning:

"There is a leopard. Let's hunt it so we can feast upon it."

Location still matters: The protoword may be accompanied by a pointing gesture to locate the leopard. But social coordination matters, too: Other gestures may follow to pantomime how each hunter should move to attack the prey. (Of course, just as we may utter several sentences in each turn of a conversation, so might the users of a holophrastic protolanguage utter more than one protoword in each turn.) Human sentences rarely involve such life-or-death importance as vervet alarm calls. But we have wants and desires, and so we may benefit if we have new ways to communicate them. This raises a chicken-and-egg problem of why others would want to satisfy our desires. But, as Dunbar (1996) notes, other primates exhibit behaviors like grooming that may underlie more general forms of reciprocity, while de Waal (2006) provides examples of "altruism" in apes.

The vervet monkey's leopard call is instinctive and involves the anterior cingulate gyrus and midbrain, whereas the lateral brain (centered on the F5 mirror system ≈ protoBroca's area) supports both the invention of new protowords and the emergence of combined utterances.

A leopard in the forest may be very hard to spot, so that what seems at first to be a leopard may turn out to be only the dappling of the leaves. This points up the utility of negation. If that first glimpse was wrong and no leopard was there, it would be a most useful "invention" to provide some way of signaling this, to call off the escape or hunt. Canceling different courses of action may have involved idiosyncratic expressions—for example, abruptly stopping one's run in the scavenging example—but the beginning of a general notion of negation was born and the linguistic means to express it. This is just one example of taking language beyond the here and now of request/command and description. On this view, many ways of expressing relationships that we now take for granted as part of language were discovered by individual humans, *Homo sapiens*, and were "postbiological" in origin. Adjectives, conjunctions such as *but*, *and*, or *or* and *that*, *unless*, or *because*, and so on would have been postbiological in this sense.

Recall the Just So story from Chapter 6 where we spoke of a holophrase such as *grooflook* or *koomzash*. I was *not* implying that early protolanguages were necessarily spoken, nor that they had a phonology (duality of patterning) in the sense of a small set of elements from which all protowords were constructed—whether a repertoire of basic handshapes, motions, and locations for protosign or a set of vocal building blocks akin to phonemes or syllables for protospeech. Phonology came later, as I will argue in the section "Phonology Emerging." Rather, I am using a pronounceable but meaningless sequence of letters to suggest a "protoword" that has no internal structure—but is merely a conventionalized sound pattern or gesture that has come to symbolize an event, object, or action. In particular, just as there can be many variations on a pantomime that still leave its meaning comprehensible, so too would protowords exhibit some variation when used by different tribe members on different occasions. In any case, the claim in Chapter 6 was that holophrases might have encoded quite complex descriptions such as "The alpha male has killed a meat animal and now the tribe has a chance to feast together. Yum, yum!" or commands such as "Take your spear and go around the other side of that animal and we will have a better chance together of being able to kill it." (with the "go around the other side" perhaps indicated by a gesture rather than being part of the protoword itself).

Tallerman (2006) cites not only my example "Take your spear and go around the other side of that animal and we will have a better chance together of being able to kill it" but also the notion of a holophrase expressing the message "Go and hunt the hare I saw five minutes ago behind the stone at the top of the hill" from Mithen (2005, p. 172). However, Mithen's example fails my key criterion that a protoword symbolize frequently occurring or highly significant situations since his "protoword" specifies a precise time interval and the relation of an arbitrary pair of objects. When I posit that there could be a protoword for "The alpha male has killed a meat animal and now the tribe has a chance to feast together. Yum, yum!" I do not claim that (at first) there were protowords for variations like "The alpha male has killed a meat animal but it is too scrawny to eat. Woe is we" or "The alpha male has killed a meat animal but is keeping it for himself." One must not think of protohumans as having modern thoughts and just lacking the ability to express them. Protohumans would not have the idea of trying to pantomime the equivalent of arbitrary complex sentences. Rather, they would have had a small stock of protowords that would increase over the generations as pantomimes and vocal performances became conventionalized for situations of sufficient importance or frequency.[3]

But Tallerman raises another objection. She notes that the English paraphrase of "grooflook" involves five clauses and then asks, "If modern speakers engage in conceptual *planning* only at the level of a single clause—a mental proposition—how could early hominids possibly have had the lexical capacity to store, retrieve (and execute) a single lexical concept that corresponds to several clauses' worth of semantic content?" Tallerman (2007, p. 595) objects that "whereas lexical vocabulary can be stored by pairing a concept with the arbitrary sound string used to denote it, holistic utterances must be stored by memorizing each complex propositional event and learning which unanalyzable string is appropriate at each event. This task is harder, not simpler, than learning words as symbols, and therefore less suitable for an early protolanguage scenario." But there is no obvious criterion of simplicity here. An emotionally charged event like feasting after a successful hunt would be more memorable than the distinction between, say, a plum and an apple, and thus a protoword for the situation might be easier to learn than that for a category of fruit. Moreover, why is distinguishing a plum from an apple more or less "complexly propositional" than recognizing a festive occasion? If we try to describe the difference between a plum and an apple in English, we will need complex propositions. And if it is answered that "We just recognize the shape and taste—no propositions are needed," then why can't we just recognize the similarity between memorable occasions—with no propositions needed?

For another example of the conceptual complexity of words, if we recall that in Chapter 6 we defined "eat" as "Take a substance whose ingestion is necessary for your survival, place it in your mouth, masticate it and then swallow it," we see that saying "eat" is no more simple than uttering my protowords (cf. Smith, 2008). The issue is whether members of the group can recognize the similarity across many situations and associate them with a "protoword" uttered on these occasions. Indeed, any argument against the learnability of protowords is also an argument against the learnability of words of modern languages. It is like saying that no English speaker, raised in a group with the stated conventions and expectations, could master the word "wedding" because it unpacks to "Two people, probably of opposite gender, with one wearing a white wedding dress and the other a dinner suit, are having a ceremony which may have a religious and a civil component; and they are vowing to love and cherish each other for the rest of their lives, and there are lots of guests and...." The fact that weddings can also take many other forms only reinforces my point about the complexity of experience that can condense around a single (proto)word. The point for "wedding," as for protowords, is that it taps into a range of situations that occurs with enough frequency or emotional charge that its use by the "speaker" may be triggered by some part of its semantic content and may in turn elicit other semantic content on the part of the "hearer" without requiring that either unpack the whole semantic package of lived (or other) experience associated with the protoword. A possible critique of this is to distinguish *denotation* of a sign as "the specific, literal image, idea, concept, or object that the sign refers to" and its *connotation* as the figurative cultural assumptions that the image implies or suggests, involving emotional overtones, subjective interpretation, sociocultural values, and ideological assumptions. One might then say, "*Wedding* denotes 'ceremony initiating a quasi-permanent pair-bond' with all the stuff about churches and dinner-jackets as connotation and not part of its meaning." However, there is no clear borderline here—what may seem peripheral connotation to one speaker may be central to the denotation of a word to another speaker. And, as concepts and protowords were being formed together, there was no language to build a dictionary and prescribe that it specified *the* denotation of each protoword. This is a point to which we shall return in our discussion of metaphor.

On the *holophrastic view*, early protolanguage got started by accumulating holophrases. Following the earlier work of Wray, I suggest that one (not the only one, as will become clear) of the major mechanisms whereby the increasing subtlety of protolanguages laid the basis for the emergence of languages was through the repeated *discovery* that one could gain expressive power by *fractionating* holophrases into shorter utterances conveying components of the scene or command (and then, of course, further conventionalizing the pieces). Wray (1998, 2000, 2002) suggests how the fractionation of such protowords might occur. Let's return to an example from Chapter 6 (elaborated from Arbib, 2005a): Imagine that a tribe has two unitary utterances concerning fire—packing into different "protowords" the equivalent of, say, the English sentences "The fire burns" and "The fire cooks the meat"— that, by chance, contain similar (not necessarily identical) substrings (e.g., a part of a pantomime, or part of a sound pattern) that become regularized so that for the first time there is a sign for "fire." Perhaps the original utterances were "reboofalik" and "balikiwert," and "falik" becomes the agreed-on term for *fire*, so the utterances become "reboofalik" and "falikiwert" At this early stage, the gestural or sound patterns suggested by the notations *reboofalik* and *balikiwert* might not be composed from a fixed stock of syllables—rather, they would just be two patterns with parts that are similar but not identical. However, the sort of regularization involved in merging *falik* and *balik* into a common pattern may be seen as a move toward creating a phonological stock for the emerging protolanguage. We may write the results as *reboo falik* and *falik iwert*, indicating the fractionation of each protoword by breaking it into two strings separated by a space. By the same token, fractionation in a gestural or vocal performance must be accompanied by some change in the performance that signals in a perceptible fashion the difference between the unfractionated and the fractionated string. Such signals might have been quite idiosyncratic at first, but as the number of fractionations increased, conventions would have emerged for marking them. This would contribute to the emergence of phonology.

But how can an arbitrary segment, whether gestural or vocal, come to stand as a symbol for a class of entities or an individual member of a class? This may seem perfectly natural to users of language, but no call or gesture in the entire arsenal of nonhuman communication systems has this property. Our answer came in stages:

a) We argued that pantomime could allow the communication of ideas about actions, objects, and events. This was a breakthrough at the level of the freedom to create novel associations.

b) We then argued that both economy of expression and ease of understanding would create the pressure for conventionalization, yielding both gestures that simplified pantomimes and complementary gestures that could serve to reduce ambiguity in the original pantomimes.

c) This ability to link meanings (perhaps as much connotative as denotative) to protowords extended to protospeech as well as protosign, with the two becoming complementary long before speech became dominant in most human societies.

d) But now complex imitation comes into play—the ability to observe a complex behavior and seek to divide it into parts *even when the goal of a part is not immediately apparent*. This was the phenomenon of overimitation that set humans apart from apes but that, we argued, was crucial in expanding the repertoire of socially learnable skills. Let's see how this ability makes fractionation possible. When considered individually, each of *reboofalik* and *balikiwert* has no discernible parts. But once the similarity of *falik* and *balik* is noticed, *reboo falik* and *falik iwert* become candidates for variations on a single communicative action. But what is being communicated? There was no prior community for which *falik* was a meaningful protoword, and so the meaning had to emerge (for the first time) through a consensual process.

Two cogent objections have been made to the last step of this scenario: One is that similar substrings might also occur in protowords that have nothing to do with fire, and the other is that a holophrase could correspond to many different expressions in English. The first problem confronts the compositional account as well—a child learning English must learn that "tar" is a semantic unit within "get tar" but not so within "target." For the child learning a modern language, prosody may provide relevant cues—but related conventions were unlikely to apply to early protolanguages. Indeed prosody might well have emerged with fractionation in a gestural or vocal performance since the shift from the unfractionated to the fractionated string would have to be signaled in some way. Such signals might have been quite idiosyncratic at first, but in due course conventions would have emerged for marking them. Furthermore, part of the early learning, for the aforementioned scenario, is that *falik* means *fire* in the context of *reboo* and *iwert*. The accumulation of all the contexts for any given unit can start to produce the principles of modern syntax. Jackendoff (2002) gives a related account, though not within the framework of the fractionation of holophrases.[5]

As for the second objection, a protohuman might think (without breaking the thought into words) of "reboofalik" as meaning "Wood gets hot," and "balikiwert" as meaning "Hot wood makes meat soft." Thus, it would be a contingent fact whether the common segment in the two holophrases would be interpreted as "fire" or "wood" or "hot." However, this does not invalidate the process of fractionation. Once the use of *falik* caught on, it would be a matter of subsequent usage as to which meaning would become more prevalent. For example, if the use of *falik* were to catch on in warning someone of a thermal spring, then the sense of "hot" might come to predominate over that of "fire." This mutability is, of course, still preserved in modern languages, as the meaning of words may change over the decades or centuries. My favorite example of this—from the book *Our Language* by Simeon Potter (1950, p. 116), which I read in high school—is that, when King James II saw the new St. Paul's Cathedral designed by Sir Christopher Wren, he described it as *amusing, awful,* and *artificial.* An insult? Quite the contrary. At that time, those words meant *pleasing, awe-inspiring,* and *skillfully achieved,* respectively.[6]

Let's consider a variant of the *reboofalik/balikiwert* example in the domain of pantomime. It is ahistorical, since it concerns doors, and doors did not exist when protolanguage was emerging from pantomime, but let's persevere. If I pantomime "he is opening the door," there will (contra Stokoe, 2001) be no natural separation of noun and verb. Suppose that the pantomime for *open the door* had become conventionalized by positioning the hand near the body, then making a hand-turning motion followed by a movement of the hand away from the body, while the pantomime for *close the door* became conventionalized by positioning the hand away from the body, then making a hand-turning motion followed by a movement of the hand toward the body. What is crucial to this example is that no part of the pantomimes is a symbol for the noun *door* or the verbs *open* or *close.* It is only the full performance that conveys the notion of a door being *opened* or *closed.* In this case, the common element to the two performances is the hand-turning motion, and over time this might be fractionated from the two unitary utterances to become the symbol for *door,* even though it was in no way a pantomime for *door* when the overall (preconventionalization) protoword was originally performed. Secondly, once *door* is fractionated out, then one is invited to attend to the rest of the original protoword as a new, complementary protoword—yielding *open* and *close.*

And now something even more important happens. The similarity between *door* + *open* and *door* + *close* opens the possibility of generalization to the construction *door* + *X,* where *X* can be the protoword for any action one might employ with a door, or the construction *Y* + *open* where *Y* symbolizes anything that might be opened. We also see how, even at this primitive stage, protolanguage invites generalizations that might otherwise have never been made—for the very existence of *Y* + *open* invites one to consider operations on nondoors that are like opening a door and yet (consider *opening* one's eyes) are nonetheless very different. The power of metaphor seems to be an unavoidable concomitant of the recombination of symbols in novel constructions to express meanings that were not covered in the prior repertoire of holophrases.

Similarly, in the *reboofalik/balikiwert* example, some tribe members might—if *fire* had become the agreed-on meaning for *falik*—eventually regularize the complementary gestures in the first string to get a sign for *burns*; later, others regularize the complementary gestures in the second string to get a sign for *cooks meat.* However, the placement of the gestures that have come to denote "burns" relative to "fire" differs greatly from those for "cooks meat." It thus requires a further convention to regularize the placement of the gestures in both utterances—localized "constructions" emerge to maintain the earlier set of meanings and then extend them as new protowords come to be used as slot fillers. In this way the two utterances would make the transition to non-unitary utterances or protosentences—say *reboo falik* and *iwert falik*

The key point is this: As fractionation yielded new symbols selecting components from a hitherto holophrastic meaning, so did the beginnings of syntax stir as ways of putting together these new meanings also emerged. In this way, complex imitation (recognizing variants of an action as ways of combining subactions in flexible ways that achieve subgoals under varying circumstances) would become increasingly applicable to communication.

Intriguingly, this process still occurs to the present day, and it will be demonstrated in Chapter 12. There we will see that signers of Nicaraguan Sign

Language not only came to fractionate a pantomime of rolling downhill into separate signs for *roll* and *descend* but also developed a specific construction to express simultaneity. Thus, the sequence *roll descend* could mean "descend then roll," whereas repetition of *roll* in *roll descend roll* indicates that the rolling and descending were simultaneous.

As another example of the transition from holophrases, let's return to the scenario exemplified by Figure 8-2: In American Sign Language (ASL), the signs for AIRPLANE and FLY use the same airplane-like handshape, but the choice of hand movement to distinguish them—a small movement back and forth for AIRPLANE, a single long movement for FLY—is purely conventional (Supalla & Newport, 1978). We can be sure that our distant ancestors did not communicate about airplanes, but—as noted earlier—the need to distinguish *bird* and *flying* from the holophrastic *bird flying* (so that one could, for example, indicate a *dead bird*) would have provided another pressure for the move to find protowords to express components of a holophrase. The argument is that there had to be a stock of holophrases large enough for disambiguation to become necessary—as in distinguishing *bird* as a generic concept for a creature in flight to the specifics of a bird that could engage in other activities of interest to the tribe. To convey the notion of *dead bird* might initially require a combination of the accepted protoword for *flying bird* with a pantomime of, for example, the bird fluttering to the ground and lying still. This lengthy performance would become conventionalized as a new performance that overlaps that of *flying bird* and then the two might support the invention of a protoword, at last, for *bird*, which might be part of an overlap, or perhaps come to adopt the original pantomime as now meaning *bird* rather than *flying bird* with separate modifications for *flying* and *dead*, akin to our ASL example.

An interesting objection takes us back to the section "Teaching 'Language' to Apes" of Chapter 3. If apes can learn some use of word-like symbols when taught to do so, why wouldn't our ancestral species have invented words—in roughly the modern sense, akin to nouns and verbs—directly, rather than developing holophrases first, as argued on the holophrastic view of protolanguage? The short answer is that wild apes don't invent these vocabularies; humans do. We thus have to ask how "the wild-state human" (before there were words) got to the "language-state human" (who used words routinely). To say that apes can be taught a few *fragments* of a human language that they did not invent reinforces our understanding that the impact of a new culture, or of cultural evolution, can reveal potentialities of the underlying neural system that would not otherwise have become manifest.

In short, then, the case still stands that commands and "socialization messages" with meanings such as those posited for *grooflook* or *koomzash* could have been crucial elements of protovocabulary. Moreover, such inventions need not have been made with any great frequency. Over deep time (perhaps tens of millennia), protowords were devised for only a sparse set of such situations. Perhaps, at first, at most two or three "frequently occurring situations" would be added to the "nameable" by an entire tribe in any one generation. Only with the development of enough protowords to support fractionation would the roots of protosyntax be formed, yielding a set of localized "constructions" to maintain and—as new protowords come to be used as "slot fillers"—extend the earlier set of meanings. With this, words got categorized by their ability to "fill the slots" in a certain range of constructions. It is the ability for complex imitation that makes these processes possible. In the case of protohumans, this could lead to the invention of new (proto)words and constructions. In the case of the modern child, in a community in which the use of nonholophrastic words and constructions is long-established, it provides the basis for understanding what the community already knows—that sound patterns can be dissected into strings of words and that these words can be grouped by constructions. The constructions become of greater or more focused applicability both on a historical timescale, as new words and constructions are invented over the course of many generations, and on a developmental timescale, as the child has more experience of using fragments of the ambient language to understand and be understood.

The process of fractionation continues even in modern language as words get decomposed to yield new words or word-stems: "helicopter" yields "copter," even though it was formed as "helico + pter (wing)"; "cybernetics" yields "cyber-," even though its etymology involves the stem "cybern-" (as in "govern"); web + log → blog, and kangaroo → roo → roobar (a device on the front of Australian country vehicles for protection in case of a collision with a kangaroo); hamburger (= bun typical of Hamburg) → cheeseburger, veggieburger, and so on.

There is no demand (whether in protolanguage or modern language) that decomposition always occurs, only that it sometimes occurs. The holophrastic hypothesis posits a process that may take many tens of millennia, so there is no requirement that such forces act reliably or with great accuracy. Indeed, languages still beget new languages on a timescale of centuries. Note, however, the difference between processes that occurred before protohumans were cognitively aware of the idea of protolanguage—they had implicit rather than explicit knowledge—and processes occurring in a language-aware, literate society.

Kirby (2000) employed computer simulations to show that statistical extraction of substrings whose meanings stabilize can yield surprisingly powerful results—it is not the odd coincidence but the statistical patterns that yield effects across many generations. However, it seems unlikely that true languages could develop straightforwardly from protolanguages if all "real words" had to be foreshadowed by widely distributed fragments of protowords. I thus see what might be called *the Wray-Kirby mechanism* as part of the answer but not the whole one. We have already discussed the *flying bird* example. Other mechanisms could also produce composite structures. To elaborate upon an example from Chapter 9, a tribe might, over the generations, develop different signs for "sour apple," "ripe apple," "sour plum," "ripe plum," and so on but not have signs for "sour" and "ripe" even though the distinction is behaviorally important. Thus, $2n$ signs are needed to name n kinds of fruit. Occasionally, someone would eat a piece of sour fruit by mistake and make a characteristic face and intake of breath. Eventually, some genius gets the idea of mimicking this act as a warning to some other tribe member that the fruit he is about to eat is sour. If a conventionalized variant of this gesture becomes accepted by the community, then a sign for "sour" has extended the protolanguage. A step toward language is taken when people begin to use the sign for "sour" + the sign for "ripe X" to replace the sign for "sour X" for each kind X of fruit—and then only $n + 1$ words were needed instead of the original $2n$.

I use the word "genius" advisedly. I believe that much work on language evolution has been crippled by the inability to imagine that things we take for granted were in no way a priori obvious, or to see that current generalities were by no means easy to discern in the particularities that they embrace. Consider, for example, that Archimedes (c. 287–212 b.c.e.) had the essential idea of the integral calculus, but that *it took almost 2000 years* before Newton (1642–1727) and Leibniz (1646–1716) found notations that could express the generality implicit in his specific examples, and thus unleash an explosion of mathematical innovation. I contend that (proto)languages, like mathematics, evolved culturally by such fits and starts.

The *sour* story also exemplifies possibilities beyond those suggested by Gentilucci's apple-cherry experiments for the emergence of protospeech on a protosign scaffolding. The posited symbol for *sour* is a vocal-facial gesture, not a manual gesture, and thus could contribute to a process whereby protolanguage began to use protospeech symbols to enrich protosign utterances, after which an increasing number of symbols would have become vocalized, freeing the hands to engage in both praxis and communication as desired by the "speaker." The ability to create novel sounds to match degrees of freedom of manual gestures (we suggested that rising pitch might represent an upward movement of the hand) could have helped create the early vocal repertoire, as would a coevolved ability to imitate novel sound patterns with onomatopoeia—creating symbols that mimic natural sounds, as in "bow-wow" for *bark* or *dog*, or "burble" for the sound of a stream—yielding vocal gestures not linked to manual gestures. However, articulatory gestures alone do not have the rich ad hoc communicative potential that pantomime provides with the manual gesture system. I reiterate the claim that it became easy to share a wide range of meanings once the mirror system for grasping evolved in such a way as to support pantomime, and that the need for disambiguation then created within a community a shared awareness of the use of conventional gestures as well as iconic gestures—whereas onomatopoeia seems to be far more limited in what can be conveyed.

Just as the one word *sour* halves the number of fruit names to be learned, so does fractionation of a holophrase to yield a noun-like element and a verb-like element greatly extend what can be expressed with a limited repertoire of words. Just m "nouns" and n "verbs"—$m + n$ in all—make possible $m*n$ (noun, verb) combinations. The transition to *Homo sapiens* thus may have involved "language amplification" through increased speech ability coupled with the ability to name certain actions and objects separately, then the ability to create a potentially unlimited set of verb-argument structures and the ability to compound those structures in diverse ways. Recognition of hierarchical structure rather than mere sequencing—exploiting the prior praxic capacity to recognize and exploit a hierarchy of subgoals in complex action recognition and complex imitation—provided the bridge to constituent analysis in language.

Nowak et al. (2000) analyzed conditions under which a population that had two genes—one for unitary utterances and one for fractionated utterances—would converge to a situation in which one gene or the other (and thus one type of language or the other) would predominate. But I feel that this misses the whole point: (1) It assumes that there is a genetic basis for this alternative, whereas I believe the basis is historical, without requiring genetic change. (2) It postulates that the alternatives already exist as a basis for the process of selection. I believe it is necessary to offer a serious analysis of how both unitary and fractionated utterances came to exist, and of the *gradual process* of accumulating changes that led from the predominance of the former to the predominance of the latter. (3) Moreover, it is not a matter of either/or—modern languages still make wide use of unitary utterances. However, Nowak et al.'s analysis can become useful if we think of it in the context of cultural rather than biological evolution, giving us a handle on the balancing out of different social schemas, rather than genes, under different patterns of language use.

Just as important as fractionation and the use of "boutique" constructions to reassemble the pieces—with the added power of also assembling similar pieces—is the transition from constructions based on the use of a new word in the protolanguage to generalization across a whole set of constructions. A sign such as that for "sour" could be added to the protovocabulary before any "adjective mechanism" existed. It might take hundreds of such discoveries before someone could regularize their commonalities and invent a general construction with a slot defining the precursor of what we would now call adjectives. Such a construction would be a step toward the emergence of a true language from the protolanguage. However, adjectives are not the "natural category" they may appear to be. As Dixon (1997, p. 142 et seq.) observes, human languages may have either of two kinds of classes of "adjectives": (1) an *open* class with hundreds of members (as in English) or (2) only a small *closed* class. Languages with small adjective classes are found in every continent except Europe. Igbo, from west Africa, has just eight adjectives meaning *large* and *small*; *black/dark* and *white/light*; *new* and *old*; and *good* and *bad*. In such a language, concepts that refer to physical properties tend to be placed in the verb class (e.g., "the stone heavies"), and words referring to human propensities tend to be nouns (e.g., "she has cleverness").

The salient point is that adjectives are a syntactic category—and syntactic categories are, by definition, only available in a form of language that has syntax. Yet we have said that protolanguage does not have syntax and therefore cannot have a category of adjectives. Nouns and verbs are also syntactic categories, so on this account protolanguage would not initially have had nouns or verbs, either. Instead, there would be an increasing number of words for describing objects and other words for describing actions, but these two classes of words would not yet have become unified in terms of two distinct forms of syntactic processing.

As a step that might eventually prove to have been in this direction, semantic categories defined with respect to two different constructions might be merged into a single category to provide a shared set of "slot fillers" for the two constructions, and this would continue as further similarities were observed and generalizations were made. The merging of categories from different constructions—for example, things one might want versus things one might hug—may blur the original semantic cues as to what may enter into the earlier constructions, and so the set of "fillers" for a specific "slot" would no longer be a semantic category, and we must regard it as a syntactic category by default. As a result, my hypothesis is that syntactic categories were an emerging property as protolanguages grew in complexity as measured by the increasing number and generalized applicability of their constructions. Very small grammars became larger and more powerful through the cultural evolution of protolanguages. There was thus no point at which one could say of a tribe "Until now they used protolanguage but henceforth they use language." Rather than positing

(i)   The alingual state → words → syntax (in two huge steps)

I argue for the scenario

(ii) The alingual state → words → words sorted into categories + ways to put words together based on those categories, with words and syntax emerging *together* in a huge number of small interdependent steps → an expanding vocabulary and not only more "idiosyncratic" constructions but also constructions of increasing generality with the consequent emergence of broad syntactic categories.

These are mechanisms whereby the virtues of a compositional description might emerge—with the consequent demand for a range of constructions to disambiguate combinations once the combinatorics began to explode. The spread of these innovations rested on the ability of other humans not only to imitate the new actions and compounds of actions demonstrated by the innovators but also to do so in a way that related increasingly general classes of symbolic behavior to the classes, events, behaviors, and relationships that they were to represent. Indeed, consideration of the spatial basis for "prepositions" may help show how visuomotor coordination underlies some aspects of language (cf. Talmy, 2000), while the immense variation in the use of corresponding prepositions even in closely related languages—English speakers go *to* the city, whereas Italian speakers go *at* the city (*á citta*)—shows how whatever basic functionally grounded semantic-syntactic correspondences might have constituted the primitive meaning of a given preposition have long been overlaid by a multitude of later innovations and borrowings. Protolanguages provided increasingly many names for classes of objects, actions, situations, commands, greetings, and more, but none of these demanded (on the holophrastic account) a preexisting stock of words from which they were composed.

Phonology Emerging

Duality of patterning (Chapter 2) refers to the patterning of language at two levels:

(i) meaningless elements (e.g., syllables or phonemes in speech; hand shapes and motions in sign languages) are combined into meaningful elements (morphemes and words); and
(ii) these elements are combined into larger meaningful units, which may themselves be subject to further meaningful combination.

I will use the term "phonology" for the system described as level (i). The examples make clear that the term makes no commitment to the type of meaningless units involved. We have just discussed various mechanisms whereby predominantly holophrastic protolanguages could have become more and more compositional. But where did phonology come from? Hockett (1960, p. 95) observes:

There is excellent reason to believe that duality of patterning was the last property to be developed [in the evolution of language], because one can find little if any reason why a communicative system should have this property unless it is highly complicated. If a vocal-auditory system comes to have a larger and larger number of distinct meaningful elements, those elements inevitably come to be more and more similar to one another in sound. There is a practical limit [. . .] to the number of distinct stimuli that can be discriminated [. . .].

We may vary the pantomime of opening a door as much as our hand-shape may vary to accommodate different handles and their movement, and with many further variations. Conventionalization of such a pantomime into protosign will capture aspects of one, or just a few, of the many possible performances rather than being built from constituents. Similarly, the early utterances of protospeech might echo the movements of a protosign; or come closer to the vocalization of a cat than the "meow" that invokes the phonology of English. I would agree, then, with Hockett, while adding another modality: "If a gestural-visual system comes to have a larger and larger number of distinct meaningful elements, those elements inevitably come to be more and more similar to one another in appearance." This too would provide the pressure for segmenting protowords into pieces which could then be replaced by an increasingly conventionalized system of "meaningless units" of the kind listed in (i) earlier.

However, duality of patterning need not be the last property to be developed, since there is nothing in the aforementioned argument that rests on the complexity, or even the existence, of *syntax*. All that is required is the existence of so large a (proto)lexicon that words run the risk of confusion without the invocation of some form of (vocal or manual) phonology. Note, too, that the use of phonology need not be all or none. Rather, it would at first be piecemeal, as efforts were made to better discriminate the production of similar protowords with distinct meanings. This might lead to a stage in which many protowords were at least, in part, "nonphonological" while meaningless units were exuberantly overgenerated in further conventionalization of other protowords. But this would set the stage for a process wherein the stock of these units would be winnowed, while more and more units would be reduced to "phonological form."

A major theme earlier was to argue for a spectrum of protolanguages increasing in complexity, rather than for one stable protolanguage. A possible sequence of protolanguage development over tens or thousands of generations might involve (a) attaining a vocabulary of perhaps a hundred protowords without phonotactic structure; (b) beginning to develop "phonemes" both to solidify chance similarities and to make it easier to distinguish utterances;

and then (c) an expanding spiral of increasing (proto)vocabulary and better defined phonotactic structure until the latter gets locked in.

As we saw in Chapter 9, MacNeilage (1998) proposed that various phonological "gestures" emerged from the opening and closing of the primate jaw, making it possible to get consonants and vowels. The lexicon then grew in tandem with the emerging set of consonant and vowel segments. But where is the adaptive pressure for "phonological evolution" unless one already has an open set of vocalizations whose semantic range can be expanded by developing consonants and vowels? I argued that a stock of protowords must be in place—and the set must be expanding—to provide the "pressure" for developing a phonological inventory. It may well be that the development of an articulatory system adequate to the demands of (proto)language phonology involved a Baldwin effect (see "Evolution is Subtle" in Chapter 6) in which case it is a challenge to understand which changes were "Baldwinian" and which were historical in nature.

Even Abstract Language Has Roots in Embodiment

Our introduction of *Beyond the Here and Now* (Properties 6 and 10 of "Protolanguage Versus Language" in Chapter 6) made two points:

1. Language involves many powerful devices that extend the range of communication but that might not be considered as touchstones to the definition of language. Thus, if one took a human language and removed all reference to time, one might still want to call it a language rather than a protolanguage, even though one would agree that it was thereby greatly impoverished. Similarly, the number system of a language can be seen as a useful, but not definitive, supplemental tool. Nonetheless, the ability to talk about past and future is a central part of human languages as we understand them.
2. These features of language would be meaningless (literally) without the underlying cognitive machinery—in this case the substrate for episodic memory provided by the hippocampus and the substrate for planning provided by frontal cortex (Chapter 5). Thus, the neurolinguist must not only seek to learn from the syntactic perspective how time is expressed in a variety of languages but also seek to understand how these verbal structures are linked to the cognitive structures that give them meaning and, thus, presumably, grounded their evolution—irrespective of what autonomy the syntactic structures may have when severed from the contingencies of communication.

Suddendorf and Corballis (2007) have examined this ability to go beyond the here and now under the heading of "mental time travel." Noting that memory systems differ in the degree of flexibility they offer, they argue that similar flexibility of mechanisms allowing prediction of future situations provided a crucial selective advantage—arguing further that the adaptive advantage of the various memory systems depends on what they contribute for future survival. They see episodic memory as the most flexible part of a more general network supporting mental time travel, stressing that its ability to "go back in time" is crucial to our ability, with varying accuracy, to foresee, plan, and shape future events. This selective advantage is immensely strengthened as language provides more and more expressive tools to share these memories and plans as humans in a given group work together toward some common end.

I have suggested that syntactic structures are scaffolded on preexisting understanding of object-action schemas. But most sentences (like this one) do not describe action-object events. Explanation of the full range of sentence structures is more the task of historical and comparative linguistics and cognitive grammar than of an action-oriented linguistics, evolutionary or otherwise. However, a critique of an argument of Bickerton (1995) may indicate why I think that the transition from object-action frames to verb-argument structures may be seen as grounding the development of sentences of increasing abstraction.

Bickerton (1995, p.22) notes that a sentence like "The cat sat on the mat" is far more abstract than the image of a particular cat sitting on a particular mat. An image does not bring in the sense of time distinguishing "The cat sat on the mat" from "The cat is sitting on the mat" or "The cat will sit on the mat" (note how various conditions "beyond the here and now" are expressed in these sentences, yet their meaning relates to the same remembered or imagined experience). An image does not distinguish "The cat is sitting on the mat" from "The mat is underneath the cat." All this is true, and we must reflect these distinctions in characterizing language. For example, we might relate the focus of a sentence (where prosody plays a crucial role not obvious in the written words) to the focus of attention in vision. However, Bickerton creates a false dichotomy when he asserts that "it is not true that we build a picture of the world and dress it out in language. Rather, language builds us the picture of the world that we use in thinking and communicating." The idea that language builds our picture of the world—rather than contributing to its richness—is misguided for it ignores the role of visual experience and then of *episodic memory* (linking episodes in temporal and other relationships) and *expectations* in building the rich perceptions and cognitions (cognitive form) of which sentences (phonological form) are just a précis. There is no claim that the relationship is one to one. Bickerton's approach leaves little room for understanding how the ability to *mean* that a cat is on the mat could be acquired in the first place. The state of the individual's schema network is vastly richer than a linear sequence of words. This does not deny that language can express what pictures cannot, or vice versa. Perception is *not* invertible—even if I see an actual cat on an actual mat, I am unlikely to recall more than a few details (consider the transition from an actual scene to a semantic representation of a few salient agents, objects, and relations, and from that to a verbal description, as set forth briefly in "A Visually Grounded Version of Construction Grammar" in Chapter 2). And what one sees is knowledge based: for example, a familiar cat versus a generic cat, or recognizing a specific subspecies. There is an intimate relation between naming and categorization.

But let's get more abstract. Bickerton (1995, p. 22–24) argues that one cannot picture "My trust in you has been shattered forever by your unfaithfulness" because no picture could convey the uniquely hurtful sense of betrayal the act of infidelity provokes if you did not know what trust was, or what unfaithfulness was, or what it meant for trust to be shattered. "In the case of trust or unfaithfulness, there can be nothing beneath the linguistic concept except other linguistic representations, because abstract nouns have no perceptual attributes to be attached to them and therefore no possible representation outside those areas of the brain devoted to language." However, the words themselves (i.e., the sequences of letters on the page or spoken phonemes) do not convey "the uniquely hurtful sense of betrayal." For this we require that they "hook into" an appropriate body of experience and association, which not all people will share—each word is the tip of the schema iceberg. Words must link into the network that itself links to nonverbal experience, both perceptual and behavioral (cf. the discussion of a person's knowledge as a "schema encyclopedia" in Chapter 2). But, of course, this does not entail that we cannot understand a sentence if we have not personally experienced what it is about. The power of compositional semantics is that we can put words together to create novel meanings (e.g., "a clown balancing a 3 foot high skyscraper constructed entirely of blue ice cream on the end of his nose"). We also come to understand words through inductive experience of hearing or seeing those words used in sentences linked to diverse contexts. But in the end, certain words must be grounded in embodied experiences as must some, at least, of the contexts that give meaning to an entire utterance to yield (by a process akin to complex imitation) a fragment of the meaning of a novel word.

Given this, an image (whether static like a picture, or extended in time like a video clip) may tap into a similar network of experience. Consider a scene from a movie of one person turning away with an expression of disillusionment and despair from the sight of another engaged in lovemaking. The words and the images have complementary strengths—the words make explicit the key relationships, and the image provides a host of details that could be only supplied (if indeed they were deemed relevant) by the piling on of more and more sentences.

If one recalls a beautiful sunset, then it may be that "The sunset where we saw the green flash at Del Mar" will *index* the scene in one's own thoughts or for communication with others, but the words alone do not recapture the beauty of the scene by forming an image of the setting and the colors of the sky.

Many would argue that one does not fully understand "hurtful sense of betrayal" unless one to some extent feels something of the emotion concerned, a feeling that involves a multiplicity of brain regions unlinked to language (see our brief discussion of the possible role of a mirror system in human empathy in Chapter 5) and the memory of particular unhappy episodes of one's own experience.

As an exercise, let me try to link the sentence "My trust in you has been shattered forever by your unfaithfulness" back to the schema network anchored in action and perception. I look at the definitions of the words and see how they are—eventually—rooted in behavior, noting the necessary role of metaphor (more on this in the next section) in the use of "shattered," and in the use of "your" to indicate both possession of an object and possession of a disposition.

My trust in you is rooted in the schema *A trusts B*, which expresses something like the behavioral disposition of A toward B that "If B tells A that C is the case, then A acts on the assumption that C is true." I do *not* argue that my mental states are rigidly constrained by such a definition. Rather, the above definition is shorthand for a whole range of behaviors and expectations that constitute "trusting."

B is faithful to A is defined socially by a set of behaviors *prescribed* and *proscribed* for B by nature of his or her relationship to A. Infidelity is then detected by, perhaps, repeated failure in a prescribed behavior or, possibly, even one example of strongly proscribed behavior.

That an object is *broken* is, in the grounding case, testable either perceptually (the recognizable structure has been disrupted) or behaviorally (the object does not behave in the expected way). *Repairing* is acting upon a broken object in such a way as to make it look or perform as it is expected to. An object is *shattered* if it is broken into many pieces—in such a way that we can recognize that repairing the damage (making the object functional again) would be difficult or impossible. Clearly, metaphorical extension is at work here—an important bridge from the embodied to the abstract.

Shattered forever then asserts that repair is impossible—there is no set of operations such that at any future time the object will function again, introducing the element of time and the *semantic extension of schemas from the here and now of action and perception*. But note, too, that *planning* and *expectations* are implicit in behavior. Moreover, our notions of future time rest on extrapolation from our experience of past times in relation to the expectations we held at even earlier times.

Having said all this, note the many "inventions" required to go, historically, from simple wants and actions to a language + thought system rich enough to express the aforementioned sentence; and note, too, *the long path a child must go through in coming to understand what these words mean.* Of course, the path (another metaphor) sketched earlier does not begin to exhaust the meaning of the sentence, and this can only be done by consideration of the embodied self. To say my "trust is shattered" also implies a state of emotional devastation that needs the empathy of another human to be fully understood.

This account is little more than a caricature, but it serves to reinforce the view that the use of language is rooted in our experience of action within the world, enriched by our ability to recall past events or imagine future ones and expanded by the cultural history of our society as reflected in our own personal experience as embodied and social beings. Yes, language gains its richness by giving access to new meanings made possible by the compositional semantics of previously available words, but only in some cases can a dictionary definition exhaust the novel meaning. Thus, while many linguists follow Chomsky in seeing an autonomous syntax as the essence of language, I argue that neither the cultural evolution of language nor the child's acquisition of language—new words, new constructions, and the ways we use them in communication—can be divorced from the embodied experience of language and cognition in their mutual interaction.

The Role of Metaphor

As indicated by this last example, the genius of language is that it supports metaphorical extension whereby words and constructions gain meaning in new domains yet may remain intelligible because they can be linked step by step back to earlier domains of discourse (from *shattered trust* back to *shattered object*)—until in time these new uses may themselves become conventionalized. Our discussion of the "awful" St. Paul's highlighted the dynamics of meaning-change. On first exposure, such dynamics seem implausible—if words are continually changing their meanings and gain their meaning within large schema networks that may differ from individual to individual, how can we hope to communicate? The answer is that we can usually isolate the effects of meaning change in parts of the semantic network and ignore them or pull them in as necessary for sufficient understanding. And, of course, understanding is rarely perfect, but we usually (alas, not always) ask for clarification before much damage is done by a particular failure to understand what another is saying.

Searle (1979, p. 132), in his book *Expression and Meaning*, distinguishes the "literal meaning" of a sentence from its "utterance meaning." Literal meaning is entirely determined by the fixed meanings of words and the syntactic rules of the language; utterance meaning is a local and variable matter, depending on speaker's intentions on particular occasions. However, an analysis of metaphor suggests that even in the absence of contextual knowledge, the notion that words have fixed meanings from which the literal meaning of a sentence can be constructed is, at best, a limiting case. Thus, following Arbib and Hesse (1986), I argue for a nonliteralist theory of meaning and metaphor that is compatible with an account of language as rooted in the dynamics of schemas.

The *Oxford English Dictionary* defines a metaphor as "the figure of speech in which a name or descriptive term is transferred to some object different from, but analogous to, that to which it is *properly* applicable." (My italics.) For example, physical "point" is transferred to denote a quality of an argument or a joke. But what is this notion of "proper"? It suggests that there really is some "universal concept" defined quite apart from the usage of a particular human group and that the "proper" use of the word was its association with just one such a priori concept. An alternative can be found in Wittgenstein's (1953) notion of a *family resemblance* in which (for example, "the Churchill nose") enough pairs of objects in the class resemble each other in some relevant respects so that these resemblances can form as it were a chain-like structure. Thus, a particular pair of members of the class may themselves have little resemblance so long as they are connected by intermediaries on a chain in which adjacent elements do resemble each other. One may look for family resemblances in other groupings, such as Roman archeological remains, psychological types, schools of painting, and so on. When words are used metaphorically, exactly the same process of meaning chains is at work. The "point" of a joke shares with the "point" of a pin some of its physiological effects; the "point" of an argument shares some properties with the point of a joke, and some with the point of a pin, but not necessarily the same ones. Indeed, language of necessity must contain general terms that classify together objects that are in detail different. As John Locke (1690, Bk. III, Ch. III, pp. 2 and 3) put it, "it is impossible that every particular thing should have a distinct peculiar name ... Men would in vain heap up names of particular things, that would not serve them to communicate their thoughts."

We thus hold that language works by capturing *approximate* meanings, with degrees of similarity and difference sufficiently accessible to perception to avoid confusion in ordinary usage. Who bothers to discriminate *every* potential shade of red by a descriptive term, even if one is an artist or gardener or house decorator? Within this perspective, metaphorical shifts of meaning depending on similarities and differences between objects are pervasive in language, not deviant, and some of the mechanisms of metaphor are essential to the meaning of any descriptive language whatever. Hesse and I captured this in the slogan that "all language is metaphorical."

But what then of the sorts of relative distinction we normally make between what we call the literal and the metaphorical? *Literal* use enshrines the use that is most frequent or familiar. It is the easiest to manage, to learn, and to teach—but what is easy to teach in one society may be more than obscure in another, so that even English-speaking children raised in different societies may regard different meanings as the literal one. Thus, when and where I was a child, the radio in the living room was referred to as "the wireless" and so reference to this concrete object in our living room gave "wireless" what was for me its literal meaning, long before my understanding that the original literal meaning of the word was "without wires," based on the notion that sound was transferred electronically from the broadcasting studio with no wires to bridge from there to our house. The literal meaning—as in the case of the wireless in the living room—is often susceptible to ostensive definition, but as such it depends on the environment in which "ostension" can occur. The (culturally contingent) literal meaning is the one generally put first in dictionary entries, where it is followed by comparatively "dead" metaphors ("point" of a pin probably comes before "point" of an argument), and more novel "live" metaphors may be omitted altogether. All this makes clear why the analysis of metaphor apparently has to start from "literal" language already understood, but it does not in the least imply that the semantic bases for the two sorts of expressions are radically different.

When a metaphor becomes entrenched in a language, it may become simply a new literal usage as in "spirits" for whisky, "leaves" for the pages of a book, or "fiery" for a person's temperament. In fact, almost any interesting descriptive term can be shown etymologically to be a dead metaphor—a fact that supports our family resemblance analysis, once the orthodox distinction between "literal" and "metaphorical" is discarded and "dead metaphors" are accepted as being pervasive in language. The thesis that "all language is metaphorical" highlights the fact that explicit use of metaphor and simile are themselves based on the most fundamental linguistic fact of all, namely that linguistic reference always depends on perceived similarities and differences.

Lakoff and Johnson (1980, p. 4) examined many examples of extended metaphors in language such as "Argument is war" revealed by such phrases as "Your claims are *indefensible*," "He *attacked every weak point* in my argument," and "His criticisms were *right on target*." Or consider the alternative metaphor that "Argument is negotiation," with its accompanying "Can we meet each other on common ground?" "What compromises are possible?" and "I cannot sacrifice my most basic assumptions." There is no "fact" to which "argument" corresponds that has the natural character of "war" or "negotiation." The extended metaphors are not in that sense true or false but are appropriate or inappropriate, more or less revealing, more or less useful, depending on the context of application and their coherence with evaluative judgments made about particular situations. Meaning is constituted by a network, and metaphor forces us to look at the intersections and interaction of different parts of the network. In terms of the metaphor, we can find and express deeper analogies between diverse phenomena. Unfortunately, of course, in the case of bad metaphors we may find that we are misled by them.

It may be possible as a first approximation to describe the developed use of language by a compositional semantics in which we explain how the words fit together to provide sentences. But in the acquisition of language, and in describing language change, we must proceed in the reverse direction as well. We can only give meanings to novel word uses if we can grasp the sense of the overall sentences in which they are used, and we have enough information about other portions of that sentence *and its context and associations* to make some reasonable hypothesis about their new roles. As we noted in *The Parable of the Parma Painting* in Chapter 1, inferring the meaning of an utterance of language need not be a simple, direct translation from "syntactic form" to "semantic form" but may be an active process calling on diverse knowledge sources to negotiate what appears to be a satisfactory interpretation. We may use our *estimate* of the overall meaning of an utterance to *guess* the meaning of a novel word therein, possibly guided by the internal structure of the word— but also guided by the social interaction (recall *The Story of the Stairs*) within which the utterance is embedded. Today, we can often catch a new word in the web of words we already know—whereas in our more distant past it was pantomime that helped establish a new protoword. But even now, interaction with the physical world may be necessary to go from a verbal definition to a rich understanding of what indeed a new word means. Just try to define cat to a child.

Parity Revisited

To close this chapter, let's circle back to two items, reproduced here in somewhat edited form, from our discussion of criteria for language readiness in Chapter 6:

Symbolization: The ability to associate symbols (communicative actions) with an open class of episodes, objects, or praxic actions.

Parity: What counts for the speaker (or producer of one or more symbols) must count, frequently, as approximately the same for the listener (or receiver).

At first, the symbols may have been unitary utterances (holophrases), rather than words in the modern sense, and they may have been based on manual and facial gestures rather than being vocalized. The idea of openness here is that symbols are no longer innate, and that members of a community can invent and share new means for the exchange of ideas and social cues. The parity principle for communicative actions is reminiscent of the role of the *mirror neurons* for grasping and other actions discovered in the macaque brain—such a neuron fires both when the monkey executes a specific action and when it sees a human or other monkey performing a similar action. We have charted a key role for complex action recognition and imitation for the "lifting" of these two properties from protolanguage to language.

What then of the claim that "all language is metaphorical"? Don't the properties of symbolization and parity imply that each symbol has a fixed meaning, and that mirror neurons support parity by allowing the mental state of a speaker (or signer) generating the symbol to be uniquely decoded by the hearer to register the intended meaning? No. All that is required for parity is that the meaning inferred by the hearer is *close enough* to that intended by the speaker *often enough* that there is an overall increase in the utility of their interactions because those symbols are available. This "close enough" may relate to delight in some shared social situation; it may have the purpose of directing attention to some interesting aspect of the environment; or it may serve to coordinate action to mutual benefit or, in cases of altruism, to the immediate benefit of just one person. In addition, we have stressed that mirror neurons are formed through learning, so that what activates corresponding mirror neurons in a community may depend on both physical and social interactions yet vary somewhat between individuals.

But we are in danger of falling into the trap here of thinking that a mirror neuron for a symbol encodes the meaning of that symbol. But that is not the case, as can be seen by recalling Figure 8-3 in Chapter 8. There we distinguished:

- the mirror system—comprising both the appropriate mirror and canonical neurons—for neurally encoding the *signifier* (the symbol as an articulatory gesture, whether spoken or signed), from
- the linkage of the sign to the neural schema for the *signified* (the concept, situation, action, or object to which the signifier refers), such as the perceptual schemas of the VISIONS system of Chapter 1.

Parity between speaker and hearer is thus a two-fold process: It rests on the hearer both recognizing what word-as–a-phonological-entity the speaker produced as well as having sufficient experience related to that of the speaker for the schema assemblage elicited by that recognition to more or less match the speaker's intentions. And, as we have seen, this interpretation (induced schema assemblage) will be swayed by context and may result from dynamic processes in the hearer's schema network that take him or her well beyond any direct "literal" meaning.

Moreover, we have placed much emphasis in this chapter on the implications of complex action recognition and imitation in going beyond the use of single words to assemblages built up through the hierarchical application of constructions in such a way that a multiword utterance built up using the constructions of the language's grammar can induce understanding in the hearer in such a way that parity is more or less preserved. Preliminary efforts to express this in computational terms were sketched in "A Visually Grounded Version of Construction Grammar" in Chapter 2. Let us relate this to the way in which both the dorsal and ventral streams in primate cortex are able to marshal perceptual schemas to provide a working model of the state of the organism in relation to its world that can be used as a basis of action.

In discussing the "what" and "how" pathways of Figure 4-4 in Chapter 4, I suggested that the perceptual and motor schemas of the dorsal stream include highly parameterized information adequate for the detailed control of action, whereas the ventral stream has a range of schemas more closely linked to *understanding* a situation and thus marshaling a wide range of information to decide on a course of action. The success of the organism requires close integration of the two systems (as exemplified in the FARS model, Fig. 4-11)—the well-controlled execution of an action is useless unless the planning of an action has determined the extent to which, in the current circumstances, it is desirable (as determined by planning via the ventral system) and executable (as determined by the assessment of affordances by the dorsal system).

As just noted (recalling Fig. 8-3), Saussure's (1916) analysis of language distinguished the signifier from the signified. When we see or hear a word we can look at it as form, the *signifier*, devoid of meaning. We can simply write or pronounce it *as an action* and recognize a similar action made by others, as indeed we do for nonwords like *gosklarter*. However, in normal language use, the motor act is linked to a meaning, the *signified*. Thus, a French speaker saying *cheval* and an English speaker saying *horse* have in mind the same kind of equine quadruped to serve as the signified. We now go further to discuss the linkage of neurons encoding the signifier to neurons encoding the signified, though a less precise terminology will often be employed. As Hurford (2004) notes, only those concepts that relate to actions that the self can perform should be expected to correspond to mirror neurons *for the actions themselves*, and relatively few words are associated with such concepts. This may at first sight seem to run counter to any approach to grounding language mechanisms in a system rooted in mirror neurons. The resolution is to stress that *the Mirror System Hypothesis views mirror neurons for words as encoding the signifier but not in general the signified.* Mirror neurons *for words* encode the articulatory form (or written form, or gestural form in a signed language) but must be linked to other neural networks for the encoding of meaning. Thus, the mirror system for language can be involved in the execution and recognition of a signifier, for example, *parliament*, without any requirement that it signifies an action in the speaker or hearer's repertoire.

Does this mean that we must each have mirror neurons for the tens of thousands of words in our vocabulary, so that learning a new word requires training new neurons? Not if one interprets this as requiring that each word have an associated set of neurons that fire when and only when that specific word is heard or uttered. But recall the assertion ("Introducing Mirror Neurons," Chapter 5) that, rather than viewing each mirror neuron as coding for a single action, it seems more plausible to regard mirror neurons as, to the extent that their activity correlates with actions, doing so as a *population code* with each neuron expressing a "confidence level" that some feature of a possible action—such as the relation of thumb to forefinger, or of wrist relative to object—is present in the current action. As such, hearing a novel word may link to its pronunciation on an effortful phoneme-by-phoneme basis, but to run the word trippingly off the tongue requires practice, as does the linkage of the unique population code for the word to the encoding of the signified—and even more synaptic change is required if a novel signification must be learned. Such population coding may help explain why hearing a word may elicit associations not only with words that sound similar, but also with a variety of related meanings, so that context may strongly modulate the processes of competition and cooperation that elicit the particular meaning we extract from an overall utterance on a particular occasion.

With this, consider Figure 10-1. The lowest box corresponds to concepts/ signifieds. The middle box is a *dorsal* stream, including a mirror system for articulatory expression (signifiers in the form of words-as-motor-entities), which, we claim, evolved from (but is not coextensive with) the mirror system for grasping (the top box). Together, the two lower boxes serve communication integrating hand, face, and voice. The lowest box shows concepts for diverse actions, objects, attributes, and abstractions are represented by a *ventral* network of concepts-as-schemas stored in long-term memory (with our current "conceptual content" formed as an assemblage of schema instances in working memory). Analogously, the "Mirror for Words" contains a network of word forms in long-term memory and keeps track of the current utterance in its own working memory (recall Fig. 2-11 in Chapter 2).

What may be surprising is that the arrow linking the "Mirror for Actions" to the "Mirror for Words" in Figure 10-1 expresses an evolutionary relationship, not a flow of data. Rather than a direct linkage of the dorsal representation of

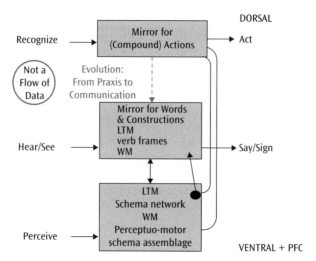

FIGURE 10-1.   Words as signifiers (articulatory actions) link to signifieds (schemas for the corresponding concepts), not directly to the dorsal path for actions. The basic scheme is enriched by compound actions and constructions. LTM, long-term memory; PFC, prefrontal cortex; WM, working memory. (Based on Figure 4 from Arbib, 2006b).

the action to the dorsal representation of the articulatory form, we have two relationships between the dorsal pathway for the "Mirror for Actions" and the schema networks and assemblages of the ventral pathway and prefrontal cortex. The rightmost path of Figure 10-1 corresponds to the connections whereby inferotemporal cortex and prefrontal cortex can affect the pattern of dorsal control of action (recall the FARS model from Fig. 4-11 in Chapter 4). The path just to the left of this shows that the dorsal representation of actions can only be linked to verbs via ventral schemas. This general scheme might be supplemented by direct connections in those special cases when the word does indeed represent an action in the person's own repertoire, but there are scant data on how generally such connections might occur.

The dorsal-ventral division shown in Figure 10-1 is reminiscent of that postulated by Hickok and Poeppel (2004) in their analysis of cortical stages of speech perception. The early stages involve auditory fields in the superior temporal gyrus bilaterally (although asymmetrically), but this cortical processing system then diverges into two streams:

- A *dorsal stream* mapping sound onto articulatory-based representations, which projects dorso-posteriorly. It involves a region in the posterior Sylvian fissure at the parietal–temporal boundary (area Spt) and ultimately projects to frontal regions. This network provides a mechanism for the development and maintenance of "parity" between auditory and motor representations of speech.

• A *ventral stream* mapping sound onto meaning, which projects ventro-laterally toward inferior posterior temporal cortex (posterior middle temporal gyrus) that serves as an interface between sound-based representations of speech in the superior temporal gyrus (again bilaterally) and widely distributed conceptual representations.

An experience my wife had shortly after arriving in California from Australia may illustrate the distinction. She had to take a hearing test and, much to her indignation, failed. She asked the doctor to explain, because she believed her hearing was fine. The test required her to listen to a series of words and repeat each one after she heard it. She had proceeded by using the ventral stream, recognizing each word, then repeating it in her own accent (compare the indirect pathways via the lexicon or praxicon in Fig. 7-4 in Chapter 7)—and the doctor had graded her as incorrect when the American and Australian pronunciation did not match. Understanding this, she took the test again, doing her best to fake the pronunciation she had heard (dorsal stream; direct pathway), and aced the test.

Our ability to generate and recognize complex actions (and the mobilization of these skills in complex imitation) takes us beyond the mere perception and articulation of words, to underpin the ability to mobilize words and constructions to generate and recognize utterances that capture aspects of the brain's schema networks that embody our knowledge and understanding, and our perception, memories, and plans for the future.

One must not conflate how processes operate in modern languages already equipped with a range of abstract syntactic categories and function words with what we try to infer was their operational mode when protolanguages emerged with increasing complexity. Based on the aforementioned analysis of constructions and bricolage, I have argued that protolanguage did not start with any set of universal syntactic categories, whether nouns and verbs or others. Rather, constructions initially yielded semantic categories, but as these were generalized they lost their semantic moorings. In the next chapter we will look briefly at how a modern child now acquires language to chart both commonalities and differences with the experiences of our ancestors as languages emerged from protolanguages. In Chapter 13, we will study the process of *grammaticalization*, which still operates in language change, suggesting that it began to operate as soon as there were constructions to operate upon, helping to create a variety of constructions as protolanguages became more complex and languages began to emerge.

11

How the Child Acquires Language

We have now seen the key process whereby languages got started. The emergence constructions at first imposed semantic categories on the proliferating words of an emerging lexicon, and constructions themselves became subject to processes of merging, generalization, and extension. As a result, word categories became increasingly divorced from the semantic moorings defined by filling the slots of very specific simple constructions and instead became increasingly syntactic as they expanded to fill the slots of the more general constructions. This chapter complements the preceding account by looking at present-day language acquisition to see how processes that were operative in getting language started may still apply as children come to master the language that is already around them. In Chapter 12, we will look at how the same processes may underlie what happens when a community of deaf people, and the speaking people with whom they interact, invents a whole new sign language in the course of just two or three generations. Then, in Chapter 13, we will look at processes of historical change that have shaped and changed languages in recent centuries.

Each of these three chapters gives a very brief sample of topics whose treatment could occupy many volumes. Our aim is not comprehensiveness but, rather, to introduce ways to use available data as a basis for assessing what capabilities the language-ready brain must possess to support the processes seen in language acquisition, language emergence, and language change, seeing how these support our claims about the processes established through biological evolution that make possible the transition from protolanguages to languages charted in the previous chapter.

Language Acquisition and the Development of Constructions

For most children, learning language is inseparable from learning about the world and how to interact with it—the child learns what actions each object makes possible (the *affordances* of the object; i.e., a bottle is to grasp and to drink from at the same time as she is extending her set of *effectivities*, the basic repertoire of actions on which further actions may be based through interaction with those around her). The child learning to talk (or sign) is also learning the functional significance of the environment (objects, events, physical layout/ place), and this is inseparable from opportunities for action. In some cases, the child will learn actions before learning words for them; in other cases the child may recognize actions and the words for them long before (if ever) she masters the actions herself (as in *bird flies*). Her range of effectivities expands as she gains skill by participating in new activities; and this is accompanied by a growing understanding that her body is like that of others, and thus that she may learn to do what the caregiver does to achieve similar benefits or avoid risks. At an early stage, caregivers direct attention to give infants crucial practice in what to notice and do and when to do it, though the extent of such explicit guidance varies from culture to culture ("A Cooperative Framework" in Chapter 7). Moreover, these activities enable the child to grasp important prerequisites for communicating with language—such as knowing that words refer, that words have an effect on the receiver of a message, and that caregiver and child may achieve a (more or less) shared understanding of ongoing events. All this corresponds to the properties of symbolization, intended communication, and parity that were established as criteria for language readiness in Chapter 6.

Children can learn certain things for themselves by trial and error. However, by directing the child's attention to her own effectivities in relation to affordances in the environment (and helping the child acquire new ones), the caregiver greatly narrows the search space for learning and consequently enhances the speed and extent of learning. We defined *complex action recognition* as the ability to recognize another's performance as a set of familiar movements designed to achieve specific subgoals, and *complex imitation* as the ability to use this as the basis for flexible imitation of the observed behavior. This extends to the ability to recognize that such a performance combines novel actions that can be approximated by (i.e., more or less crudely imitated by) variants of actions already in the repertoire. The young child is acquiring the basis for these skills as she develops a basic set of actions and a basic set of composition techniques (of which forming a two-element sequence is perhaps the simplest).

It requires several years for a child endowed with the neural mechanisms of a normal human brain and interacting within a human language community to become fluent in a specific language. Let me turn to one specific model of language acquisition to exemplify the way in which individuals may come to interiorize the social schemas that define the community to which they belong.[1] To this I add that the very diversity of human language makes it clear that, whatever the extent of biologically based universals that may unite human languages, most of what defines any specific language is rooted in a cultural, rather than biological, process of historical evolution. How does the child extract patterns from the utterances of a community of mutually intelligible speakers to form the schemas that interiorize her own version of the language?

In describing language acquisition we stress communication as primary and note that it leads to development of a system whose regularities can be *described* by a grammar regardless of whether that grammar plays a causal role in the mechanisms of language production and perception. The model of language acquisition due to Jane Hill (Arbib, Conklin, & Hill, 1987; Arbib & Hill, 1988; Hill, 1983) starts not from innate syntactic categories and constraints but from the observation that the child wants to communicate and likes to repeat sounds at first and, later, words and sentences. Hill modeled data she had gathered from a 2-year-old child, recording how the child interiorizes fragments of what she hears to build what we would now call constructions, based on the child's current concerns and interests. Over time some constructions merge with others, some fall into disuse, some gain complexity, and the lexicon grows and is categorized in tandem with the development of these constructions. However, and this accords well with our schema-theoretic basis (Bartlett, 1932), when a 2-year-old child "repeats" a sentence, she does not repeat the sentence word for word, nor does she omit words at random. Rather, the child's behavior is consistent with the hypothesis that she already has some schemas in her head and that an active schema-based process is involved in assimilating the input sentences and generating the simplified repetitions. Recalling Figure 10-1, note that we may distinguish the perceptual and motor schemas that are encoded in the brain as signifieds from the neural encoding of the signifiers by constructions that may encode concepts as lexical items or specify ways to hierarchically construct an utterance (recall also Figs. 2-10, 2-11, and 2-12 in Chapter 2).

Hill studied Claire, a 2-year-old girl responding to adult sentences, once a week for 9 weeks to provide a specific database to balance the general findings in the literature. Intriguingly, Claire's utterances changed every week. There was no such thing as "2-year old language" to be given one lumped model. Rather, since the child was different every week, the model had to be one of microchanges, in the sense that every sentence could possibly change the child's internal structures. This is "neo-Piagetian" in that it builds on Piaget's ideas of schema change (Piaget, 1952; see "Schema Theory in Historical Perspective" in Chapter 1), but it analyzes it at a fine level, rather than in terms of fixed stages that the child must go through. At birth the child already has many complex neural networks in place that provide "innate schemas" that enable the child to suckle, to grasp, to breathe, to excrete, to feel pain and discomfort, and so to learn that to continue a certain action in some circumstances and to discontinue another action in others is pleasurable. Once the child begins to acquire new schemas, she changes the information environment of old schemas so that they can change in turn. As noted in Chapter 7, there is no fixed set of "primitive actions"—schemas that are "basic" at one stage of life may disappear as they become subsumed in schemas that see more frequent use at a later stage.

Certainly, language rests on some innate substrate (whatever it is that makes the human brain language-ready). And we know that language is degraded in specific ways when there is damage to certain portions of the brain. What is at issue is to determine what is the initial structure that the (highly adaptive) substrate of the brain gives to the child. Does it give her the concept of noun and verb, does it give her certain universal principles and parameters, or does it give, rather, the ability to abstract sound patterns (or gestural patterns) and to associate such patterns with other types of visual stimulation or patterns of action? Hill's model suggests that, at least for certain limited portions of a child's linguistic development, general mechanisms of schema change can yield an increasing richness of language without building upon language universals of the kind postulated in Chomsky's Universal Grammar.[2]

Initially, the child will use only a single word, but the word may well serve as a holophrase—a whole utterance whose pieces have no separate meaning for the child. Thus, the sound patterns that we write as *want milk* and *milk* may have the identical meaning that the child wants milk—but at a stage where the child has no meaning for *milk* save as part of the consummatory act that it involves (and certainly no general concept of *consummatory act!*). However, eventually, the child begins to fractionate its utterances, so that *milk* can be talked of outside the context of wanting, and *want* can be applied to different things in the child's world.

Contrast this with Chapter 10's account of how languages got started. In both cases, the claim is for a transition from holophrases via fractionation and recombination to words bound by constructions, with the latter opening up a range of meanings beyond those of the original holophrase. The key difference, however, is that the words and constructions did not exist until the early humans invented them, whereas the modern child may *perceive* a holophrase, but its decomposition into words is a social given that she has to learn but not invent.

Back to the modern child. Hill studied how the child's "grammar" may change starting from this two-word stage, and she kept the grammars she hypothesized free of any characterization of the more adult grammar that the child's language use will eventually approximate but that is not yet present. Hill's description of grammar consists of constructions that represent relations.[3] In the beginning, every construction consists of one invariant word, the relation word, and one slot with an example slot filler, for example, *want milk*, in which *want* is the relation word and *milk* is the slot filler. Given such a construction, Hill's model shows how the child may come to produce an entire set of two-word sentences in which any object of her desire for which the child knows the lexical label may be substituted for the word *milk*. Thus, she may express *want doll, want blocks, want juice*; the number of utterances being limited only by her vocabulary for objects that she may want. At this stage, the slot will accept only a small set of slot fillers, based on the meaning of the relation word—the very limited semantic category of "wantable things."

The model begins by forming a different construction—and thus a different semantic category—for every individual relation word. The concepts encoded in the constructions will express relations of interest to the child that are related to her needs or that describe instances of movement or change that attract her attention. As the child relates fragments of adult utterances to situations of interest to her in her environment, constructions for expressing the stated relations are added to the grammar, and the items in the lexicon are tagged according to the way in which they might combine with relation words. In this way *word classes are constructed based on potential for word use*, and it is by means of the word classification process that constructions are generalized.

The *initial* "2-year-old grammar" of the model comprised basic schemas for words, basic schemas for concepts, and the basic constructions that provided a grammar marked by a richness of simple patterns the child had already broken out of experience, rather than the grand general rules that we would find in the grammarian's description of adult language. And what was "built in" were not grammatical rules but rather processes whereby the child could form classes and try to match incoming words to existing constructions, using those constructions to generate the response. In particular, the model explains how categories akin to those of "noun" or "verb" might arise through the developmental aggregation of words into diverse classes, rather than being imposed as innate categories within a biologically specified Universal Grammar.

Figure 11-1 shows the components of Hill's model. The model takes as its input adult sentences together with indications (provided by the modeler, where relevant) of the physical context in which the sentences are uttered. Output from the model is a representation of child-like sentences repeating or responding to the adult input in accordance with the current state of the model's linguistic capacity. The child's knowledge is represented by dynamic data structures encoding the child's lexicon, the child's grammar, the conceptual knowledge of the child, and the physical context of the dialogue. The model is given a basic lexicon and a set of concepts with a mapping between

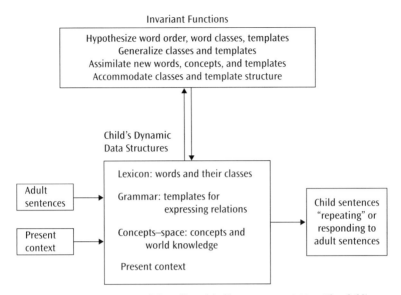

FIGURE 11-1.   Basic components of the Hill model of language acquisition. The child's knowledge is represented by dynamic data structures encoding the child's lexicon, the child's grammar, the conceptual knowledge of the child, and the physical context of the dialogue. (From Arbib et al., 1987, p. 122.)

the two. No assumptions have been made about the ultimate form of the adult grammar nor about what must be built into the model, but a precise account is kept of the knowledge and processes found necessary even for this elementary level of language understanding and production. Processes attend to the adult input and use rules of salience to focus on examples within the adult data that are used as the basis for language growth. The input data are in no way especially coded for the model but are generally taken from language acquisition corpora of adult-child dialogue. The model uses its language experience (i.e., the processing of the input sentences) to build a grammar that is at first a flat grammar but that eventually evolves into a grammar that may be described, if one chooses, by a set of recursive context-free phrase structure rules. The model embodies five assumptions:

1. The child has schemas for and talks about relations.
2. The child has schemas for and employs word order in her utterances.
3. The child employs processes of concatenation and deletion when, for example (see below), two two-word constructions are concatenated and then a repeated instance of a shared word is deleted to yield a three-word construction.
4. The child forms classes of concepts and classes of words.
5. The classifying process causes successive reorganizations of the information stored.

We posit a process of *classification through word use* whereby words that are used in similar ways come to be assigned to the same class, thus extending from members of the class to further members of the class certain patterns (constructions) of word use. The initial grammar is given by a set of constructions, consisting of a "relation" and a "slot," which is free of any characterization of the adult grammar that will emerge but is not yet present. Hill observed a brief stage in which Claire concatenated two-word constructions with a common word, as in

little bear baby bear

but these soon give way to such three-word constructions as

little baby bear.

Such four-word utterances with repeated lexical items occurred so briefly that Hill hypothesized that the three-word utterances were arrived at (1) by concatenating the two constructions "little bear" and "baby bear" and (2) by collapsing the concatenated relations into a single three-word utterance by deleting the first occurrence of the repeated word. Some evidence that the concatenation best captures the semantics of such three-word utterances in the young child is given by the finding of Matthei (1979) that the young child interprets "the second green ball" as "the ball that is second and green." In fact, several children, when presented with an array in which the second ball was not green, actually rearranged the balls in order to make the situation conform to their interpretation of the words.

From an adult sentence such as "Daddy gave the toy to the boy" the model might initially respond with a single word such as *toy*. A subsequent presentation of the same sentence might cause the model to acquire a construction for *gave toy* where *gave* would be classified as a relation word and *toy* as a slot filler. Yet another presentation of the sentence might cause the model to learn the different ordering for *Daddy gave* where *Daddy* was a slot filler, and eventually the construction (*slot1 gave slot2*) might be learned for *Daddy gave toy*. What is learned in each presentation of the input depends upon the language experience of the model and what has been learned so far. Thus, learning is highly dynamic in that each time the same input sentence is presented to the model a different set of constructions and additional lexical class information may be applied, and possibly modified.

No information is given about word classes in initializing the model, but hearing sentences such as "Mommy gave the toy," "John gave the book," and "Sue gave the puzzle" would eventually cause the model to put *toy, book,* and *puzzle* all together in a class of words that stand for possible objects of the relation-word *gave*. Note that it would not matter if the input sentences were far more complex than those used here for illustration. If the model is focusing on the word *gave*, then a sentence such as "Mommy gave the toy to Sue while she went into the store to buy groceries" would have just the same effect as the short sentences used previously. Where William James speaks of "buzzing, blooming confusion,"[4] we would talk of ignorable details. By this process word classes are derived from the model's ability to produce language. The process results in a multiplicity of overlapping and intersecting word classes. The model requires schemas for word classification and construction classification in order to grow, but the actual classes remain flexible. Processes of generalization eventually also permit the classifying of relation words that might permit, for example, *giving* and *bringing* to be relation words that could be classed together as words that have similar syntactic properties. Successive reorganizations of the grammar and the lexicon occur as learning takes place. Thus, the early constructions grow into the more powerful constructions introduced in Chapter 2 as the key to a more flexible view of grammar than one based on Universal Grammar. In this fashion, the model suggests one way in which language based initially on cognitive knowledge can grow into a syntactic system that will be increasingly independent of its semantic and cognitive foundations.

Hill's model thus provides a certain set of innate mechanisms that could drive the child's acquisition of a certain body of language. However, these mechanisms do not explain how it is that language eventually becomes nested or recursive in the sense that certain language structure can repeatedly incorporate simpler forms of that structure in increasingly elaborate constructions. Hill outlined what those mechanisms might be but did not study them in depth. It does not appear that the elaboration of the model would force one to build in the structures that Chomsky would claim to be innate. Since humans can learn language, in its full sense, and other creatures cannot, we must conclude that infants are endowed with learning abilities that are more powerful than those of other animals and that make the construction-based learning of language possible.[5]

Perceiving Spoken Words: A Dog Detour

We now switch from children to dogs, seeing what studies of perception by dogs of words spoken by humans suggest about "symbol perception" in a species for which there is no use of language as such. Kaminski, Call, and Fischer (2004) investigated the ability of a border collie named Rico to acquire the relation between a word and the object to which the word refers. Rico had been gradually familiarized with an increasing number of items and associated words by his owners and had learned the spoken labels of over 200 items, which he correctly retrieved upon request. Kaminski et al. verified that Rico was indeed able to retrieve items without any cue other than the familiar spoken label by having the dog receive the spoken command in one room, then retrieve the object from among several in an adjacent room where he could not see his master and thus could not receive the master's unconscious cues. Then, to assess Rico's learning ability, Kaminski et al. introduced a distinct novel name and a distinct novel item. In the first trial of a session, the owner situated in one room asked Rico to go to another room and bring back a familiar item by giving the name familiar to him. In the second or third trial he used the novel name—in response to which, in 7 out of 10 sessions, Rico retrieved the one novel item among the familiar items placed in the next room. Four weeks later, given names for which he had correctly retrieved the novel target item in the earlier sessions, Rico retrieved the correct object in 3 out of 6 sessions and brought only an unfamiliar item in the other 3 sessions. These results demonstrate that Rico has both

- *exclusion learning* (also known as emergent matching; Wilkinson, Dube, & McIlvane, 1998): the ability to associate a novel name with an item because it is not already named, rather than through explicit pairing of the name with the item, and
- *fast mapping*: the ability to learn a new association on one trial (or a very few trials) rather than through a large number of conditioning trials.

These findings raise two different questions: (a) Are these mechanisms of fast mapping and exclusion mapping used by apes in so-called language learning, and (b) do Rico's abilities suggest that the human child learning words makes use of these general mechanisms that (because of their availability to Rico) appear not to be specific to language?

Dogs appear to have been evolutionarily selected for attending to the communicative intentions of humans (Hare, Brown, Williamson, & Tomasello, 2002). Moreover, Rico is a border collie, and border collies are working dogs able to respond to a large number of commands from a human for, for example, herding sheep. Thus, although dogs are far off the evolutionary path of the primates, the fact that they have been so successfully domesticated suggests there may be a process of convergent evolution as humans and dogs have come to live together so successfully in so different a relationship from that of, say, humans and cats. Such a process has no part in the evolution of nonhuman primates, and so one must accept—in answer to (a)—that not all the mechanisms apparently available to Rico may operate as effectively in the brains of apes. Indeed,

Rico's "vocabulary size" is comparable to that of "language-trained" apes, dolphins, sea lions, and parrots (Hillix & Rumbaugh, 2003; Miles & Harper, 1994; Pepperberg, 2008), but Rico's word-learning abilities appear to surpass those of nonhuman primates such as chimpanzees, for which Seidenberg and Petitto (1987) were unable to demonstrate this sort of fast mapping.

On the basis of Rico's performance, Kaminski et al. (2004) argue that the seemingly complex linguistic skill of word learning seen in human children may be mediated by simpler cognitive building blocks—fast mapping and exclusion learning—that are also present in other species. However, Bloom (2004) stresses the differences between Rico and a human child. Rico is 9 years old and knows about 200 words, whereas a human 9-year-old knows tens of thousands of words and can learn more than 10 new words a day (Bloom, 2000). Children's word learning is highly robust, and they can learn words from overheard speech, even if nobody is trying to teach them. Rico, in contrast, learns only though a specific fetching game. Children can understand words used in a range of contexts; Rico's understanding is manifested in his fetching behavior. For a child, words are symbols that refer to categories and individuals in the external world (Macnamara, 1982). When children learn a word such as "sock," their use may at first be limited to a specific context, but with further experience they are able to use the word in a wide range of contexts. One might say that what the child first learns, and what Rico can only learn, is a protoword rather than a word. The protoword becomes a word only through its ability to be used flexibly as part of a construction. A word is a word because it can be used as an element of language, rich in constructions. On this basis, neither Rico nor Kanzi (Chapter 3) have words, but they do have protowords that support rudimentary communication with humans.

However, anticipating the objection that Rico may interpret "sock" as a holophrase for "fetch the sock," Kaminski et al. (2004) note anecdotal evidence that he indeed understands that words refer to objects since he can be instructed to put an item into a box or to bring it to a certain person. The shepherding abilities of border collies show that their ability to learn words is not limited to small fetchable objects, but their skills are consistent with the assertion that Rico's vocabulary is restricted to one-word commands—though, notably, these are clearly triadic and referential (to use the terminology of Chapter 3)—rather than diverse forms of syntactically structured sentences. By contrast, children can use words in diverse ways, and they can produce words as well as understand them. Given such reservations, Bloom (2004) asserts that "it is too early to give up on the view that babies learn words and dogs do not," though we might counter that babies learn only protowords, and it is only through processes such as those charted by Jane Hill that they become words.

Capabilities

Our quick look at a model of language acquisition linked to Construction Grammar, and our detour into the learning of commands by dogs, lends support to the view that a word becomes a word, as distinct from a protoword, because it is part of a language system that can combine it with other words to make new meanings. To this it might be objected that there are some words we use only in a single linguistic context, such as *petard* in *hoist on his own petard*, to which it may in turn be countered that while this is true, once we know that a petard is "a small bomb used to blow up gates and walls when breaching fortifications," it has the potential for use in other constructions (as in the present sentence) even though we seldom or never exercise it. Indeed, the idiom is a freezing of words that were once joined together by live constructions but have now come to form a holophrase. However, unlike the holophrases that were first employed by our distant ancestors who had only protolanguage and that were unitary utterances with no internal word-like parts, these are "language-laden" holophrases that combine words (whether familiar or unfamiliar) into an idiosyncratic whole.

What links early and modern humans is that when the young child first extracts a string of one or two words from those spoken around him, they constitute a *holophrase to the child,* and the child must begin to understand how different such utterances may be assembled by employing a process of fractionation followed by the development of constructions to reassemble the pieces (but with the ability to combine other pieces as well) before these pieces can become words, and the original holophrases be perceived as phrases. I thus claim that the same basic mechanisms may have served both protohumans inventing language and modern children acquiring the existing language of their community. These mechanisms comprise the following:

1. The ability to create a novel gesture or vocalization and associate it with a communicative goal.
2. The ability both to perform and perceive such a gesture or vocalization. This would improve with experience as its use spread within the community, as would sharpening of the perception of occasions of use by members of the community.
3. Commonalities between two structures could yield to "fractionation," the isolation of that commonality as a gesture or vocalization betokening some shared "semantic component" of the event, object, or action denoted by each of the two structures. This could in time lead to the emergence of a construction for "putting the pieces back together," not only allowing recapture of the meanings of the original structures but also with the original pieces becoming instances of an ever wider class of slot fillers.

Our discussion of Rico makes clear that the modern child's ability to master the circumambient language, especially the explosion in the acquisition of vocabulary that occurs in most cases between the ages of 2 and 3, is supported by two mechanisms that facilitate and speed up learning: *exclusion learning*, the ability to associate a novel name with an item because it is not already named, and *fast mapping*, the ability to learn from that new association in one trial (or very few). This ties in with our original view of complex imitation—it is not the ability to repeat something one has just observed, but rather the ability to add a skill of moderate complexity to one's repertoire after observing another repeat it on several occasions.

When it comes to modern languages, the early mastery of the phonology of a language (something that protolanguages would have lacked before their complexity drove the emergence of duality of patterning) is a key skill—it provides a relatively small set of actions that can be used to analyze a novel word on hearing it or seeing it signed, and then use that analysis to perform the word with moderate success in the context in which it was earlier used. Mastery of the nuances of the word's meaning and increased fluency with its pronunciation may then involve further experience, as is the case with any skill. As the stock of words expands, so does it make possible the learning of new constructions, in which a "slot filler" involves not the use of a single word but rather the use of a class of words that emerged, in the spirit of Hill's model, through use of language rather than being predefined as part of an innate syntax.

Ontogeny does *not* in this case recapitulate phylogeny. Adult hunters and gatherers had to communicate about situations outside the range of a modern 2-year-old, and protohumans were not communicating with adults who already used a large lexicon and set of constructions to generate complex sentences. Nonetheless, I argue that biological evolution created the brain mechanisms that made the cultural evolution of language possible in the past and support both language acquisition and the emergence of new languages in the present day.

12

How Languages Emerge

We have sought to understand the interplay of biological and cultural evolution in yielding modern humans with their rich, flexible, and diverse languages, delimiting the innate capabilities of the human brain that allow human children to master language in a society whose caregivers had evolved to develop those capabilities. Most humans are born with adequate hearing and acquire speech as their primary mode of communication, but the Mirror System Hypothesis shows how the brain evolved to support language as a multimodal system of production and performance that involves voice, hands, and face. This makes us receptive to the lessons that can be learned when voice is ineffective. In this chapter, we analyze the recent emergence of two new sign languages: Nicaraguan Sign Language (NSL) and Al-Sayyid Bedouin Sign Language (ABSL). Researchers use the study of different "cohorts" (NSL) or generations (ABSL) of signers to gather insights into processes of language change. Understanding the tradeoff between innate capabilities and social influences in the emergence of NSL and ABSL will ground an understanding of how these modern social influences may differ from those available to early humans at the dawn of language and yet—just as we did in comparing how languages got started and how modern children acquire them—we will argue that analysis of the mechanisms that supported the rapid emergence of these new sign languages can expand our understanding of how protolanguages became languages on a far longer time scale.[1]

Nicaraguan Sign Language developed in just 25 years in concert with the development of a community of deaf Nicaraguans. It has been claimed that NSL arose "from scratch" (Pearson, 2004) in that the community of deaf Nicaraguans who developed it "lacked exposure to a developed language" (Senghas, Kita, & Özyürek, 2004). This chapter will critique this claim as the basis for analyzing what innate capabilities of the human brain and what social factors supported the dramatic development of NSL. The key issue is this: Did deaf Nicaraguans "invent language"—as the claim that NSL arose out of nothing might suggest—or did they "invent *a* language," in which case we must understand how knowledge of other languages affected the development of NSL?

Laura Polich spent the year of 1997 in Managua, and during that time interviewed many people in and associated with the Deaf community. The resultant book, *The Emergence of the Deaf Community in Nicaragua: "With Sign Language You Can Learn So Much"* (Polich, 2005) provides a historical record and a glimpse of key individuals involved in the emergence of NSL. The result is an invaluable complement to the linguists' cohort-by-cohort analysis of specific linguistic features of NSL. Polich documents that in 1979 there was no Deaf community in Nicaragua, yet there was a formal organization of deaf adults by 1986. Noting the increased opportunities for adolescents and young adults to get together that made the 1980s different from the 1950s, Polich hypothesizes that adolescents and young adults played important roles in the formation of the Deaf community and its sign language.

Al-Sayyid Bedouin Sign Language (ABSL) has arisen in the last 70 years in an isolated endogamous Bedouin community in the Negev desert of Israel with a high incidence of genetically based deafness (Scott et al., 1995). However, unlike NSL, ABSL developed within the family structures of a preexisting socially stable community. As a result of the recessiveness of the gene for deafness in this group of Bedouin, there are many deaf individuals distributed throughout the community. This means that hearing members of the community have regular daily contact with deaf members and that, consequently, signing is not restricted to deaf people. Furthermore, new signers are born into an environment with adult models of the language available to them, though this was obviously untrue of the first generation, and not necessarily true of older second-generation signers since although the first generation were around they were not necessarily close by or frequently interacted with.[2]

Early Experience With and Without Hearing

Most humans are born with adequate hearing and acquire speech as their primary mode of communication. Generally, deaf people have hearing losses in the severe to profound range and can detect only the loudest of sounds, if any. For them, the auditory signal cannot be the primary input.[3] However, 95% of deaf children are born to hearing parents and soon become communicative outsiders in their families (Karchmer & Mitchell, 2003). By contrast, people for whom profound hearing loss occurs after adolescence are most likely to consider oral language their primary form of communication and not to identify with the signing community.

Human babies from a very early age are receptive to sensory input that will later be used linguistically. Babies with hearing are able to recognize their mothers' voices within the first few days of life, and sighted babies pay early attention to the movements of caregivers' faces and their eye gaze (DeCasper & Fifer, 1980; DeCasper & Spence, 1991). The newborn hearing infant exhibits effects of some months of auditory exposure while in the womb, and by 6 months after being born the infant will exhibit language-specific responsiveness to auditory input (e.g., Japanese infants can initially respond to the distinction between /l/ and /r/ sounds but eventually lose this ability). By 9 months the infant will respond best to the syllabic structure of the ambient language so that an English infant will become attuned to CVC as well as CV syllables (C = consonant; V = vowel), whereas Japanese infants become attuned to a restricted range of "moras," syllables of the CV form or /-n/. By 1 year of age, the hearing child will increasingly use vocal production to express herself using something like words, complementing innate vocalizations like crying and laughing. However, it is worth stressing that even the hearing child makes extensive use of gesture in the transition to speech, as does the deaf child learning to use sign language, noting the distinction between a relatively free-form gesture and a conventionalized sign (Capirci & Volterra, 2008). Iverson et al. (1994) found that gestures were more prevalent than (vocal) words in the children they observed as 16 month olds, whereas the majority of children had more words than gestures by 20 months of age. Moreover, Capirci et al. (1996) observed that, at both ages, the most frequent two-element utterances were gesture-word combinations; and production of these combinations increased significantly from 16 to 20 months even as the use of two-word utterances increased sharply.

Deaf babies exposed to a sign language have been documented to follow similar linguistic milestones to hearing children exposed to a spoken language (Lillo-Martin, 1999; Meier, 1991; Newport & Meier, 1985) and become members of a Deaf community in which a sign language is the primary form of communication (the capital D in Deaf here indicates membership of such a community, as distinct from the loss of hearing). This strengthens the argument that the brain mechanisms that support language are multimodal, rather than evolving to primarily support the vocal-auditory modality. However, it is not uncommon for a deaf child who has only auditory exposure to language at six years of age to have an oral language very different from that acquired by typically hearing children. Even with specialized training in oral language, a deaf child's ability to understand auditory language and use oral expression is greatly delayed compared with the progress made by normally hearing children, and many deaf children never develop recognizable spoken language.

But deaf children raised by nonsigning parents do develop *home sign*, which is a rudimentary form of communication with family members though far from a full-fledged language (Goldin-Meadow, 1982). Typically, such a child will have a small "vocabulary" of home signs together with just a few strategies for combining signs into longer messages. Since this development does not rest on "direct input" from either a spoken language or a sign language, home sign will differ from child to child. I put quotes around "direct input" since it bears on the issues we will consider in distinguishing the evolution of the first languages in (proto)human prehistory from the emergence of new languages in the present day. First, there is no direct input from *sign language* because the home signers are children of speaking parents who do not know sign language. However, there is the input from seeing gestures—both deictic gestures and more descriptive gestures—used as part of speech acts. Reinforcement of the child's own gestures depends on the responsiveness of other family members to the messages they are meant to convey—as in the notion of the idea of *human-supported ritualization* introduced in Chapter 3 and revisited in Chapter 8. Such gestures do not themselves constitute a language, but they do teach the child that pointing and pantomime can be used to communicate just as they do in the development of a hearing child (recall the earlier discussion of the use of gesture by 16- and 20-month olds). The "input" from *speech* is even less direct. But the fact that family members can be seen to take turns to speak and gesture, sometimes to no apparent end, but in other cases with clear links to emotional impact or achieving instrumental goals, creates an understanding of the general notion of dialogue conducted by a blend of gesture and facial expression. Moreover, a child's caregiver will provide a structured environment such as pointing at specific objects or actions as well as pictures in picture books that—even though the child cannot hear the spoken names of what is in the picture—encourages the understanding that objects and actions, and so on, do have names. In some cases, the child can adapt a caregiver's gesture to provide such a name; in other cases, a more or less ritualized pantomime will serve, but this process is far slower and more limited than for children to whom the names are supplied in speech (if the child can hear) or sign language.

Home signers can combine a few signs to form what Goldin-Meadow calls a "sentence," though one must note that these are very simple in structure compared to the range of sentences seen in full human languages. However, these "sentences" do exhibit some basic "grammatical properties." Goldin-Meadow and Mylander (1998) find consistent word order among home signers (even those in different cultures): They regularly produce two-gesture strings in which actions appear in final position (O-V, object-verb; or S-V, subject-verb), with intransitive actors and patients more likely to appear in such strings than transitive actors.

Goldin-Meadow (2005) argues that home sign systems display properties of language that are what she calls *resilient* (see Table 12–1, based on Goldin-Meadow, 2003—though I have not included all the properties she descries in home sign). However, home sign does not exhibit what she calls *fragile*

Table 12-1   The Resilient Properties of Language

The Resilient Property	*As Instantiated in Home Sign*
Words	
Stability	Sign forms are stable and do not change capriciously with changing situations.
Paradigms	Signs consist of smaller parts that can be recombined to produce new signs with different meanings.
Categories	The parts of signs are composed of a limited set of forms, each associated with a particular meaning.
Arbitrariness	Pairings between sign forms and meanings can have arbitrary aspects, albeit within an iconic framework.
Sentences	
Underlying frames	Predicate frames underlie sign sentences.
Deletion	Consistent production and deletion of signs within a sentence mark particular thematic roles.
Word order	Consistent orderings of signs within a sentence mark particular thematic roles.
Inflections	Consistent inflections on signs mark particular thematic roles.
Language use	
Here-and-now talk	Signing is used to make requests, comments, and queries about the present.
Displaced talk	Signing is used to communicate about the past, future, and hypothetical.
Narrative	Signing is used to tell stories about self and others.
Self-talk	Signing is used to communicate with oneself.
Meta-language	Signing is used to refer to one's own and others' signs.

Source: Adapted from Goldin-Meadow, 2005.

properties of language, such as techniques for marking tense. She suggests that fragile properties do not fall within the province of an individual child developing a communication system without the support of partners sharing the system. Segmentation and sequencing of motion events have been observed in home signers exposed only to unregimented co-speech gestures. One home signer produced the sequence *flutter descend* to describe snowing (see Figure 3 in Goldin-Meadow, 2003). But what else could he do? He retrieves a sign "flutter" that does not exhaust what he perceives about the situation, and then produces another, "descend." This is not really compositionality but relates to the mere concatenation of signs—one may encounter a new situation that resembles a situation for which a sign already exists, then be dissatisfied with the "gaps" left by that sign. If another sign is available to cover the gap, at least in part, then that may be uttered, too. This is much weaker than being able to marshal constructions to put together words to express the cognized relations in a situation. Thus, more attention needs to be given to the sentencehood of the "sentences" that underlie the generalizations in Table 12-1. As a caution, note the later statement that "second-generation ABSL signers consistently produce sentences in which predicates appear in final position, but unlike home signers, they produce longer sentences with two or more nominals appearing before the predicate," showing that the "sentences" referred to in Table 12-1 are much much simpler than the reader versed in English might expect them to be. Again, one might argue with the claim that "words" in home sign are more than "protowords" (recall the discussion of the child's earliest "words" in Chapter 11), disputing that these signs are differentiated by the noun, verb, and adjective grammatical functions they serve, rather than the semantic functions of object, action, and attribute. The full structure of home signs deserves a much fuller analysis than I give it here. However, the key point for us is that home sign is far, far more limited than the sign languages that emerged in Nicaragua and in the Negev Desert.

Nicaraguan Sign Language

A Brief History

Before the 1970s, deaf Nicaraguans had little contact with each other (Polich, 2005; Senghas, 1997). Most deaf individuals stayed at home, and the few schools to which they had access treated them as mentally retarded. During this period the home sign systems developed by different deaf Nicaraguans varied widely in form and complexity, but no sign language emerged (Coppola, 2002). An expanded elementary school for special education of the deaf was opened in 1977 followed by a vocational school in 1981, both in Managua, Nicaragua. About 50 deaf students were initially enrolled in the program, growing to more than 200 by 1981 and increasing gradually during the 1980s. Students continued their contact outside school hours, and by the mid-1980s deaf adolescents were meeting regularly on the weekends (Polich, 2005). It is important to note that instruction was conducted in Spanish, though with limited success. I will return to this point later. But here, let's focus on the emergence of NSL.

From the start, the children began to develop a new, gestural system for communicating with each other—in part by consolidating the different home signs each had developed. The gestures expanded over time both in their number and by the addition of constructions, to form a rudimentary sign language (Kegl, Senghas, & Coppola, 1999). As the years passed, the early collection of gestures developed into an expressive sign language, NSL. Through continued use in and out of school, NSL has grown with successive innovations being learned naturally as new children enter the community each year (Senghas & Coppola, 2001). As of 2005, there were about 800 deaf signers of NSL, ranging from 4 to 45 years of age. Annie Senghas (2003) argued that changes in its grammar first appear among preadolescent signers, soon spreading to subsequent, younger learners, but not to adults. This statement seems a little strong—a successful innovation would presumably spread to most children currently in school, regardless of whether they were younger than the innovators. Nonetheless, the fact remains that most adults do fail to master innovations in NSL made by a cohort 10 years younger—just as many hearing adults around the world fail to develop a taste for the music currently popular with teenagers. This pattern of transmission, when combined with the rapid and recent expansion of NSL, has created an unusual language community in which the most fluent signers are among the youngest.[4] Note that while NSL is the first language for these children it is not quite a native language, since they start learning NSL when they enter school around age 6.

Emerging Patterns of Motion Description in Nicaraguan Sign Language

To exemplify what has been learned about the development of NSL, I will focus on one study (Senghas et al., 2004) that exploited the difference between older signers, who retain much of NSL's early nature, and younger signers who produce the language in its expanded, most developed form. They did this by comparing the signed expressions of 30 deaf Nicaraguans, all of whom had been signing NSL since the age of 6 or younger, grouped into cohorts according to the year that they were first exposed to NSL: 10 from a first cohort (before 1984), 10 from a second cohort (1984 to 1993), and 10 from a third cohort (after 1993). Their signed expressions during description of motion were compared to the co-speech gestures produced by 10 hearing Nicaraguan Spanish speakers while speaking Spanish.

Figure 12-1 shows two examples of hand movements made while describing a clip from a Tweety and Sylvester cartoon (see McNeill, 1992 for more on this methodology for the study of hand gesture).[5] In this clip, the cat, Sylvester, having swallowed a bowling ball, proceeds rapidly down a steep street in a wobbling, rolling manner. (A ball would roll down the hill, the cartoon cat with a ball inside wobbles down the hill, but English speakers tend to say that the cat rolls down the hill.) The complex motion event of "rolling" down a hill includes a *manner* of movement (rolling) and a *path* of movement (descending). These characteristics of motion are simultaneous aspects of a single event and are experienced as a unity. The most direct way to iconically represent such an event would be to represent manner and path simultaneously. However, languages will often

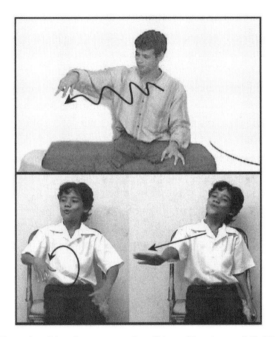

FIGURE 12-1.   Examples of hand movements describing rolling down a hill. (A) This
example shows the co-speech gestures of a Spanish speaker in which manner (rolling) and
path (trajectory to the speaker's right) are expressed together. (B) A third-cohort signer of
Nicaraguan Sign Language expresses manner (circling) and path (trajectory to signer's right)
in two separate signs in sequence. (From Senghas et al., 2004. Reprinted with permission
from AAAS.)

encode manner and path in separate elements. English, for example, uses the
sequence "rolling down" to represent manner (rolling) and path (down).

Senghas et al. (2004) found that all of the Spanish speakers' gestures and
73% of the first-cohort NSL signers' expressions included manner and path
simultaneously as exemplified in Figure 12-1A. By contrast, for second- and
third-cohort signers little more than 30% of these expressions were of this
type. Manner and path were more often expressed in succession as exemplified
in Figure 12-1B. This then provides dramatic evidence of an *emergent* feature of
NSL: The Spanish speakers that signers could observe, and most of the related
signing by first-cohort signers, did not separate path and manner in describing such an event. Yet as second and third cohorts learned the language in
the mid-1980s and 1990s, they rapidly made this segmented, sequenced
construction their preferred (but not exclusive) means of expressing motion
events. Thus, *NSL is not a copying of Spanish co-speech gestures* but here exhibits
a novel conventionalization. (It should also be noted that many sign languages
do express manner and path simultaneously.) As Slobin (2005) observes,

however, we should also note (1) that 73% of the first-cohort NSL signers and more than 30% of second- and third-cohort signers used the strategy employed by Spanish speakers, and that (2) 27% of the first-cohort NSL signers did separate path and manner. Thus, at least some of the original signs were strongly influenced by the co-speech gestures of the surrounding community, while the innovation of the separation of path and manner was achieved by some individuals in the first cohort. What we see in the later cohorts is its increasingly wide adoption.

There is a drawback to this innovation. If manner and path are expressed separately, it may no longer be clear that the two aspects of movement occurred within a single event. *Roll* followed by *downward* might mean "rolling, then descending." However, a key finding of Senghas et al. (2004) is that not only did NSL signers come to fractionate path and manner, they also developed a way to put the pieces back together again. NSL now has the X-Y-X construction, such as *roll-descend-roll*, to express simultaneity. This string can serve as a structural unit within a larger expression like *cat [roll descend roll]*, or it can even be nested, as in *waddle [roll descend roll] waddle*. The X-Y-X construction appeared in about one-third of the second- and third-cohort expressions they recorded in response to the bowling ball video clip, but it never appeared in the gestures of the Spanish speakers.

This example shows that the general process of following fractionation with a construction to put the pieces back together, and then be available to combine other pieces as well, that we posited (Chapter 10) to be operative in the evolution of protolanguages is still operative in the modern brain when the need to expand a communication system demands it. The need to find a form to express a certain meaning can catalyze the invention of new constructions, but a sign language can seek forms different from those of spoken languages. Which of the possible forms takes hold is a social matter, rather than a consequence of general learning principles.

Design Features Versus Innate Rules

But perhaps individuals would not need to discover the idea of language in their interactions with others if the brains of *Homo sapiens* were genetically endowed with a Universal Grammar that "prewired" all possible syntactic rules in the infant human brain. While researchers studying NSL and ABSL have been relatively circumspect in making claims for the implications of their research, science journalists discussing the work have not been so restrained. For example, Juliana Kettlewell (2004) claims that the work of Senghas et al. (2004) proved that NSL follows many basic rules common to all languages, even though the children were not taught them, suggesting that this shows that some language traits are not passed on by culture but instead arise due to the innate way human beings process language.

These claims are misleading if (as seems natural) we understand a "language rule" as the sort of rule of syntax that (some suggest) would be defined by setting parameters in the Principles and Parameters version of Universal Grammar. On the other hand, the statement seems correct if we take it as "language rules" (1) that as holophrases fractionate so will constructions emerge to allow recapture of the meanings of the holophrases and (2) that novel constructions provide the space for the creation of new words to fill their slots in new ways, yielding novel semantico-syntactic categories. Exercising these skills lies in the domain of "design features" (Hockett, 1987) rather than parameters of a putative Universal Grammar. The child does not have language or grammar "in its head (or genes)" when it is born, but it does have crucial learning abilities that link a capacity for complex imitation to communication as well as to praxis. I am happy to agree that:

> …such learning processes leave an imprint on languages—observable in mature languages in their core, universal properties—including discrete elements (such as words and morphemes) combined into hierarchically organized constructions (such as phrases and sentences). (Senghas et al. 2004, p. 1781)

with the caveat that we must distinguish the perhaps relatively rare discovery of novel constructions to add expressive power from the ability to readily learn such innovations once they have been made.

In the Mirror System Hypothesis, complex imitation—an analytical, combinatorial learning mechanism—is argued to evolve within the domain of praxis. Byrne's "feeding programs" (Byrne, 2003) show that gorillas can indeed learn hierarchical and conditional structures, but this requires a long, drawn-out process of "imitation by behavior parsing" (Chapter 7). My suggestion is that the ability to more rapidly acquire novel behaviors was a crucial evolutionary step that preceded the emergence of protolanguage, let alone language. The Mirror System Hypothesis posits that the next crucial turning point came with pantomime—the transition from praxis to communication—but that the ability for conventionalization that yielded protosign as embedded within a "cultural system" required neurological innovations (witness the signers who lose signing but not the ability to pantomime; Corina et al., 1992; Marshall, Atkinson, Smulovitch, Thacker, & Woll, 2004).

The Emergence of the Nicaraguan Deaf Community

As noted earlier, until the late 1970s deaf students in Nicaragua were placed in special education classes where they were outnumbered by mentally retarded students and were unable to form a community. But then a vocational school was established that kept adolescents and young adults together "at a time when they were carving out their identities and craving a peer group in which to try out and enact their abilities to be social actors" (Polich, p. 146).[6] Note here the crucial notions of *social actor, peer group,* and *creating one's identity.* The process that Polich charts is the transition from a deaf person in Nicaragua having no peer group and thus having the passive social role of an outcast, to a person with a language that empowered him or her to be a true social actor within the Deaf community created by the enriched communication that came with the expanding capabilities of NSL. This process, as Polich shows, was catalyzed by a number of individuals, some deaf and others hearing, intent on opening up to the deaf the social opportunities that most hearing people could take for granted. For example, Ruthy Doran, a hearing person who not only taught the deaf children at the vocational school but also did much to create a social environment for them, told Polich:

> There wasn't a sign language [around 1980]...But we were able to understand one another. We would [...]...use a lot of the gestures that everyone around here (in Nicaragua) uses and we had a set of some signs that the students made up. (They aren't used now.) We had special signs like for the days of the week that we had used with each other for years, and they had learned new signs [...]...which they taught me. And when everything else failed, we would write words down, or else act it out. (Polich, pp. 77–78)

Another teacher, Gloria Minero, remembers great diversity in the signs used before 1987:

> there was a lot of rudimentary gestures and ASL signs and mimicry, which are not "signs" but more "iconic." There wasn't much structure—that came later. (Polich, p. 89)

Thus, in its early stages the community being formed was influenced by the gestures of the surrounding community and included hearing people who spoke Spanish. And note the huge cultural input that goes into something like having a sign for each day of the week—a long way from the more-or-less spontaneous gestures of home sign. Even those who could not speak had at least a small vocabulary of written Spanish and the group had access to some signs of American Sign Language (ASL). Of course, using a few signs of ASL is very different from knowing ASL as such—just as a tourist in Paris may be able to say "Bon jour" and "Merci" but not know French. However, note the difference between the true statement "In the early 1980s, many deaf Nicaraguans knew no grammar" and the false statement "In the early 1980s, no deaf Nicaraguans knew grammar." The impressive achievement of creating this new language, NSL, did not have to rest solely on innate capabilities of the human brain (which distinguish us from other primates, for example) but could indeed exploit the cultural innovations of existing language communities (though, as the work of Annie Senghas and others shows, the NSL community keeps moving beyond this basis in creating new words and constructions).

In Nicaragua in the 1970s and beyond, most language teaching for deaf children was oral training based on Spanish, which was successful for relatively few students. It thus was a revelation when, in 1983, Ruthy Duran and two other teachers visited Costa Rica and saw how sign language was used there to augment an oral program (Polich, Chapter 7) and that signs could constitute a fully expressive language. However, they were unable to get approval for the use of Costa Rican sign language for instruction in Managua. Instead, the full use of sign language had to await the development of a sign language within Nicaragua. The point here, however, is that the *idea* of sign language was available to some members of the nascent community, even though the full use of such a language was not. Meanwhile, Spanish speakers played a crucial role in the early development of NSL and the Nicaraguan Deaf community, although their input became increasingly marginal as both the language and the community became more powerful.

Gloria Minero encouraged the students to develop an association of deaf persons to work for more education and increased jobs for its members, assisting work on a constitution and bylaws. The official founding of the association came in 1986. Thus, while many of the deaf Nicaraguans could not speak Spanish, there were enough who did and could work with their hearing mentors to help develop a document written in Spanish. The original name was Associación Pro-Ayuda e Integración a los Sordos (APRIAS), the Association to Help and Integrate the Deaf. This reflects the original aim of the association, which was integrationist—to aid deaf members to join mainstream society through speaking. However, as the use of sign language grew among APRIAS members, they came to appreciate the communication possibilities it opened for them, and the emphasis shifted away from speech. Communicative outsiders in their own homes, they became part of a developing community within APRIAS. The crucial point that Polich establishes is *the virtuous circle of developing a language and a community that uses that language.* The joy of conversation provides powerful social bonds. Through such conversation, one has the chance to gain fluency in available signs and to share experiences that drive the invention and spread of new signs and constructions to tell others about those experiences. Polich found that it was only after APRIAS formed, probably not until 1989 and 1990, that the idea took hold that sign language could become the major medium of communication among deaf persons (rather than being used as a secondary system while placing primary emphasis upon oral communication).

However, whatever the importance of the community, each aspect of the language has to meet two conditions: (1) a specific individual or dyad used it for the first time (or the first time that they and others knew about) and (2) others, understanding its meaning, came to adopt it for their own use. Of course, as more people came to use it, the sign or construction may have shifted its "pronunciation" as well as its meaning. It is thus worth noting what Polich has to say about Javier Gómez López, whom many deaf adults who attended early APRIAS meetings credit with teaching sign language to all the others. Javier's interest in sign language began when he was given a sign language dictionary during a trip to Costa Rica in the late 1970s. He would seek out anyone who knew a sign language or had access to a dictionary of any kind in order to improve his vocabulary, and he would simultaneously teach what he learned to other deaf Nicaraguans. It is unclear how he managed to learn the language first while simultaneously teaching others. Perhaps he was more enthusiastic about signing, used it more consistently, and was patient about teaching what he knew to those less fluent. Moreover, Javier was active in the workshops in the years around 1990 in which groups of members of the association discussed which signs should be adopted as the "correct" versions that members should use.[7]

In 1990, the Royal Swedish Deaf Association sent representatives to visit APRIAS. This was apparently one of the earliest major contacts between APRIAS and individuals who not only advocated the use of sign language and expected deaf individuals to enter the world of employment but who also had a cultural conception of deafness as a difference rather than a defect. The Swedes urged the deaf members to rethink the value of oral skills and to value more deeply the sign language that they were using with each other. The new slate of officers for APRIAS elected on November 4, 1990 marked an important shift from an integrationist philosophy to one celebrating the deaf as a community and center of social agency for the deaf, with therefore no special need to integrate as oral individuals into the general society. The catch, however, is that oral Spanish is needed to find good jobs, and very few deaf people in Nicaragua have anything beyond low-paying jobs.

In 1991, the Swedes began to finance the collection of entries for a professionally published sign language dictionary. They also financed professional sign language instruction for teachers of the deaf and for teaching basic literacy classes to deaf members of the association. This makes clear that, at least from 1990 onward, the Nicaraguan Deaf community was in no way isolated. Note, however, that the Swedes did not teach Swedish Sign Language. Rather, while helping the Nicaraguan systematize what they had achieved in the early stages of creating NSL, they also provided models of expressiveness of sign language that spurred Association members to extend NSL. Indeed, Annie Senghas (personal communication) observes that the second cohort studied both Spanish dictionaries and ASL videos as a basis for devising new signs to expand NSL. But, although NSL exhibits some lexical influences from other sign languages, it shows enough distinctness of syntax and vocabulary to be classified as a separate sign language. Note that English, French, and German have distinctive phonologies—a hearing person doesn't need to speak these languages to recognize which language is being spoken on the basis of its distinctive "melody." In the same way, each sign language has its distinctive "phonology" in that certain handshapes recur as part of many signs, whereas others are not used in that sign language though they are fine in another; and similarly for the way the hands are moved within space, and manual gestures coupled with facial gestures. Thus, because NSL had already gained some distinctive "melody" of its own, the aim was not just to finger spell Spanish words and copy foreign signs, but rather to find equivalent signs with the look and feel of NSL. While NSL exhibits some lexical influences from Costa Rican, American, Swedish and Spanish sign language, it is not simply one of these languages. NSL shows enough variants in syntax and vocabulary that it can be classified as a separate sign language.

This supports the argument that the first "signers" (when in fact there was no such language as NSL, just a host of diverse, limited precursors) had the "Language is all around, I just can't hear it" cues that supported the creation of a community in they could learn the creations of others and begin to build an expanding vocabulary and shared set of constructions. The communal emergence of the new sign language from the mishmash of varied home signs and gestures increased just when adolescents and young adults began to remain longer in the educational system and began to increase their after-school contact. Polich argues that (1) being at an age when participation as an independent social actor is important interacted with (2) the formation of a group whose identity was based upon deafness, and both of these interacted with (3) the need for a communal sign language. All three elements seem to be needed, and they did not arise one at a time but developed together as a system.

However, the dynamics change as the fruits of the efforts of the first signers present a system of some complexity—perhaps somewhere between a protolanguage and a full language—to younger children. The deaf 6-year-olds now enter an educational system in which a changing NSL provides their first language environment, marking a passage from the constricted use of home sign.

Al-Sayyid Bedouin Sign Language

Since most deaf children in Nicaragua have hearing parents, and almost none of these have any knowledge of NSL, it is true that families do not play for NSL the role they play in transmission of most human languages—including ABSL. In this section, we use findings on ABSL to sharpen the lessons we gleaned from the study of NSL. First, let's summarize the history and context of the language as set forth by Sandler et al. (2005).

The Al-Sayyid Bedouin group, in the Negev region of present-day Israel, are descendants of a single founder, who arrived 200 years ago from Egypt and married a local woman. The group, now in its seventh generation, contains about 3,500 members, residing in a single community. Frequent consanguineous marriages have led to very strong group-internal bonds and group-external exclusion. About 150 people[8] with congenital deafness have been born into the community within the past three generations, all descended from two of the founders' five sons. All deaf individuals show profound neurosensory hearing loss and are of normal intelligence. In striking contrast to the deaf in Nicaragua, the deaf members of the community are fully integrated into its social structure and are neither shunned nor stigmatized. Both male and female deaf members of the community marry, and almost always to hearing individuals (since 2005 there have been two marriages of deaf people to other deaf people).

Many of the hearing members of the community communicate by means of the sign language with siblings and children of deaf individuals and other members of a household (which may include a large extended family), often becoming fluent signers (Kisch, 2004). In other words, the sign language is a second language of the village with deaf infants born into an environment with adult models of the language available to them (Sandler et al., 2005).

Signers readily use ABSL to relate information beyond the here and now, such as descriptions of folk remedies and cultural traditions, some of which are no longer in force. Sandler et al. (2005) state that they have documented personal histories of deaf members of the community and witnessed conversations in ABSL about topics as diverse as social security benefits, construction techniques, and fertility. Wendy Sandler, one of the four linguists who have studied ABSL (the others are Mark Aronoff, Irit Meir, and Carol Padden), gives her view of the relevance of their study of language emergence to the study of language evolution in the following terms (personal communication, September 2010; lightly edited):

> My team and I believe that we can learn something useful about the way
> in which human language developed originally by studying emerging sign

languages of the ABSL type. This belief is born of specific findings about ABSL, many of which have come as a surprise to us. For example, we find that the development of conventionalization in the form of words, the convergence on shared lexical items, the development of phonology (Sandler, Aronoff, Meir, & Padden, 2011), the emergence of complexity in prosody and syntax (Sandler, Meir, Dachkovsky, Padden, & Aronoff, 2011) as well as morphology are all much more gradual than would be expected either on the Universal Grammar view or on the view that the language is influenced by the surrounding hearing community. We also find that embodiment (Meir, Padden, Aronoff, & Sandler, 2007) plays a unique role in the development of sign language lexicons (one not found in spoken language). Further studies have focused on distinguishing pragmatic from syntactic word order (Padden, Meir, Sandler, & Aronoff, 2010) and assessing social factors in language emergence and development (Meir, Sandler, Padden, & Aronoff, 2010). This means that even in a community of communicators with modern brains and in a cultural context of a fully-fledged (but largely inaccessible) language, the development of language as we know it is best seen as a self-organizing system, influenced by the physical transmission system, cognitive and communicative factors, and also social factors such as community size and type and amount of interaction. We surmise that at the dawn of human language, structure also emerged gradually, and possibly along similar lines of development—though it may well have taken a lot longer.

My one quibble will be to assess in more detail their rejection of the view that the language is influenced by the surrounding hearing community.

Word Order in Al-Sayyid Bedouin Sign Language

Sandler et al. (2005) studied the second and third generations of signers—the first generation of signers consisted entirely of four siblings, all of whom are now dead. They focus their report on eight signers of the second generation, seven deaf and one hearing, all then in their 30s and 40s, except one in her 20s, but note that preliminary results from the third generation, ranging from teenagers to young children, reveal interesting differences between the systems of the two generations. They generated their corpus by presenting two tasks to the second generation of signers: (1) spontaneous recounting of a personal experience and (2) descriptions of single events portrayed by actors in a series of short video clips designed for field elicitation by the Language and Cognition Group at the Max Planck Institute for Psycholinguistics (Nijmegen, The Netherlands). All responses were videotaped, translated by a hearing signer from the same generation, and transcribed. The transcriptions consist of glosses for each individually identifiable sign production. Signs for actions or events were classified as the predicate nucleus of a sentence; other signs were classified as noun (N) arguments, adjectives, numerals, and negative markers, based on their meanings. Subjects, objects, and indirect objects (IO) were identified depending on their semantic roles in a clause and the standard mapping of these roles onto syntactic positions (Jackendoff, 1987).

Sandler et al. (2005) found that the grammatical relation between subject (S), object (O), and verb (V) was fixed at a very early stage in the development of ABSL, providing a convention for expressing the relation between elements in a sentence without relying on external context. However, the particular word orders in ABSL differ from those found both in the ambient spoken languages in the community and in Israeli Sign Language (ISL; Meir & Sandler, 2008). Therefore, the emerging grammatical structures should be regarded as developing as part of the emergence of ABSL. Moreover, Sandler et al. (2005) further claim that these grammatical structures are "a reflection of a basic property of language in general," a claim that we must scrutinize.

Most strings could be parsed unambiguously using semantic criteria, but in some cases prosodic criteria played a crucial role. Manual criteria at the intonational phrase boundary included holding the hands in place, pause and relaxation of the hands, or repeating the final sign in the constituent; nonmanual cues included both a clear change in head or body position and a concomitant change in facial expression (Nespor & Sandler, 1999). For example, one signer, in describing his personal history, produced the following string: MONEY COLLECT BUILD WALLS DOORS. The first prosodic constituent is MONEY COLLECT meaning "I saved money," confirming that it is an O–V sentence. The semantics indicates that WALLS and DOORS are patients related to the verb BUILD. BUILD WALLS DOORS was parsed using a prosodic break between BUILD and WALLS. This break involved holding the hands in position at the end of BUILD, and then moving the body first forward, then up, then enumerating the things being built, WALLS and DOORS. The spontaneous translation of the string by a consultant was: "I saved some money. I started to build a house. Walls, doors."

This string is instructive because of the potential ambiguity and the atypical word order of the chosen interpretation, but the vast majority of sentences in their data were unambiguous and straightforwardly (S)O–V. Either subject or object may be unexpressed, resulting in S–V or O–V strings. For example, in the observed description of a video clip showing a woman giving an apple to a man, WOMAN APPLE GIVE; MAN GIVE ["The woman gave an apple; (she) gave (it) to the man"], the first clause is S–O–V, and the second clause is IO–V. Another signer responded to the same clip with the following string: WOMAN GIVE MAN TAKE, that is, two S–V sentences. This generation of signers had little or no contact with ISL, whose word order appears to vary more widely in any case (Meir & Sandler, 2008), so the S-O-V is not inherited from ISL.

Moreover, the basic word order in the spoken Arabic dialect of the hearing members of the community, as well as in Hebrew, is S–V–O. Nonetheless, the only hearing subject in their study—bilingual in Arabic and ABSL—uses the S–O–V word order in his signing. Hence, the robust word-order pattern exhibited by the data exhibit an independent development within ABSL. Sandler et al. (2005) speak of "a pattern rooted in the basic syntactic notions of subject, object, and verb or predicate," but it is not clear from their data that ABSL signers are relying on these syntactic relations rather than the semantic relations between action, agent and theme, and so on.[9]

Like home signers, second-generation ABSL signers consistently produce sentences in which predicates appear in final position, but unlike home signers, they produce longer sentences with two or more nominals appearing before the predicate. And, indeed, second-generation ABSL signers are exposed to sign language from an early age and have more opportunity for extended sign language interaction with peers and adults than home signers.

As noted earlier, home signers show consistent word order appearing early in their gestural productions (Goldin-Meadow & Mylander, 1998). Although these children have no contact with other deaf signers, they regularly produce two-gesture strings in which actions appear in final position, and home-signers tend to omit signs for S, the subject. Indeed, when hearing speakers who know no sign language are asked to use their hands and not their mouths to communicate, the same O-V order arises despite the fact that their natural spoken language uses the S-V-O order (Goldin-Meadow, Yalabik, & Gershkoff-Stowe, 2000).[10]

The conclusion, then, is that language systems that are developed without input from conventional language appear prone to exhibit O-V order, at least in their early stages: "Here is the object; now see what is being done to it." Perhaps it is not too fanciful to compare this to the order of processing required in the MNS model of the mirror system (see Fig. 5-3 in Chapter 5): It requires that attention be directed to an object and its affordances before the network can recognize what action is being directed toward the object.

Phonology Emerging in Al-Sayyid Bedouin Sign Language

In Chapter 10, I quoted Hockett (1960, p. 95) to the effect that

> If a vocal-auditory system comes to have a larger and larger number of distinct meaningful elements, those elements inevitably come to be more and more similar to one another in sound. There is a practical limit [...] to the number of distinct stimuli that can be discriminated.

while noting that this would apply equally well to the expanding vocabulary of protosign as to that of protospeech. This quote was also used by Aronoff et al. (2008) in exploring the significance of ABSL for the discussion of protolanguage. As we have seen, they show that ABSL "has a robust basic syntax and a rich communicative repertoire" but they do present cases in which different people will use different signs for the same concept (a phenomenon that also happens with spoken languages without a written tradition). For example, the sign for "tree" or "banana" may remain close to pantomime though the signs used by different family members may be similar. This seems consistent with the hypothesis on the evolution of phonology, "Phonology Emerging," in Chapter 10. We saw that sign language has duality of patterning, but here the elements are a limited stock of handshapes, positions in signing space, and movements. Sandler, Aronoff et al. (2011) offer a detailed treatment of the issue of duality of patterning and the emergence of phonology, and they agree with Hockett that duality/phonology emerges when the message set gets too big for holistic signals. However, they note that sign languages may be able to get more mileage out of holistic signals that do not conform to the phonology because of the advantage of iconicity in creating interpretable signs as distinct from spoken words.

The Accrual of Constructions in Nicaraguan Sign Language and Al-Sayyid Bedouin Sign Language

Sandler et al. (2005) view the appearance of the S–O–V word order conventionalization in ABSL "at such an early stage in the emergence of a language [as] rare empirical verification of the unique proclivity of the human mind for structuring a communication system along grammatical lines." However, the "grammar" demonstrated in the earlier ABSL examples is very simple, and it should not be overinterpreted. What is remarkable is that the order of constituents was not taken over from that used by the Arabic-speaking members of the community. How did that occur? The earlier discussion of why the X-Y-X construction of NSL differs from Spanish constructions offers some clues. My hypothesis is that ABSL and NSL differ from home sign because:

- The existence of a community provides more opportunities to use signs and choose signs, so that some get lost to the community while others gain power by being widely shared—that is, "natural selection by learning"
- Since knowledge of another language is possessed by some members of the community, they seek to translate this knowledge into the new medium (as proven for the lexicon in the case of signs for days of the week entering the lexicon during the early stages leading up to the emergence of NSL), but few attempts to capture a given property will become widespread in the community.

If a language does not have a conventionalized word order, a sentence such as "Kim Jan touch" is ambiguous; it can mean either that Kim touched Jan or that Jan touched Kim. Once languages have had time to accrue such mechanisms as verb agreement, marking properties of subject or object, or case marking on noun to indicate their relation to the verb, the roles of participants can be made clear, even without consistent word order. In the absence of such mechanisms, word order is the only way to disambiguate a message linguistically. Thus, Sandler et al. (2005) insist that of even greater significance than any particular word order is the discovery that, very early in the history of the emergence of ABSL, a conventionalized pattern emerges for relating actions and events to the entities that perform and are affected by them. The S–O–V order they observed in ABSL is the most common word order in languages generally, according to Dryer's (1996) comprehensive survey of spoken languages. Newmeyer (2000) hypothesizes the S–O–V was the order for the original language "Proto-World" (though other authors doubt that there was one original language in human prehistory). He also hypothesizes that this protolanguage had inflectional affixes that marked the grammatical roles of sentence constituents, in addition to word order. ABSL, however, has no inflection of any sort.

Sign languages make use of "signing space" to make spatial relations clear (see Fig. 2-2 in Chapter 2) in a way that is denied to speech which is temporal without being spatial. Moreover, unlike speech, the manual modality makes it relatively easy to invent forms that can be understood by naïve observers (e.g., indexical pointing gestures or iconic miming gestures). As a result, communication systems can be invented "on the spot" in the manual modality. But (to revisit a question we confronted for NSL) has ABSL arisen de novo with *no influence* from any established language, either signed or spoken? I would answer "No." ABSL developed in a community in which the deaf were integrated with Arabic speakers, and the latter already had the use of a language. The problem was to find ways to express what they wanted to say in sign. As the earlier examples suggest, the challenge was to find low-energy ways to express these thoughts in a new medium. The resulting system had many novel features not present in Arabic, but this is very different from asserting there is *no influence*. Let me illustrate this with an example from English. The French expression "Respondez s'il vous plait"—"Reply, please (literally: if it pleases you)"—has passed into English as the abbreviation RSVP, spoken according to the English pronunciation of these four letters of the alphabet. This form is now used as both a noun and verb, and most people who use it do not know that it contains "please" as part of its meaning—hence the expressions "Please RSVP" or "Please send your RSVP to X." Despite this, it would be mistaken to deny that RSVP derives from French influence. But it does demonstrate that once a sign is introduced into a language by those who do know its etymology, it can take on a life of its own once adopted by those unaware of, or choosing to ignore, this etymology, and who thus can be quite free in the way they assimilate it to the structures of their own language.

There is a crucial distinction here. "Influence" and "borrowing" are different phenomena. All languages borrow words, but we would not say that Carib influences English because the word *hurricane* is borrowed from Carib. French influence would be something like changing the order of adjective and noun— *boy good* instead of *good boy*. But the discussion of X-Y-X in NSL is free from Spanish influence on NSL, while the S-O-V of ABSL runs counter to Arabic influence. But I am *not* claiming that Spanish influenced NSL or that Arabic influenced ABSL. I am saying that the speakers accelerated the development of each sign language *because they had the notion that words could be combined to express complex meanings and thus injected their clumsy attempts to express these compound meanings in the realm of gesture.* The presence of such performances provided invaluable grist for the mill of language emergence, but the emergence of specific constructions suited to express these compound meanings was internal to the emerging sign language community, just as was the conventionalization of signs to express word-like meanings.

The existence of Spanish *and its co-speech gestures* in the NSL environment contributes, I have suggested, to the "communicative idea" that deaf children then seek to express in the absence of speech, even though certain signs and constructions would in some cases displace the original gestural patterns. Indeed, Russo and Volterra (2005) note that Senghas et al. (2004) provided no information about the extent of the influence of gestures of hearing people during the early stages of acquisition of the deaf learners and about the influence of spoken and written languages such as Spanish or English (see Capirci & Volterra, 2008 for further development of these ideas). They note that Fusellier-Souza (2001, 2006), studying the "emerging sign languages" (ESL) spontaneously developed by deaf individuals in Brazil who were isolated from any Deaf community, in which case there was a strong continuity between the gestures used by the hearing population and the lexicon of the emerging sign languages. However, each of the three deaf people (two male, one female) Fusellier-Souza studied had a speaking person with whom he or she developed his or her own sign language, unique to this dyad. Moreover, each person developed a role within the broader Brazilian society and developed strategies for communication with other people. In some sense, then, an "emerging sign language" is better thought of as a "dyadic sign language" (DSL) to reflect the fact that it is the product of a community of at least two, but not necessarily more than two, people within their own lifetime. A DSL thus exhibits what can happen to home sign when, though isolated from an existing sign language, it has the crucial property that it is shaped by *exceptional* input from speaking members of the surrounding community (in this case, the other member of the dyad). We might say that a DSL is a "super home sign" as distinct from a home sign truncated either because the young child becomes a member of a Deaf signing community at a relatively early age (as happens with the current NSL community) or the child is treated as retarded and no one makes the effort to communicate with the child beyond the basics that can be conveyed in the child's early home sign (as was the case for many deaf children in Nicaragua prior to the formation of a special school for deaf children). Fusellier-Souza (personal communication, December 2007, slightly edited) reports that:

> two of my subjects (Ivaldo & Jo) have always worked in contact with hearing Brazilian people of their settings. When they are not in communication with their privileged hearing interlocutor, the communication with other hearing people is characterized by a kind of "exolingue gestural communication" based on face-to-face interactions, shared knowledge, use of the iconicization process activating the intent of the speaker to "say by showing" (using highly iconic structures, gestures of the hearing culture and loads of pointing for referential constructions). None of my deaf informants mastered written Portuguese. However, I've observed that Ivaldo uses his arm as a kind of board on which to use specific written forms of Portuguese (city name abbreviations, numbers, short names) in order to communicate with his hearing interlocutor. It's a clever strategy showing the use of functional writing despite extremely limited knowledge of written language.

A DSL thus lacks the systematization that results when a larger Deaf community converges on a shared set of signs but nonetheless reflects active engagement with speakers, akin to what I have suggested was operative in the presystematization stages of ABSL and NSL. Fusellier-Souza, who adopts the theoretical framework of the French linguist Christian Cuxac (see, e.g., Sallandre & Cuxac, 2002), stresses the role of iconicity in the autonomous development of signs, seeing it as playing an important role in different linguistic levels (phonetic, morphemic, lexical, syntactic, semantic, discourse). Here we may recall the crucial role of pantomime in the Mirror System Hypothesis, while also recalling that many processes serve to "erode" iconicity. Indeed, many signs in ASL make explicit the effects of bilingualism. For example, the ASL sign for BLUE is a nativized form of the finger spelling of B.[11] Russo and Volterra (2005) stress that the way in which young signers are exposed to gestural, vocal, or written language in the first years of acquisition may strongly affect their language competence (Bates & Volterra, 1984; Volterra & Erting, 1994), so that differences between generations of signers may be attributable to the different communicative inputs to which they were exposed. ABSL and

NSL reflect the merging of many people's contributions over multiple cohorts or generations and this process continues.

The Influences of Culture and Community

As we have seen, the Nicaraguan and Bedouin sign languages did not develop in a vacuum, but owe a debt to multiple influences. The language and the community appear to have grown in tandem. Polich's (2005) history of NSL shows the importance of adolescents and influential individuals in shaping the NSL of the first cohort. Thus, while young signers may better support the spread of innovations, this does not imply that all the innovations result from 6-year-olds regularizing the relatively poorly formed signs they see around them, though such regularization by young signers is certainly one factor in the emergence of the new sign language.

In discussing NSL, Senghas et al. (2004) assert the following:

> Our observations highlight two of the learning mechanisms available during childhood.
>
> a)   a dissecting, segmental approach to bundles of information; *this analyti-cal approach appears to override other patterns of organization in the input,* to the point of breaking apart previously unanalyzed wholes.
> b)   *a predisposition for linear sequencing; sequential combinations appear even when it is physically possible to combine elements simultaneously,* and despite the availability of a simultaneous model. [My italics.]

The analytical process of (a) is akin to our basic process of fractionation, though the statement of (a) omits mention of the complementary formation of constructions. As a caveat to (a), however, note that languages do resist decomposition when the compound is in frequent use. Thus, in English we say *kick* instead of *hit with the foot* and *punch* for *hit with the fist* but still have the decomposition *hit with a/the X*, where X is a less common instrument or where the foot or fist requires special emphasis—but even here, *He punched him with his left fist* seems better English than *He hit him with his left fist*. As a caveat to (b), note that many sign languages (including ASL) do make use of simultaneity—the path of the hand while signing a verb may be modified to express qualities that in English would be expressed sequentially by adding an adverb, and the form of the hand performing the predicate may be linked to the type of specific object acted upon.

Indeed, Senghas et al. themselves note that many sign languages use simultaneous combinations in addition to sequential ones—but then add that children acquiring ASL initially break complex verb expressions down into sequential morphemes (Meier, 1987; Newport, 1981), rather than producing multiple verb elements together in the single, simultaneous movement found in adult models. However, I suggest that this is a matter of attention and skill. Clearly, language must be learnable. The issue is where the specificity of learning lies. Language is a vast tissue of cumulative inventions that must (1) be made for the first time as well as (2) modified and (3) passed into vogue before (4) they become part of the language as passed on to successive generations. Some compounds are easy to imitate; others are hard. Speaking children first progress toward speech by mastering sounds that involve differential control of one articulator and only later master differential control of multiple articulators simultaneously (see Studdert-Kennedy, 2002 for data consistent with this view). Complex imitation is cumulative—the set of familiar actions available for the decomposition of novel actions grows with experience. Moreover, deaf children within a Deaf community (as distinct from those creating home sign) do not acquire signs by ritualizing pantomime, but rather emulate the signs themselves as entities within a communicative system—but pantomime and other gestures may serve to clarify what the novel gesture means. If a child sees a complicated sign, he or she will successfully mimic one or two features at first. I would thus suggest that what might look like breaking complex verb expressions down into sequential morphemes may be a matter of motor simplification rather than a linguistic reanalysis. Breaking complex skills into pieces and then learning how to gracefully reconstitute them is a general property of motor learning, and it should not be counted as a design feature specific to language.

Decades or Millennia?

Does the rapid rise of ABSL and NSL imply that once the brain of *Homo sapiens* achieved its present form, a mere two or three generations sufficed for emergence of a full human language? To the contrary, it has been argued (Noble & Davidson, 1996) that the brain of *Homo sapiens* was biologically ready for language perhaps 200,000 years ago, but, if increased complexity of artifacts like art and burial customs correlate with language of some subtlety, then human languages as we know them arose at most 50,000 to 90,000 years ago. If one accepts the idea that it took humans with brains based on a modern-like genotype 100,000 years or more to invent language as we know it, one must ask what advantage the NSL and ABSL communities had that early humans lacked. Recall the earlier hypothesis that ABSL and NSL differ from home sign because

i) The existence of a community provides more opportunities to use signs and choose signs, so that some get lost while increasingly many gain power by being widely shared.

ii) Those members of the community with knowledge of another language seek to translate this knowledge into the new medium.

Polich (2005) has shown us how NSL developed as the medium for community building even as the growing community supported the development of the language. But I claim that what catalyzed this development to take place in 20 years, more or less, was the overlap with a surrounding community in which language was already established and the changed awareness that the deaf could aspire to the formation of a community of their own. ABSL developed within an existing community as people—deaf and hearing—developed new forms of communication that enabled the deaf to become active members of that community. Even the relatively isolated home signer learns from his family that things can be freely named, and he recognizes the success of speech acts of others even if he cannot understand what is being said. Note, however, that the home signers studied by Goldin-Meadow do not remain isolated. Within a few years almost all are instructed within an oral or sign language. Contrast the different scenario for "dyadic" sign languages in Brazil.

Nicaraguan children (like home signers and the first generation of deaf Al-Sayyid Bedouin) lived in a world of many distinctive objects, both natural and artificial, and could see that something more subtle than pointing could be used to show which object was required. Moreover, some of the first NSL cohort had at least basic knowledge of Spanish, while the Al-Sayyid Bedouin community always integrated deaf and hearing people in the same extended family; thus, the speakers who already knew how to express something of their needs, or share their interest in the current scene, in Arabic would be motivated to try to convey these same ideas by pantomime and the development of increasingly conventionalized gestures.

Do the data on NSL suggest that if a group of babies were raised in isolation from humans with language, then in a few biological generations some critical mass of children—let's say 30 or so—would be enough to develop a language?[12] Must we reject the idea that it took human brains 100,000 years or more to invent language as we know it? Or is it the case that the Nicaraguan deaf children had an advantage that early humans lacked? I adopt the latter view. The advantage is the knowledge that things can be freely named and the knowledge that languages do exist. Certainly, the Nicaraguan children could not hear, but they could see the lip movements that indicated that their families could communicate their needs and requests. In addition, they lived in a world of many distinctive objects, both natural and artificial, and could see that something more subtle than pointing could be used to show which object was required. Moreover, some had at least basic knowledge of Spanish and had both seen and performed a variety of co-speech gestures. They were thus motivated to try to convey something of their needs or to share their interest in the current scene, by pantomime and the development of increasingly conventionalized gestures. By contrast, early humans shared a community but had no models of successful language use. For us, as modern humans, it seems almost inconceivable that the very *idea* of language is something that has to be invented. However, to take a related example, we know that writing was only invented some 5,000 years ago. Yet we have every reason to believe that no changes in brain genotype were required to support literacy, though the syndromes of dyslexia show that not all human brains are equally well prepared to match speech to writing, and the experience of literacy does indeed change the organization of the brain (Petersson, Reis, Askelof, Castro-Caldas, & Ingvar, 2000). Yet, once one has the *idea* of phonetic writing, it is a straightforward exercise to invent a writing system—as has been demonstrated by many Christian missionaries who wanted to bring literacy and the Bible to a people who had language but no writing. Even more pertinently, around 1820, Sequoyah, a Cherokee who knew very little English and could not read it, invented—inspired solely by the *idea* of writing—a successful syllabary with 86 characters to represent the sounds of the Cherokee language (Walker & Sarbaugh, 1993).

In view of all this, I doubt that a few children on a desert island would develop much beyond a rudimentary communication system of a few vocal and manual gestures and some conventionalized pantomime unless they had hundreds of generations in which to create culture and the means to discuss it. But they *would* have the brains to support such inventions once they were developed across many generations, whereas other creatures would not.

13

How Languages Keep Changing

We have seen (Chapters 10 and 12) the key process whereby languages get started—the emergence of more and more constructions first imposes semantic categories on the proliferating words of an emerging lexicon, and then constructions themselves became subject to processes of merging, generalization, and extension. In this process, word categories became increasingly divorced from the semantic moorings defined by filling the slots of very specific simple constructions and instead became increasingly syntactic as they expanded to fill the slots of the more general constructions. We also saw (Chapter 11) how processes that were operative in getting language started may also apply as children come to master the language that is already around them. This chapter complements these accounts by studying a few of the processes of historical change that have shaped and changed languages in recent centuries to suggest that they were operative in ancient times as protolanguages climbed the spectrum toward more and more features of modern languages. But first we look briefly at the archeological record of the making of stone tools to set some possible dates for the different stages posited in the Mirror System Hypothesis.

Before There Were Languages

Human cultures are far more diverse and complex than the "cultures" of any other species. This rests on increased dexterity, learning skills, and cognitive capacity in individual humans (Whiten, Horner, & Marshall-Pescini, 2003), which in turn support the increased "ratcheting" of human cultural transmission (Tennie, Call, & Tomasello, 2009; Tomasello, 1999). Moreover, the kind of social interaction we are familiar with at present requires nonprimitive languages. These observations support the notion of coevolution of language and social structure, with borrowing between cultures involved in both. The evolution of language would have added new dimensions to the life of early humans. They would have been more equipped to cooperate together in all aspects of life and to plan joint activities. This could have been the trigger for the development of a more sophisticated lifestyle, new forms of food gathering and preparation, leading to population increase and expansion into new territories. Here we see niche construction at work as a process of cultural rather than biological evolution, as niches reflect social schemas (as given by the development of agriculture, trade, cities, and so on—each providing a physical and social niche made possible by a shared set of cognitive representations) and then become part of the selective pressure for the adoption of new social schemas.

There is today no language that could be called primitive in the sense of having just a few hundred words and only a little grammar. Indeed, tribes with a limited material culture generally have an intricate social structure with an articulated system of classificatory relationships and communal obligations. For example, we noted earlier the complexity of linguistic structures reflecting kinship structures common in the Australian culture area but unknown elsewhere (Evans, 2003). Other complex systems may include pronouns with several number distinctions such as separate pronouns for "you (singular)," "you two," "you all," and sometimes also "you few" and two different pronouns for "me and you" and "me and someone else, other than you." However, *it is by no means the case that all languages are exactly equal in complexity* (Dixon, 1997, p. 75, footnote 8). Any one language may have greater overall grammatical complexity and/or a communicative advantage in a certain sphere as compared to another. When a pidgin (an impoverished second language shared by two or more linguistic groups) crystallizes into a Creole (which becomes the first language of a group), within just a couple of generations it becomes a linguistic system comparable in complexity to any well-established language. Given this rapidity, Dixon supports the hypothesis of sudden development in the evolution of language—for him, the first emergence of language was like an explosion. The human mind would have been mentally ready for language, and then it would have been invented, almost as a complete system. One would not get to 5,000 words in one generation, but Dixon suggests that each generation added appreciably to the vocabulary they learned from their parents.

Against this, one must note that the modern formation of new languages generally follows from a language that already has a large stock of concepts and grammatical devices. My claim is that there was a long accumulation of innovations across a spectrum of protolanguages that yielded something like modern languages by a process of bricolage over tens of millennia.

As noted previously, many archaeologists argue that humankind developed language at most 100,000 years ago (Noble & Davidson, 1996); but others believe that languages were used by species of *Homo* prior to *Homo sapiens*. However, nothing has been said in the preceding chapters about the time line for the various changes in the evolution of *Homo* that are associated with the biological evolution of the language-ready brain after the last common ancestor of chimpanzees and humans. In this section, I will use data on stone tools from the archeological record to calibrate the Mirror System Hypothesis. We sample the record of Paleolithic stone tool making, focusing on Stout's (2011) analysis of the hierarchy of processes apparently involved in Oldowan and Acheulean tool making, but with a somewhat different analysis informed by the brain modeling of Chapters 4 and 5.[1]

Oldowan Tool Making

The earliest known stone tools (Semaw, 2000) are assigned to the Oldowan Industry (ca. 2.6–1.4 million years ago) and consist of sharp stone flakes struck from cobble "cores" by direct percussion with another stone (the "hammerstone"). They consist of choppers, bone breakers, and flakes that may have been used to break open the bones of animals to extract the protein-rich marrow. The key innovation lay in flaking stones to create a chopping or cutting edge. Typically, many flakes were struck from a single core stone.

Even the basic act of striking a flake demands more than the appropriate grasp of hammer stone and cobble. For example, when producing a stone flake, the part of the hammerstone that is intended to strike the cobble becomes the end effector for the strike. As Bril et al. (2010) emphasize, expertise is exhibited not only in the overall organization of the behavior but also through increasingly skillful execution of single actions (which rests on extended practice). For example, in present-day studies, only experts at detaching stone flakes from a flint core through a conchoidal fracture regulated their actions according to changes in hammer weight in a manner that left kinetic energy unchanged. Their expertise was manifested in their mastery of the interactions between functional parameters.

As Stout (2010) observes, Oldowan stone making includes the following: (1) *procurement of raw materials* (both core and hammerstone—though one may start with a hammerstone retained from a previous occasion, and then either select a core from a pile at hand or conduct the preliminary search and evaluation until a suitable core is found) and (2) the repetition of *flake detachment* as often as is desired or possible with the given core and hammerstone. The latter involves four steps: select an affordance for detachment on the core; position the core for ease of access to the affordance; hold the hammerstone and position it relative to the affordance; and strike the affordance with the appropriate part of the hammerstone. Stout represents this by a tree diagram with six nested levels, ranging from the overall goal of flake production to specific manipulations of the core and hammerstone. However, I think the working memory requirements are more economical than this suggests. Given the overall goal of making a stone flake, the script reduces to the following: Do I have a hammer-stone? Do I have a core? Is there an available affordance for flake detachment? If so, proceed with flake detachment. If not, back up as far as needed.

Some early Oldowan assemblages exhibit systematically biased patterns of flake detachment that are underdetermined by the morphological variability of Oldowan cores, suggesting (Stout, Semaw, Rogers, & Cauche, 2010) a learned tendency to select targets in relation to the position of previous detachments (e.g., laterally adjacent, alternate face, same plane, etc.). Nonetheless, the stasis of Oldowan tool making suggests transmission of a few basic discoveries rather than emergence of a general skill for tool making. Here we see a parallel with the limited call set of any group of chimpanzees, which seems quite distinct from the takeoff in innovation in protolanguage once the ability to create protowords becomes explicitly available to the community. The range of Oldowan tools seems comparable to those of modern chimpanzees. Boesch and Boesch (1990) assessed tool use for three wild chimpanzee populations, finding 12 types of tool use in Mahale, 16 in Gombe, and 19 in Taï, where 6 types of tool making had been observed. Sticks were used and prepared at all three sites. However, Taï chimpanzees performed more modifications before using them and were the only chimpanzees seen to pound objects with tools and to combine two different tool uses to get access to one food item. For example, their Figure 1 shows an adult female cracking a hard panda nut with an 8-kg hammerstone while an adult male uses a small stick to extract kernel remains from a piece of nut opened and partly eaten by the female.

Acheulian Tool Making

The Acheulian tool industry consisted of axes, picks, and cleavers. It first appeared around 1.5 million years ago and is associated with *Homo erectus*. The key innovations are the shaping of an entire stone to a stereotyped tool form, as well as chipping the stone from both sides to produce a symmetrical (bifacial) cutting edge. This activity required manual dexterity, strength, and skill. However, the same tools were also used for a variety of tasks such as slicing open animal skins, carving meat, and breaking bones. The Early Acheulean (ca. 1.6–0.9 million years ago) can be characterized by elaborate flake production and by the emergence of large cutting tools, while Late Acheulean (ca. 0.7–0.25 million years ago) sees production of blanks as the basis of more sophisticated shaping to achieve different tool forms.

For Stout (2010), all the Early Acheulean forms of elaborate flake production reflect the key innovation of modification of the core to enable subsequent flake detachments as an explicitly preparatory action, rather than as a by-product of primary flake detachment. *Procurement of raw materials* (both core and hammerstone) is as before, but now the extra stage of *core preparation* is involved: This is like Oldowan flake detachment, but now the criterion is not to produce a final flake but rather to convert a less desirable cobblestone into a desirable cobblestone plus a remainder. Then flake detachment is practiced repeatedly with the manufactured core, after which core preparation is repeated until the possibilities of the original core are exhausted. Since the stone "remembers" the repeated applications, the limits to repetition are physical rather than involving cognitive limits on working memory.

Two large cutting tool forms typical of the earliest Acheulean sites are pointed "hand axes" produced on large (>10 cm) flakes and relatively thick, and pointed "picks" typically produced from cobbles. The production of such tools involves both structured flaking and the further innovation of intentional shaping. The production of large flakes (called "blanks") suitable for shaping into a hand axe was a key innovation of the Early Acheulean, and it involves an elaboration of raw material procurement into a multicomponent quarrying process. Blank production requires a heavier hammerstone and much greater force than Oldowan flake production, and the largest cores would have necessarily been supported on the ground instead of in the hand. This requires the use of additional small boulders or cobbles to brace the core in an appropriate position (Toth, 2001). These fundamental differences in perceptual-motor organization make Acheulean blank production qualitatively different from Oldowan flaking (Semaw, Rogers, & Stout, 2009).

This coordination of production elements requires that the tool maker develop the skills of not only (1) selecting a cobblestone from (a fragment of) which a tool of a given type could be produced (e.g., a hand axe or pick—both these forms can occur at a single site) but also (2) forming a stable visual representation of the shape of the tool to be produced on this occasion and associated lower level actions. The crucial point is that the choice of affordances for each blow would now be based on this imagined final shape, rather than the independent selection of a place on the cobble as offering a suitable affordance for striking off a flake. Relatively broad criteria for forming a blade support the visualization of the desired shape of the axe or pick and then the use of this to guide the choice of affordances. Modern toolmakers (e.g., Pelegrin, 1990) describe shaping in terms of the pursuit of local subgoals resulting in the successive approximation of an overall target form. For example, a short series of flakes might be aimed at creating an edge, followed by a reappraisal of the overall form, selection of the next appropriate subgoal and so on. This increases the hierarchical complexity of the process, but the key change is the novel demand on working memory—namely to keep in mind the desired form and use this to evaluate the next flake. This could, but need not, involve an intermediate level of "finish this edge first."

We may note here not only the relevance of the FARS model (Chapter 4) but also the importance of the role of visualization in setting the goal. The challenge is not so much increased hierarchical complexity as in the ability to maintain the visual goal even as one rotates the cobble to find new affordances then changes it by removing further flakes. The core itself, as it changes, structures behavior by its relation to a visualized final form of much greater specificity than "a decent core" or "a decent flake." Note that even in Oldowan tool making, the perceptual side—judging a suitable affordance with respect to the current goal—goes "hand in hand" with exercising the motor side, the appropriate effectivity.

As Stout (2010) emphasizes, this technology shows substantial variation: At one Olduvai site (1.33 million years ago) large cutting tools were produced using a consistent "rhomboidal" strategy of unifacial removals from opposite sides of tabular quartz blocks, while at other sites in Gona, Ethiopia (1.6 million years ago) and West Turkana, Kenya (1.7 million years ago), variable combinations of unifacial and bifacial removals from two or three worked edges were used to fashion trihedral "picks" from lava cobbles. However, given the great separation in space and time between Olduvai 1.33 million years ago and West Turkana 400,000 years earlier, the evidence points to *very* slow cultural evolution rather than variations of a shared technique in any one Early Acheulean community.

The technological transition to the Late Acheulean occurred before 0.5 million years ago (Clark, 2001). It involves the appearance of smaller, thinner, more regular and symmetrical large cutting tools thought to require the use of a "soft hammer" technique during production. The 0.7 million-year-old site of Isenya in Kenya (Roche, 2005) provides one of the earliest reported examples of such tools and also provides examples of "cleavers." These require predetermined blank production to yield a long, sharp cleaver bit on the blank prior to any shaping. This process elaborates Early Acheulean blank production. Late Acheulean methods are transitional to subsequent Middle Stone Age prepared-core flake production strategies, with the main shifts being a reduction in size (likely related to the introduction of hafting in the Middle Stone Age) and a further diversification of methods.

In characterizing this new technology, Stout (2010) emphasizes three innovations: (1) the choice of soft versus hard hammer stones (there is thus an explicit preparation of a "tool kit" of hammers, rather than just seeking a hammerstone at large); (2) a repertoire of products beyond just the hand axe and pick; and (3) platform preparation (preparation of the surface to be struck; not to be confused with the "stand" for holding the core mentioned earlier). The production of the thinner, more regular large cutting tools characteristic of the Late Acheulean involves a more elaborate shaping process (Edwards,

2001). Examples of well-thinned Late Acheulean large cutting tools have been described from Europe, Western Asia, and Africa in a variety of raw materials. Various different sized hammer stones may be required for different subgoals within the shaping process. Together with selection of a hammer appropriate to the intended percussion, platform preparation becomes part of a new structural unit, "complex flake detachment," which may be substituted for simple flake detachment and combined iteratively to achieve subgoals during shaping and especially thinning. Of particular relevance here is the issue of automatization: The initial increase in the depth of the action hierarchy (simple flake detachment becomes a subschema of complex flake detachment) becomes reversed as the coordinated control program for complex flake detachment becomes automatized, and thus it can be treated as a unitary action within the overall process.

The Emergence of Homo Sapiens

By 200,000 years ago, the technology was in place to create a variety of tools, since the rough blank could follow a pattern that ultimately became cutting tools, serrated tools, flake blades, scrapers, or lances. Furthermore, these tools could be used with other components to form handles and spears, and as tools to make other tools such as wooden and bone artifacts.

Archeology in Europe has found instances of human art in the forms of beads, tooth necklaces, cave paintings, stone carvings, and figurines from 40,000 years ago. This period in tool manufacture is known as the Upper Paleolithic, and it ranges from 40,000 years ago to the advent of agriculture around 12,000 years ago. Sewing needles and fish hooks made of bone and antlers appear, along with flaked stones for arrows and spears, burins for working bone and ivory, multibarbed harpoon points, and spear throwers made of wood, bone, or antler (Mithen, 2007; Wynn, 2009; Wynn & Coolidge, 2004).

However, McBrearty and Brooks (2000) stress that we must not read too much into the European provenance of much of the relevant archeology. Proponents of the "human revolution" theory claim that modern human behaviors arose suddenly, and nearly simultaneously, throughout the Old World ca. 50,000–40,000 years ago and some would link this to reorganization of the brain accompanying the origin of language. Contra this, McBrearty and Brooks document that many of the components of the "human revolution" are found in the African Middle Stone Age tens of thousands of years earlier and occur at sites that are widely separated in space and time. They thus argue for a gradual assembling of the package of modern human behaviors in Africa and its later export to other regions of the Old World. The first signs of modern behavior coincide with the appearance of fossils that have been attributed to

Homo helmei, but they argue on anatomical and behavioral grounds that *Homo helmei* should not be differentiated from *Homo sapiens*, so that the origin of our species can be linked with the appearance of Middle Stone Age technology at 250,000–300,000 years ago, following the late Acheulean.

This view is consonant with the Mirror System Hypothesis if we offer the following equations[2]:

- The Oldowan was a period during which our ancestors were still limited to simple imitation and communicated with a limited repertoire of vocal and manual gestures akin to those of a group of modern great apes.
- The early Acheulean was *transitional* between simple and complex imitation, with the transfer of skills being limited in depth of hierarchy and exhibiting little if any ratcheting. At this stage, protohumans communicated with a limited repertoire of vocal and manual gestures larger than those of a group of modern great apes but still very limited.
- The late Acheulean was the period in which complex imitation emerged, and communication gained an open-ended semantics through the conscious use of pantomime with a reliance on increasingly rich memory structures capable of holding hierarchical plans for both praxis and communication. Here we may note the emphasis on the expansion of memory in the approach to evolution of brain mechanisms supporting language offered by Francisco Aboitiz and his colleagues (Aboitiz & García, 2009; Aboitiz, García, Brunetti, & Bosman, 2006; Aboitiz & Garcia, 1997).

We could then agree on the following:

- *Homo sapiens* was the first species of *Homo* with a language-ready brain. However, it took more than 100,000 years for the developing power of protolanguage to yield the first true languages with their consequent impact on the acceleration of cultural evolution.

Further research is required to place this claim in the context of research on cultural evolution—for example, to assess to what extent it is compatible with the rather different account by Richerson and Boyd (2010) of "Why Possibly Language Evolved," rooted in their considerable work on cultural evolution extending from their classic book (Boyd & Richerson, 1985) to their recent demonstration that rapid cultural adaptation can facilitate the evolution of large-scale cooperation (Boyd, Richerson, & Henrich, 2011). A current sampling of relevant research is contained in the special issue of the *Philosophical Transactions of the Royal Society B: Biological Sciences* devoted to the proceedings of the Discussion Meeting on "Culture evolves." In their Introduction, Whiten et al. (2011) survey the various approaches to their subject. Perhaps most relevant to the basis of the Mirror System Hypothesis in comparative primatology are studies revealing that processes important in cultural transmission are more widespread in other species than earlier recognized, suggesting previously unidentified continuities between animal and human culture. Nonetheless, given the differences charted here between the communication systems of nonhuman primates, protolanguages, and languages, equal attention must be given to papers assessing the diversification of human cultures together with those exploring the impact of cultural evolution in the predispositions of human minds for cultural transmission. For example, Rendell, Boyd et al. (2011) advert to our theme of imitation by analyzing how copying affects the amount, evenness, and persistence of cultural knowledge. A crucial target for study will be to assess the way in which a modern human brain could support tens of millennia of relative stasis in tool use and (presumably) protolanguage yet yield a rapid acceleration in recent millennia. Is it cause or effect of the demographic explosion?

Protolanguages as Understood in Historical Linguistics

In Chapter 12, I put forward the idea that the pace of language change will be vastly faster in a community that contains members who already have the use of fully complex languages, as distinct from our early ancestors who had only the rudiments of protolanguage. There may have been tens of millennia in which the basic "discoveries" of language structure were made, and these then diffused over the at-that-time relatively limited extent of human habitation over further tens of millennia providing an areal family of protolanguages with enough in common to anchor the full complexity of early languages as they emerged over, perhaps, the period from 100,000 to 50,000 years before the present.[3]

In every section of the book except this one and the brief preview in Chapter 6, the word *protolanguage* means an open-ended communication system that (perhaps during the late Acheulean and on into the early tens of millennia of *Homo sapiens*) bridged between the ape-like communication systems of protohumans (e.g., in the periods of Oldowan and Early Acheulean periods) and languages as we know them today. However, in the present discussion of historical linguistics, we locate ourselves firmly within the realm of the history of human languages, and here we will use the word "protolanguage" to mean a fully developed language ancestral to a range of later languages. When the written forms of a number of languages are available, linguists can actually trace the relation of the languages. For example, it is well documented how the growth of the Roman Empire brought the Latin language to much of present-day

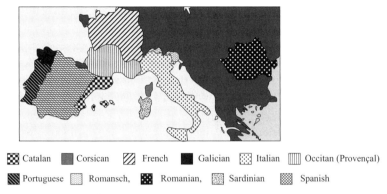

▨ Catalan	■ Corsican	▧ French	■ Galician	⠿ Italian	⦙⦙⦙ Occitan (Provençal)

▩ Portuguese ▨ Romansch, ▦ Romanian, ▨ Sardinian ▨ Spanish

FIGURE 13-1.   Romance languages in Europe.

Europe and North Africa, and how over the course of history different peoples
adapted Latin to their needs in different ways—from French to Italian to
Romanian and many other Romance languages. Figure 13-1 shows *some* of
the Romance languages in approximately the sites where, for various reasons,
a group of people varied their lexicon and their grammar over the centuries
to the point where what they spoke was better characterized as a separate
language rather than a dialect of Latin. However, it also shows the marks of
history. The Roman Empire eventually broke into two separate empires, the
Western Empire with its capital in Rome, and the Eastern Empire with its capital in Constantinople (present-day Istanbul). Greek rather than Latin became
the official language of the Eastern Roman Empire and Romania remained as
the one "island" in the East in which Latin continued as the dominant tongue,
eventually mutating into the Romanian language of today. Spanish and
Portuguese are very similar, and the two of them are more similar to Italian
than to French. All this would seem, at first, to support a *family tree* model of a
collection of related languages with "parent and child" linkages that show the
descent of the languages from a postulated single protolanguage.

There are other marks of history that Figure 13-1 does not show. For example, while much of North Africa was included in the Roman Empire, the successful spread of Islam from Arabia across North Africa effectively eliminated
the use of Latin and replaced it with Arabic as the dominant language of the
region. Thus, present-day North Africa has no "homegrown" Romance languages. Parts of Spain were also for many centuries under Muslim, Arabic-
speaking rule but were eventually reunited under Christian rulers who did
not tolerate the use of Arabic. As a result, Spaniards speak a Romance language (because of the Reconquest) but Spanish has far more Arabic-derived

words in its vocabulary than other Romance languages (the result of the years of Moorish dominance). This reminds us that a family tree shows only a small part of the history—it shows all the descendants of one person or language, but (unless it foregoes the simple structure of an "Australian tree" with a single root at the top, branching downward) it does not show the partners who made the descendants possible. However, although a person has exactly two parents each donating the same amount of genetic material, a language may have several parents each contributing in different amounts and in different ways to the lexicon and grammar of their offspring.

Another aspect of history is that, although Romance languages initially developed within the footprint of the Roman Empire in its heyday, Romance languages are now spoken around the world where they remain as the legacy of European colonialism from 1492 onward—with, for example, Portuguese dominant in Brazil and Spanish dominant in the rest of Latin America. We also have Francophone and Anglophone areas of Africa and the widespread use of English in India, reflecting the spread of French and British imperialism. Even though the empires have now dissolved and, in many cases, the European powers are now friends rather than masters of the countries they once ruled, use of the colonial language often remains widespread.

But what of the history of languages long before the rise and fall of the Roman Empire? Europe, Asia, and Africa are connected land masses in which humans have been living for tens of thousands, of years, with *Homo sapiens* radiating out from Africa, where, it is presumed, language originally developed. Archeologists have shown that humans arrived about 50,000 to 60,000 years ago in Australia/New Guinea (which was then one land mass); some 12,000 years to 20,000 years ago in the Americas, crossing from Siberia via the Bering Strait; and less than 4,000 years ago in the islands of the Pacific. It may never be possible to decide on linguistic grounds whether language developed just once (monogenesis) or separately in two or more places (polygenesis). And it will certainly never be possible for linguists to recover the structure of "protoworld" if indeed monogenesis holds. Nonetheless, it seems more likely that multiple protolanguages developed well before there were languages with anything like the richness of modern human languages.

Approximate dates have been assigned for historical protolanguages— about 6,000 years before the present has been suggested for proto-Indo-European. However, given the lack of written records, perhaps all we can say is, "We do not know" or, perhaps, "Probably some time between 5,000 and perhaps 12,000 before the present." What happened between the dawn of language and the protolanguages of modern language families such as Indo-European, some 6,000 to 10,000 years ago? Since the reconstruction process can only assume regularity in the reconstructed language, the parts of a protolanguage that are reconstructed tend to show tidy and homogeneous patterns, with few (if any) irregularities. Attested spoken languages are seldom like this—there are often one or more substrata (features from the language that the given languages replace) or superstrata (features from another language formerly spoken within the same society by a dominant group).

Every language and dialect is continually changing, but the rate at which a language changes is not constant. Generally, a language with no immediate neighbors is likely to change relatively slowly whereas a nonprestige language is likely to become more similar to a prestige language that is known to most of its speakers. When two groups of people—each speaking a distinct language—merge to form one community with a single language, this will be most directly influenced by just one of the original languages but is likely to have a sizable substratum or superstratum from the second language. In linguistics, a *substratum* is a language that has lower power or status than another, while a *superstratum* is the language that has higher power or status. Both substratum and superstratum languages influence each other, but in different ways. We shall see more of this in our later discussion of pidgins and creoles. Generally, the group with the greater prestige will be the one with the most new things. Australian aboriginal languages have borrowed from English terms for *gun, pub, church, policeman, car, shirt, trousers, mirror, work, buy,* and *muster.* But when a prestige language is an invader, it may borrow terms from the indigenous languages for local flora, fauna, and artifacts, so that English has loan words from Australian languages such as *kangaroo, wombat, budgerigar,* and *boomerang.* In many situations nouns are borrowed more freely than verbs.

German and English are closely related (sharing many grammatical forms and a high proportion of the most frequently used lexemes, including those with irregular inflections), but English has a sizable French superstratum in lexicon and to some extent in grammar and phonology. In the future the grammar and lexicon of English will undergo considerable changes in its descendants. Grammatical irregularities are likely to be lost. In addition, words of Romance origin in English vocabulary could be used at the expense of Germanic lexemes. If this were to happen, future linguists might infer a three-way split from a protolanguage into German, English, and French, rather than seeing German and English as sister languages, with English being modified by the influence of French. Conversely, when reconstructing a putative protolanguage for a given language family, the historical linguist may come out with more forms—to which a particular meaning or function is assigned—than any one language is likely to have had, such as two forms for a certain person/number combination in pronouns, for certain demonstratives or interrogatives, or for certain body parts. Indeed, attempts to reconstruct proto-Romance from the daughters of Latin would certainly not give us the Latin for which we have full written records (Schmid, 1987).

With geographical separation, the development from one language to two would be a gradual process. This is because with no contact between the groups they would not be trying to communicate with each other. If contact were reestablished at some intermediate time (before the languages were fully distinct), either speakers of the two groups would establish close relations and each accommodate its speech toward that of the other group, establishing them as dialects of one language; or each group might adopt a standoffish attitude toward the other, engineering further changes in each way of speech so that they would eventually have two distinct languages. For example, I was told by a Slovenian colleague (personal communication, January 15, 1999) that such a deliberate effort was being made to differentiate Serbian and Croatian from Serbo-Croatian as a side effect of the wars then underway in the former Yugoslavia. Different orthography can also be used to reinforce difference. For example, Spanish uses ll and ñ for the palatal lateral and nasal, while Portuguese employs lh and nh.

As Dixon (1997) notes, there are various catalysts for rapid language change. These include *natural causes*, such as changes in living conditions, fall or rise in sea levels, disease, and genetic mutation; *material innovations* such as new tools and weapons, means of transportation, and the invention of agriculture; and *development of aggressive tendencies* as when a local chief aspires to more inclusive power, or a new religion emerges that brooks no challenge. *Geographical possibilities* include expansion into uninhabited territory and expansion into previously occupied territory. Where the invaded territory consists of many small groups, each with its own language (as in the Americas and Australia), or where the numbers of the invader greatly exceed those of the original inhabitants (as in New Zealand), the original languages will decline and in time be replaced, to a great extent, by the prestige language (though attempts have been underway in New Zealand to reinvigorate and spread the use of the Maori language).[4] Where the invaded territory does have well-developed political groups, languages with millions of speakers and perhaps one or more highly developed religions, then the indigenous languages will not decline in use, but the language of the invader still becomes the prestige language, as in India. Very occasionally, the invader's language may fall into disuse, as happened with Norman French in England. Even here, though, it has provided a very significant superstratum within modern English, despite the facts that the number of Normans was relatively small and they came from a culture with no major material or religious differences from the English.

In the remaining two sections we first look at *grammaticalization* as a process of language change that may operate over time within a language, and we then turn to *pidgins and creoles* to see how a new language may emerge from contact between two or more already existing languages.

Grammaticalization

Grammaticalization is the process whereby over time information expressed in a string of words or a supplementary sentence becomes transformed into part of the grammar. It provides a crucial engine for language change.[5] The following pairs of sentences from English demonstrate the process. In each case, a particular verb used in sentence A becomes a marker for the indicated grammatical function in sentence B:

A	He kept the money.	Verb
B	He kept complaining.	Durative
A	He used all the money.	Verb
B	He used to come.	Habitual
A	He's going to town.	Verb
B	He's going to come.	Future

Moreover, in each case, there was a time in the history of English when usage A was part of the language but B was not, whereas in current English either form can be used. These examples motivate an extended view of *grammaticalization* as embracing not only the process whereby lexical forms become grammatical forms but also the transition from grammatical forms to further grammatical forms. In this way linguistic forms previously used for meanings that are relatively concrete or easily accessible can be employed for the expression of more grammatical functions.

We can formalize these examples of the A-B relation as follows (there are, of course, many other types of grammaticalization):

a. There are two items *a* (in A) and *b* (in B) in language L that sound the same, where *a* serves as a lexical verb and *b* as an auxiliary marking grammatical functions such as tense, aspect, or modality.
b. While *a* has a noun as the nucleus of its complement, *b* has a nonfinite verb instead.
c. B is historically derived from A.
d. The process from A to B is unidirectional; that is, it is unlikely that there is a language where A is derived from B.

Heine and Kuteva (2007, 2011) developed the scheme shown in Figure 13–2 for the historical emergence of linguistic categories by processes of successive grammaticalization, discussing ways in which grammaticalization theory may serve as a tool for reconstructing the cultural evolution of languages from

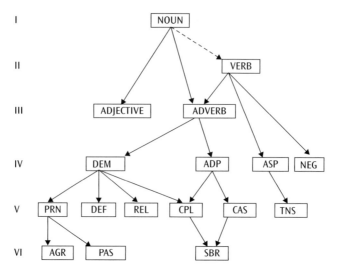

FIGURE 13-2.   A scheme for the historical emergence of linguistic categories by processes of successive grammaticalization (adapted from Heine & Kuteva, 2007, p. 111). The six levels are spelled out in Table 13-1. AGR, agreement marker; ADP, prepositions and other adpositions; ASP, (verbal) aspect; CAS, case marker; CPL, complementizer; DEF, marker of definiteness ("definite article"); DEM, demonstrative; NEG, negation marker; PAS, passive marker; PRN, pronoun; REL, relative clause marker; SBR, subordinating marker of adverbial clauses; TNS, tense marker. The dotted line indicates that there is only indirect evidence for reconstructing this development.

earlier forms, rather than the biological evolution that made protolanguages (in our usual sense) and the subsequent processes of grammaticalization possible. The exploration of all the arrows in the figure is beyond the scope of the present volume, but we have already seen in the earlier A-B pairs examples of how aspect (ASP) and tense (TNS) may have emerged by the grammaticalization of verbs (VERB). The six layers of the figure are seen as exemplifying the six stages of grammatical (cultural) evolution shown in Table 13-1. In terms of the approach in Chapter 10, however, we would not start with a Stage I of nouns alone, with verbs emerging in Stage II. Rather, we would start with protowords whose fractionation would yield constructions whose cumulative effect would be to yield categories of slot fillers akin to nouns and verbs. Moreover, as we have already stressed, what constitutes a noun and what constitutes a verb may be highly language dependent, although each will be grounded in words-for-objects and words-for-actions, respectively.

Such a table raises the question: What was the motivation for developing all these structures? Does a language *need* all of these devices, including verbal inflections, case suffixes, and so on? Our earlier discussion would argue against this. Different languages differ in their employment of important grammatical

Table 13-1   The Six Stages of Grammaticalization Posited by Heine and Kuteva

I	nouns [one-word utterances]	stone, tree
II	verbs [mono-clausal propositions]	sleep, cut
III	adjectives, adverbs [head-dependent structure]	big tree
IV	demonstratives, adpositions, aspect markers, negation—all of which provide elaboration of phrase structure	in this big tree
V	pronouns, definite (and indefinite) markers, relative clause markers, complementizers, case markers, tense markers—providing mechanisms for clause subordination, temporal and spatial displacement and so on.	the big tree that I saw
VI	agreement markers, passive markers, adverbial clause subordinators	when the fire was lit

features. German has a system of case inflections, whereas English does not; and both English and German have grammatical inflections, whereas Chinese does not. As each language has changed through history, grammaticalization can continually innovate while existing constructions may disappear. The drive is the need to communicate, but similar messages can be expressed in diverse ways.

Heine and Kuteva offer a four-stage model (Table 13–2) of context-induced reinterpretation of meaning in grammaticalization as the source meaning (as in sentences A earlier) becomes transformed into its new, grammaticalized target meaning (sentences B)—but note again that in general the emergence of the new target meaning in novel contexts need not block the continued use of the word in its source meaning in other contexts.

Heine adds to the study of grammaticalization another approach to language evolution: consideration of *parenthetical categories* as linguistic "fossils"

Table 13-2   Heine and Kuteva's Four-Stage Model of Context-Induced Reinterpretation of Meaning in Grammaticalization

Stage	Context	Resulting Meaning	Type of Inference
Initial stage	Unconstrained	Source meaning	—
Bridging context	A new context triggering a new meaning	Target meaning foregrounded	Invited (cancelable)
Switch context	A new context incompatible with the source meaning	Source meaning backgrounded	Usual (typically noncancelable)
Conventionalization	Target meaning no longer needs to be supported by context that gave rise to it; use in new contexts possible	Target meaning only	—

that, though they exist in modern languages, may tell us something of stages en route to language. Here are some English examples of parenthetical categories:

- *Formulae of social exchange*: goodbye, happy birthday, hi, never mind, sorry, watch out! well done, thank you, yes, no, no way, listen
- *Vocatives*: Peter! Mrs. Smith! Ladies and Gentlemen! My dear friends!
- *Interjections*: hey, ouch, whoopee, wow, yo, yuck

Each of these parentheticals is autonomous. It can form an utterance of its own that is not integral to the sentence grammar either syntactically or prosodically, and it forms a separate intonation unit set off from the rest of the utterance by means of pauses. Its use is optional, occurring much more often in spoken than in written discourse. On this basis, Heine suggests that formulae of social exchange, vocatives and interjections, were each important in the conceptual grammar of early languages but not integrated into a single system. Note, however, that these examples of formulae of social exchange and vocatives all employ standard words of English, whereas interjections do not. Thus, it seems plausible that in due course conceptual grammar came to incorporate formulae of social exchange and vocatives as parts of the integrated grammar of the language, whereas the interjections may augment discourse yet not really be part of the language. For example, a hand gesture of greeting and farewell might be a possible precursor for finding formulas of courtesy to bring them within language, and in some cases these formulas could be compressed to yield new words that are now within the language, as in *God be with you* → *Goodbye*, and *Ma dame* → *Madam*.

To close this section, we return to the issue of *recursion*, which we met in Chapter 6 when introducing the property we called *syntax, semantics, and recursion*. Earlier, in Chapter 2, we met a basic example of this: a noun phrase (whether just a noun, or already built up using adjectives) can be a constituent of a larger noun phrase, as in forming "rose" then "blue rose" and then "wilted blue rose." Thus, recursion arises naturally, in this very simple case, through the linkage of language to the process of scene description when we add further details or specificity to our description as we attend to further aspects of a scene. Heine and Kuteva suggest some of the further ways in which recursion may have arisen:

A: There is the car. I like that (one).	Demonstrative pronoun
Intermediate: There is the car; that (one) I like.	Demonstrative pronoun
B: There is the car [that I like].	Relativizer

Here we see a process of *integration* as *that* changes roles, taking us from juxtaposition [S1 + S2] of two separate sentences to embedding recursion S1

[S2] via the device of relative clauses, where in A the demonstrative pronoun *that* of S2 refers anaphorically to some participant of S1 but in B has become grammaticalized to a relative clause marker, while S2 becomes grammaticalized to a relative clause.

In the next example we see something like the merging of a *conceptual parenthetical* (e.g., I think, if you will, as it were, etc.) with the sentence that follows it.

A: Ann said that: Paul has retired.	Demonstrative pronoun
Intermediate: Ann said: that Paul has retired.	
B: Ann said [that Paul has retired].	Complementizer

In A, *that* serves as a demonstrative pronoun in S1, referring ahead to the content of S2. There is then a boundary shift with *that* changing from being the final element of S1 to becoming the initial element of S2. Finally, in B, *that* is reinterpreted as (hence grammaticalized to) a complementizer marking S2 as a complement clause.

How might processes analogous to grammaticalization operate before languages existed? The key is that such processes do not need a complex grammar to get started. In Figure 13–2, Heine and Kuteva posit a stage I of nouns and a stage II of verbs, though their dashed arrow indicates some perplexity concerning the transition. By contrast, as suggested earlier, we start with holophrases as our stage I with words for objects and words for actions (not yet syntactically structured as nouns and verbs) crystallizing out together in stage II. Once fractionation and the compensatory invention of constructions had yielded even a limited set of words and constructions, the effort of expressing in words novel ideas that then enter into the modification of many utterances would have provided fuel for the engine of grammaticalization, an engine that is running today in changing languages around the world.

Pidgins, Creoles, and Protolanguage

Having seen some of the ways in which grammar can change over time, we now turn to the study of pidgins and creoles to get examples of how a new language can be formed when two existing languages are brought into contact.[6]

We first examine Bickerton's theory (1984). On his account, *pidgins* have no native speakers, have limited use, and are created by adults by stripping language to a small lexicon with loss of semantic specificity *and with no syntax*. As a result, pidgins have no functional or grammatical categories, no syntax, no structured sentences, no meaningful word order, and no subordination. Instead, messages consist in stringing together just a few words from a small lexicon of multifunctional words. According to Bickerton, *creoles* are then created from a pidgin in one generation by children (native speakers) who grow up with the pidgin of their parents as their native language, and in making daily use of what is initially an impoverished linguistic model, the children expand the lexicon and add grammar to yield structured sentences with meaningful word order, subordination, and a large lexicon. Where the Bickertonian paradigm sees pidgins as highly limited in their communicative function, a Creole is a full language that can be used in all situations.

How does so dramatic a change occur so rapidly? Bickerton (1984) assessed a number of different creoles and found that the innovative aspects of creole grammar are similar across all creoles. Later, we shall see that this was due to too limited a sample of different creoles. For now, though, we note that Bickerton explained his finding by the *language bioprogram hypothesis*, namely that these grammatical innovations he found across all creoles rest on a genetically encoded "bioprogram." In expanding the pidgin, children are hypothesized to use their inborn universal principles of language, the Language Bioprogram. We can relate this hypothesis to the notion of an *innate Universal Grammar*. The Principles and Parameters model of language acquisition (see Chapter 11, Note 2) argues that a child has an innate set of linguistic principles such that learning the syntax of a language simply requires attending to a limited set of adult sentences to set the parameters for the principles. But where do these parameters come from if the child is not exposed to an adult language that provides cues as to the appropriate settings? To answer this, the *language bioprogram hypothesis* adds the claim that there are "default settings"—"unmarked options"—for the parameters that will hold unless the child experiences a rich nonimpoverished language. Bickerton then explains the similarity between historically unrelated creoles by the hypothesis that all of them manifest the unmarked options of Universal Grammar. And this hypothesis is seen as supporting the evolutionary view of the transition from protolanguage to language occurring long ago through mutations that supported the genetic specification of an innate Universal Grammar with default settings.

Tok Pisin (Talk Pidgin) is a creole (despite its name) that has long since evolved from its roots as a pidgin whereby English and German traders communicated with the natives of Papua and New Guinea. Already a creole, it has rapidly developed further since the country attained statehood with independence from Australia and needed a national language other than English to bring together tribes with a staggering diversity of different languages. In modern Tok Pisin, the vocabulary has expanded immensely as the creole has become the medium for education, local business, and even the reports of parliamentary proceedings, but some of the old strings remain in use—the English word *calf* corresponds to the Tok Pisin *pickaninny longa cow*, child belonging to a cow. In addition to expansion of the lexicon, the process of grammaticalization (e.g., transforming strings of words into grammatical markers—as we saw in the previous section) has expanded the grammar, so that *baimbai* as a separate word indicating that the sentence denotes an event that will occur *by and by* has now been reduced in form to *bai* and then moves next to the verb to become an explicit future tense marker. Romaine (1992, p. 245) offers the following possible stages for the grammaticalization of *bai*:

1. *Baimbi mi go*
   By and by I go
2. *Bai mi go*
   I'll go
3. *Mi bai go*
   I'll go

and suggests that *baimbai* began giving way to *bai* in the 1950s and 1960s.

As an alternative to the *language bioprogram hypothesis*, we now turn to an account of the relation between pidgins and creoles due to Claire Lefebvre (2010). I should add that Derek Bickerton has reviewed this section and emphasized that Lefebvre's theory is by no means dominant even among creolists who reject his own theory. I am not qualified to adjudicate between the competing theories. Nonetheless, I find her theory valuable because it illustrates how knowledge of two languages—both lexical and grammatical—may enter the formation of a creole, and thus it enriches our understanding of possible mechanisms whereby protolanguages may have gained in complexity as they were confronted with other protolanguages as tribes came to interact with each other. For Lefebvre, pidgins and creoles are not qualitatively different from one another save that native speakers are more fluent and use more complex word forms than nonnative speakers (Jourdan & Keesing, 1997), as in the *baimbai* example from Tok Pisin. Moreover, there are pidgins (still used as a second, nonnative, language) that have expanded in the same way as those native languages that are known as creoles (e.g., Mühlhäusler, 1986). The size of a language's lexicon is a function of its use. If a language is used only for restricted purposes, as when pidgins were used primarily by colonial masters to instruct laborers in a limited set of jobs, as on a wharf or a plantation, then the lexicon will be small. But this need not be the case. Moreover, where Bickerton sees pidgins as stripped bare to lexical categories, eliminating the functional categories of the contributing languages, Roberts and Bresnan (2008) surveyed 27 socially restricted pidgins and jargons and found that about half of them had some inflectional morphology that had been retained from the prior languages. Of course, this raises a terminological problem. If one defines a pidgin by its lack of syntax, then the half of the "socially restricted pidgins and jargons" that had some inflectional morphology are not pidgins but something else, perhaps even creoles. Just because some language is known by the general public as a pidgin does mean that it really is a pidgin, with Tok Pisin as a prime example. So, we will here adopt the notion of a pidgin as used only by people who have a distinct primary language while a creole is a native language derived historically from a pidgin. "Creolization" is then the process whereby the pidgin of the parents becomes the native language of their children.

The issue, then, is whether all creoles emerge from a communication system without any inflectional morphology or whether a substantial number emerge from a communication system with some prior form of inflectional morphology. In what follows, we follow Lefebvre in her theory of how a creole emerges in the latter situation. Lefebvre (2010) argues that the claim that pidgins lack syntax is most often associated with the fact that they manifest variable word orders without having the sort of case markers (as, e.g., in Latin) that indicate the roles of words that can appear in different places within the sentence. However, she notes that this fact may be based on a limited analysis that fails to keep track of the native language of different speakers of the pidgin who may use the word order of their respective native languages. For example, in China Coast Pidgin (Matthews & Li, unpublished data), the Wh-constituent is fronted in English sources, as in English—*What* thing that Poo-Saat do?— but not when following Chinese syntax—You wantchee *how* muchee? Thus, although the pidgin may appear to have no fixed word order, hence "no syntax," the variation in word order among speakers may follow from the variation observed among their respective mother tongues. The future development of the creole from this basis may then inherit one construction rather than another, with children more likely to adopt constructions that pattern after each other rather than those that differ greatly.

Atlantic creoles tend to reproduce the features of their West African substrate languages, whereas Pacific creoles tend to reproduce the features of their Austronesian substrate languages, and so on. To account for this, Lefebvre (1998, 2004) invokes relabeling, grammaticalization, and other processes that play a role in language change to explain how pidgins, and hence creoles, get their basic grammatical structure. This approach does not invoke an innate language bioprogram. Here we briefly look at her theory of relabeling. The core idea is this. Pidgin genesis involves adults who are native speakers of various languages. These speakers have no common language and instead create a "lingua franca" by relabeling the lexical entries of their native lexicons on the basis of phonetic strings adopted from the superstrate language. The resulting lexical entries have the semantic and syntactic properties of the original lexical entries but new phonological representations (though this formulation ignores the fact that if there is more than one substrate, the different syntactic and semantic elements need to be reconciled).

Each word in language A combines three elements: /phonological representation/^{A}, how the word is pronounced in language A; [semantic features]^A corresponding to what the word means when used by a speaker of language A; and [syntactic features]^A that specify how the word may be employed in the constructions of A. Lefebvre's notion is that at first, when native speakers of A using the pidgin are obliged to interact with the elite group who speak what will become its *superstrate* language, B, they will communicate better by adding /phonological representation/^{B} to the existing lexical item comprising {/phonological representation/^{A}, [semantic features]^A, [syntactic features]^A}. However, over time the original phonological representation from A may be lost, yielding the new *relabeled* lexical item

{/phonological representation/^{B}, [semantic features]^A, [syntactic features]^A}

as an element of the emerging pidgin. For example, the phonological representation /hù/ from the West African language Fongbe gets relabeled by a variant of the French /assassiner/ since both mean "to murder" to yield the Haitian Creole word /ansasinen/. However this word is not synonymous with the French word because /hù/ can mean "to mutilate" as well as "to murder," so that in Haitian Creole one can "assassinate" one's foot!

While semantically driven relabeling seems to play a key role, it is not the full story. Although we have seen that the stripping away of all syntactic features need not be the touchstone of forming a pidgin, nonetheless at least *some* features will be stripped away. But some may remain, and in many cases these will belong to the *substrate* A—and it is this role of the grammar of the substrate that provides constraints on the creation of novel constructions by the children who are its first native speakers, rather than yielding the same grammar for all creoles based on the default settings of Universal Grammar. Moreover, grammaticalization (such as the formation of *bai* from *baimbai* in Tok Pisin) can occur both before and after creolization so that the emerging language will eventually exhibit many syntactic features not preserved in the original pidgin as part of the grammar of either the substrate or the superstrate. It should also be added that different historical circumstances may yield different admixtures of semantic and syntactic features from the two languages. Syntactic features may be inherited from both languages, and there may be no general formula for what will survive into the creole once its speakers no longer have knowledge of a different native language to affect their utterances.

And Language Keeps Evolving

Language is not something whose general structure was fixed at some distant point in our prehistory. Writing greatly extended the "memory" that supports records and legends, while the printed book made access to such complexity available to a large populace, not just an educated elite.

The development of different professions yields a variety of new tools that extend the scope of the host language, whether it be the tool of numerical notation mastered by almost all speakers of the base language or the esoteric additions of legal language or mathematical argumentation that only years of specialized study can render accessible.

The rise of the computer, the World Wide Web, videogames, and smart phones renders language ever more flexible, as it comes to incorporate graphics, simulations, novel social networks, and the following of paths that respond to the whims and inclinations of the "reader." Here we see how the long-established mechanisms of the language-ready brain have supported, and will continue to support the development of new tools for language and thought, some of which merely extend languages as humans knew them centuries ago and others of which will extend our human abilities in ways that are dramatically new.

Notes

Chapter 1

1. Subsequent work has extended our computational model of visuomotor coordination in frog and toad—we call it *Rana computatrix*, "the frog which computes"—at the level of both schemas and neural networks for phenomena such as detours and path planning, avoidance behavior sensitive to the trajectories of predators, and details of snapping behavior that link neural control to biomechanics. See Arbib (1989b) for a partial review of work on *Rana computatrix*.

2. An old joke of mine: "Just because the brain looks like a bowl of porridge doesn't mean it's a serial computer."

3. For a better approximation than breaking the reach to grasp into a fast initial movement and a slow approach movement, see, for example, Hoff and Arbib (1993).

4. Building on the use of schemas to study action and perception in humans and frogs, Jeannerod (1997) surveys the role of schemas and other constructs in the cognitive neuroscience of action, whereas Arkin (1998) shows how schemas have played an important role in the development of behavior-based robots.

5. For more on the VISIONS system, see Draper, Collins, Brolio, Hanson, and Riseman (1989); Hanson and Riseman (1978); and Arbib (1989a), Sec. 5.3.

6. Looking ahead to the discussion of Construction Grammar in Chapter 2: This presentation of the HEARSAY model avoids any implication of the autonomy (or better the centrality) of syntax, and it is put in such a way that a Construction Grammar approach would be quite compatible since the phrasal hypotheses could be particular constructions (e.g., is this a *Wh*-question construction? etc.).

7. For my early work with David Caplan, see our paper (Arbib & Caplan, 1979)—mentioned in the earlier discussion of HEARSAY—and the book we coedited with the British neurologist John Marshall (Arbib, Caplan, & Marshall, 1982).

8. Our Gifford Lectures were published in 1986 (Arbib & Hesse, 1986).

9. Ochsner and Lieberman (2001) and Adolphs (2009) trace a number of strands in recent research that contribute to *social cognitive neuroscience*, including the role of a brain region called the amygdala in fear reactions and in recognizing the fearful expressions of others. See also Lieberman (2007) and Decety and Ickes (2009).

10. Petrides and Pandya (2009) offer a more subtle analysis than was available in the 1990s of the macaque homologs of Broca's area and the related connectivity

in macaque and human. These new findings have yet to be used to update the analyses reviewed in the present volume.

11. For the original statement of the Mirror System Hypothesis, see Arbib and Rizzolatti (1997) and Rizzolatti and Arbib (1998). The fullest statement of the Hypothesis, prior to this book, came in Arbib (2005a), which includes many commentaries both pro and con the hypothesis by researchers from diverse disciplines. These commentaries stimulated much of the further refinement of the Hypothesis and related subhypotheses that this book offers.

Chapter 2

1. Ferreira et al. (2002) argued that the language comprehension system creates syntactic and semantic representations that are merely "good enough" given the task that the comprehender needs to perform, rather than being complete and accurate with respect to the input. Ferreira and Patson (2007) present findings based on the recording of event-related potentials (neural activity recorded from the scalp of the listener) that show the use of simple heuristics rather than compositional algorithms for constructing sentence meaning, and for handling disfluencies with more or less accuracy. Our suggestion here is that the speaker may also provide syntactic and semantic representations that are just "good enough" to convey information to the hearer.

2. This caused a momentary pause to wonder what "bash" could be for "bashful" to mean "full of bash." I later learned from the *Oxford English Dictionary* that this *bash* is formed from *abash* by loss of the initial *a* (the process is called *aphesis*). *Abash* means "To destroy the self-possession or confidence of (any one), to put out of countenance, confound, discomfit ... or the like."

3. Jackendoff (2010) and Hurford (2011) emphasize the "primitiveness" of such compound nouns in their relative lack of compositional constraint.

4. A *metaphor* is a figure of speech in which a word or phrase is transferred to an object or action different from, but in some sense comparable to, that to which it is literally applicable—as in "This factory is a *hive* of industry." *Metonymy* involves substituting for a word or phrase another word or phrase denoting a property or something associated with it—as in "Harry is my strong right arm."

5. Studdert-Kennedy (2002) relates mirror neurons and vocal imitation to the evolution of particulate speech (see also Goldstein, Byrd, & Saltzman, 2006).

6. Marina Yaguello (1998) builds her book on linguistics around the playful use of language, and in tribute to Lewis Carroll she entitles her book *Language Through the Looking Glass*. Alas, despite the title, the book does not discuss the mirror system!

Chapter 3

1. The present chapter is based on the review article "Primate Vocalization, Gesture, and the Evolution of Human Language" (Arbib, Liebal, & Pika, 2008).

2. The evolution of the system for learning songs by male songbirds is divergent from mammalian evolution, but for the neuroscientist there are intriguing

challenges in plotting similarities and differences (Doupe & Kuhl, 1999; Jarvis, 2004, 2007). However, these challenges lie outside the scope of this book.

3. Current estimates suggest the common ancestor of humans and macaque monkeys lived around 25 million years (according to the Rhesus Macaque Genome Sequencing and Analysis group, 2007; see also Steiper, Young, & Sukarna, 2004), while Cheney and Seyfarth (2005), citing Boyd and Silk (2000), have the human/baboon last common ancestor at 36 million years ago. The common ancestor of humans and chimpanzees lived 5–7 million years ago (at most 6.3 million years ago, according to Patterson, Richter, Gnerre, Lander, & Reich, 2006).

4. See Figure 1-2 of Lieberman (1991) for similarities between the separation calls of primates. Lieberman in turn cites MacLean (1993) on the crying pattern of human infants.

5. In this volume we will treat manual gesture as playing a scaffolding role in the opening up of semantics, but the data of Ferrari et al. on mirror neurons will link in the consideration of orofacial gestures. And, of course, we will consider the relation between vocalization and speech. Building on the work on Facial Action Coding Schemes, Slocombe, Waller, and Liebal (2011) have recently called (as I do) for integrated multimodal research on language evolution: "By examining communicative signals in concert we can both avoid methodological discontinuities as well as better understand the phylogenetic precursors to human language as part of a multimodal system."

6. Peirce's trichotomy is crucial to Terrence Deacon (1997) in his important book *The Symbolic Species: The Co-evolution of Language and the Brain* in which humans are the symbolic species. However, I don't think the important issue is whether apes have symbols and whether they can be iconic but rather (as indeed Deacon argues) that humans can master immensely more symbols than other creatures and combine them in myriad ways so that symbols allow humans unparalleled flexibility for communication and thought.

7. For more examples of gestures acquired by apes through ontogenetic ritualization or social learning, see Bard (1990), Goodall (1986), Nishida (1980), Pika et al. (2003), Pika, Liebal, and Tomasello (2005), and McGrew and Tutin (1978).

8. See Hayes and Hayes (1951) and Kellogg and Kellogg (1933) for attempts to teach apes to use speech, Savage-Rumbaugh et al. (1998) for more on Kanzi, and Gardner and Gardner (1969) and Savage-Rumbaugh et al. (1998) for teaching hand signs and lexigrams to apes.

9. Since both are arbitrary with respect to the ape's experience, I would not expect a significant difference between what apes can learn with lexigrams and what they can learn with signs plucked from sign language. (The use of the verb "plucked" here is to emphasize that the ape learns how to make certain handshapes to convey meanings related to those for which something like those handshapes is employed in American Sign Language, say, but without the grammar that transforms use of the gestures into language.)

Chapter 4

1. We say something is practical if it is concerned with actual use or practice—if it is guided by practical experience. In this book the contrast is between praxis

and communication. A similar contrast is that between a practical joke—that is, actions designed to make someone feel foolish, usually for humor (at least for the trickster)—and a "normal" joke, told in words.

2. Although we shall not consider them further, we should note that the spinal cord also contains elements of the autonomic nervous system, which is concerned with the innervation of glands, and the control of the muscles of piloerection and the smooth muscles in the walls of arteries and visceral organs.

3. Readers who want to study human neuroanatomy further may wish to purchase *Sylvius 4: An Interactive Atlas and Visual Glossary of Human Neuroanatomy* (Williams et al., 2007) for download to their computer. It incorporates a comprehensive searchable database of more than 500 neuroanatomical terms that are concisely defined and visualized in photographs, magnetic resonance images, and other illustrations.

4. For more material on the topic of "Motivation and Emotion: The Motors of Action," the reader is referred to the book edited by Fellous and Arbib (2005), *Who Needs Emotions: The Brain Meets the Robot*. See especially the chapters by Kelley, Fellous and LeDoux, Rolls, and Arbib.

5. HM (Henry Molaison) died on December 2, 2008, at the age of 82. An informative full-page obituary was printed in the December 18, 2008 edition of *The Economist* weekly newspaper.

6. For the original account of Scoville's surgeries and Brenda Milner's related study of loss of recent memory after bilateral hippocampal lesions, see Scoville and Milner (1957). There are many follow-up studies, including those of Squire and Zola-Morgan (1991) and Corkin et al. (1997). Hilts (1995) provides a book-length biography of HM.

7. The source for my brief biographical account of Phineas Gage is Malcolm Macmillan's Web site devoted to Phineas Gage, *The Phineas Gage Information Page*: http://www.deakin.edu.au/hbs/psychology/gagepage/. The discussion of "The damage to Phineas Gage's brain" is based on the corresponding section of the Macmillan Web site. See also Macmillan (2000) for a great deal more about Phineas Gage, including reprints of Harlow's (1848, 1868) accounts of Gage's injuries and Bigelow's (1850) analysis thereof. A more leisurely account of Gage's accident and its aftermath is given in Chapter 1, Unpleasantness in Vermont, of Antonio Damasio (1994).

8. The FARS model was developed by Fagg and Arbib (1998), who provide full details of the model together with copious simulation results. The original FARS model relies on connections between prefrontal cortex and F5. However, there is evidence (reviewed by Rizzolatti & Luppino, 2001) that connections from PFC to F5 are very limited, whereas rich connections exist between PFC and AIP. Rizzolatti and Luppino (2003) thus suggested that FARS be modified so that information on object semantics and the goals of the individual influence AIP rather than affect F5 neurons directly. We discuss the modified conceptual model here.

9. For more on the supplementary motor area (SMA), and the distinction between pre-SMA and SMA-proper, see Rizzolatti et al. (1998).

10. For the role of basal ganglia in inhibiting extraneous actions and priming imminent actions, see Bischoff-Grethe et al. (2003). See Dominey, Arbib, and Joseph (1995) for an earlier model of the possible role of the basal ganglia in sequence learning. Lieberman (2000) discusses the role of human basal ganglia in language.

11. For further information on the auditory system of macaques, see Deacon (1992), Arikuni et al. (1988), Romanski et al. (1999), and Rauschecker et al. (1998).

12. For data on ablation of Broca's area homologs on vocalization, see Sutton et al. (1974 for monkey), Leyton and Sherrington (1917 for chimpanzee), and Deacon (1992 for human).

Chapter 5

1. For the afficionado of neural network learning, this is somewhat more subtle than mere Hebbian association of the overall trajectory with the canonical code because the methods we employed (Bonaiuto, Rosta, & Arbib, 2007; Oztop & Arbib, 2002) serve to recognize the trajectory from its initial segments "as early as possible," rather than waiting for the grasp to be completed.

2. There is one study (Mukamel, Ekstrom, Kaplan, Iacoboni, & Fried, 2010) reporting single-neuron recording during neurosurgery that tested for the mirror property with four actions (frown, smile, precision grip, power grasp) and did find some neurons with the mirror property for one or more of these actions—but they did not record from the "classical" areas in which mirror neurons have been recorded in the monkey. By contrast, there are hundreds of brain imaging studies finding "mirror system" properties in the human.

3. Another approach has been to use transcranial magnetic stimulation (TMS) of a brain region while the subject watches an action. If observation, boosted by TMS, potentiates the muscles that the observer might use in executing the action, we may hypothesize that the region contains mirror neurons for the action (Fadiga, Fogassi, Pavesi, & Rizzolatti, 1995).

4. One of the most interesting examples of "mirror neurons" of possible relevance to communication in another species is the finding (Prather, Peters, Nowicki, & Mooney, 2008) of neurons in the swamp sparrow forebrain that respond in a temporally precise fashion to auditory presentation of certain note sequences in this songbird's repertoire and to similar note sequences in other birds' songs. Furthermore, these neurons innervate structures in the striatum (an area we related in Chapter 4 to sequence learning) important for song learning. Such findings contribute to the view (not pursued further in this volume) that, despite the immense evolutionary divergence, analysis of brain mechanisms responsible for vocal learning in songbirds may contribute to our understanding of the vocal learning mechanisms supporting speech in humans (Jarvis, 2007).

5. For related critiques, see Dinstein, Thomas, Behrmann, and Heeger (2008) and Turella, Pierno, Tubaldi, and Castiello (2009).

6. Although the monkey's recognition of action may be quite rich, I would argue that human language and other cognitive abilities make human awareness very different from the monkey's (Arbib, 2001).

Chapter 6

1. Jablonka and Lamb (2005) provide an accessible introduction to EvoDevo.

2. Some authors now prefer to use the term *hominin* rather than *hominid*, but we will here use *hominid* in the stated sense. The *Oxford English Dictionary* defines a *hominin* as a member of a species regarded as human, directly ancestral

to humans, or very closely related to humans, belonging to the tribe *Hominini*. Some authors regard the tribe Hominini as including the genus *Homo* and the Australopithecines, thus making *hominin* equivalent to *hominid* in older terminology. Colin Groves (1989) groups humans, chimpanzees, gorillas, and orangutans into the *Hominidae*, and he groups humans, chimpanzees, and gorillas into the *Homininae*, while the human fossil record comprises the tribe *Hominini*.

3. For analogies between nonbiological processes of language change and the biological mechanisms of natural selection, see, for example, Dixon (1997) and Lass (1997).

4. The term "language-ready" was independently introduced in Arbib (2002) and, with a related sense, by Judy Kegl (2002) who wrote " ... all human children are born with language-ready brains that are capable of creating language and recognizing language-relevant evidence in the environment. In the absence of language-relevant evidence, the language-ready brain fails to engage in the first-language acquisition process." Kegl wrote in relation to the invention across a few decades of Nicaraguan Sign Language—an intriguing subject to which we return in Chapter 11. Where we may disagree is whether, as I suggest, humans had language-ready brains prior to the invention of languages.

5. I record my own personal debt to Chomsky in the section "My Second Lamppost: Embodied Neurolinguistics" of Chapter 1.

6. For more on co-speech gestures, see, for example, Iverson and Goldin-Meadow (1998) and McNeill (1992, 2005).

7. Note that we do not regard symbolization and compositionality as one "thing." Property 3 gave symbolism alone as a property of protolanguage. We now argue that enriching symbolism with compositionality is essential to language. There are certainly systems with compositionality but no symbolism (like birdsong) or with symbolization but no compositionality (like child speech circa 18 months).

8. Carol Chomsky (1969) traces the changes that occur in the child's mastery of syntax from ages 5 to 10.

9. For the original statement of the Mirror System Hypothesis, see Arbib and Rizzolatti (1997) and Rizzolatti and Arbib (1998). The fullest statement of the Hypothesis prior to this book came in Arbib (2005a), which includes many commentaries both pro and con aspects of the hypothesis by researchers from diverse disciplines. These commentaries stimulated much of the further refinement of the Hypothesis and related subhypotheses that this book offers.

10. For more on the "gestural origins" theory that humans had a (proto)language based on manual gestures before they had a spoken language based primarily on vocal gestures, see Hewes (1973), Kimura (1993), Armstrong et al. (1995), Stokoe (2001), and Corballis (2002).

11. Bickerton has recently given a somewhat modified account of language evolution in his book *Adam's Tongue* (Bickerton, 2009), and I have even more recently published an extended critique thereof (Arbib, 2011b).

12. Rudyard Kipling published his book of *Just So Stories* in 1902 (they are now available on the Web at http://www.boop.org/jan/justso/). In "The Elephant's Child," for example, it is explained that the elephant got its trunk because the elephant child foolishly went to the river where a crocodile pulled its nose so that it got longer and longer. The elephant child escaped, but by then had a trunk instead of

a nose. Of course, this is not the accepted evolutionary explanation! Nonetheless, it is a respectable procedure to formulate a "just-so story" if it provides a step towards rigorous testing and the development of a well-founded hypothesis, rather than being accepted just because it is an amusing story.

13. Wray (1998, 2000) suggests in more detail how the fractionation of unitary utterances might.

Chapter 7

1. For lack of vocal imitation in monkeys or apes, see Hauser (1996); for chimpanzee imitation, see Tomasello and Call (1997).

2. The iteration of basic actions until some subgoal is reached was formalized in the TOTE (test-operate-test-exit) units of the cybernetic psychology of Miller, Galanter, and Pribram (1960). In the years since, workers in artificial intelligence have come up with a variety of general problem-solving architectures. Soar is one such system for keeping track of different subgoals, spawning a new problem space in which to find plans for achieving the related subgoal (see, e.g., Rosenbloom, Laird, Newell, & McCarl, 1991—much has been done to develop Soar in the years since); another is ACT-R (Anderson et al., 2004).

3. The term "exaptation" was coined by the evolutionary biologists Stephen J. Gould and Elizabeth Vrba (1982).

4. For data showing that visual displays of parts of the face and hands activate specific brain sites in monkeys, see Gross (1992) and Perrett, Mistlin, and Chitty (1987).

5. Anisfeld (2005) and Jones (1996) argue that the "imitation of facial expressions" is even less specific, for example, that tongue protrusion and so on is merely a result of being aroused.

6. Tomasello heads a group at the Max Planck Institute of Evolutionary Anthropology at Leipzig, which combines two research themes of great interest to us. First is his long-standing collaboration with Josep Call to study the behavior of chimpanzees, bonobos, gorillas, and orangutans (primarily at the Leipzig Zoo). The coauthors of the review article (Arbib, Liebal, & Pika, 2008) that served as the basis for Chapter 3, Katja Liebal and Simone Pika, both did their Ph.D. research with this group. Second is the study of early cognitive development and language learning in human children. Much of the language work (reviewed in his book Tomasello, 2003a) can be seen as fitting into the same construction grammar framework as that developed *avant la lettre* with my Ph.D. student Jane Hill (e.g., Arbib, Conklin, & Hill, 1987; Hill, 1983) some two decades earlier; it will be described in Chapter 11.

7. The description of the dance class in Santa Fe (which I observed on September 25, 1999) is from Arbib (2002).

Chapter 8

1. I say "usually" to note that there is anecdotal evidence of rare occasions on which an ape's actions seem to go beyond the instrumental. Pat Zukow-Goldring (personal communication) states that "I [i.e., she] did observe Kanzi pointing

declaratively when I visited the Rumbaugh's. He tapped a trainer who was turned away from me on the shoulder. He then pointed back at me, so she would see that I was not following them. It was not as Mike Tomasello interpreted the situation (instrumentally) that Kanzi wanted me to come with him/them, but that he knew the routine with guests. That is, the visitor was supposed to follow at a distance: they, the trainers, wanted me to follow them. And Kanzi conveyed to them what he could see they were not noticing, so they could see that I wasn't following them."

2. Intriguingly (looking ahead to neurolinguistics), Jakobson (1956) asserts: "Every form of aphasic disturbance consists in some impairment, more or less severe, either of the faculty for selection and substitution or for combination and contexture. The former affliction involves a deterioration of metalinguistic operations, while the latter damages the capacity for maintaining the hierarchy of linguistic units. The relation of similarity is suppressed in the former, the relation of contiguity in the latter type of aphasia. Metaphor is alien to the similarity disorder, and metonymy to the contiguity disorder."

3. Dogs, for example, can learn to recognize conventionalized signs—whether spoken, or hand signals—uttered by their owners. However, they lack the ability to incorporate these utterances into their own action repertoire.

4. Figure 8-3 was inspired by comments of Hurford (2004).

5. Jim Hurford (personal communication) suggests that speech came to dominate over manual gestures in human language because of the improbability of a vocalization being interpreted as anything but a signal—as well as the property of being good for attracting attention.

6. The meaning of a word that we hear will differ greatly depending on the language context in which we hear it. For example, *affluence* in French signifies a *crowd of people*: whereas *affluence* in English signifies *a lot of something* (typically wealth).

7. Dickens's account of Laura Bridgman occurs in Chapter 3 of *American Notes* (available online at http://www.online-literature.com/dickens/americannotes/4/) and, like the book as a whole, is very much worth reading. Further details can be found in the Wikipedia article http://en.wikipedia.org/wiki/Laura_Bridgman.

Chapter 9

1. Following Arbib (2005a), we may note that the Chinese character 山 (san) may not seem pictorial, but if we see it as a simplification of a picture of three mountains, ⛰, via such intermediate forms as 山, then we have no trouble seeing the simplified character 山 as meaning "mountain." While such a "picture history" may provide a valuable crutch to the learner, with sufficient practice the crutch is thrown away, and in normal reading and writing, the link between 山 and its meaning is direct, with no need to invoke an intermediate representation of ⛰. The "etymology" of the Chinese character *san* follows Vaccari and Vaccari (1961). Of course, relatively few Chinese characters are so pictographic in origin. For a fuller account of the integration of semantic and phonetic elements in Chinese characters (and a comparison with Sumerian logograms), see Chapter 3 of Coulmas (2003).

2. For the work of Massimo Gentilucci and his colleagues in Parma, see, for example, Gentilucci, Santunione et al. (2004) and Gentilucci, Stefanini et al. (2004), and for a related discussion of language evolution, see Gentilucci and Corballis (2006).

3. Since these are Japanese monkeys, one may speculate that not only do they have a "food coo" and a "tool coo" but also a greeting call, the "hi coo."

4. See Goldstein et al. (2006) for a review of speech production from an evolutionary perspective.

Chapter 10

1. In linguistics, a *polysynthetic language*, like Navajo, is one in which a single word may contain as much information as an entire English sentence but is not holophrastic because the verb gets its complexity by affixing particles that extend the meaning again and again according to the syntax of the language. An *analytic language* (or *isolating language*) is one in which the vast majority of morphemes are free morphemes and are considered to be "words." Most languages lie somewhere in between. However, in the protolanguage literature, some authors use the terminology "synthetic" for a compositional protolanguage because meanings are "synthesized" by combining words, and "analytic" for a holophrastic protolanguage because meanings akin to those of modern English content words can only be obtained by teasing apart the meanings of protowords. To reduce confusion, I avoid the analytic/synthetic terminology for protolanguages and use the holophrastic/compositional terminology throughout.

2. Much of the present chapter is based on Arbib (2008), which is just one of the papers in a special issue of *Interaction Studies* 9(1)—since published as Bickerton and Arbib (2010)—that debates the two opposing views on the nature of protolanguage.

3. An interesting debate concerns the relation between "thought" and "(proto) language." How could we think something without the words to express it? How could we learn a new word without having already thought of the meaning to which it is to be attached? For discussion of such issues, see Carruthers (2002) and the attendant commentaries.

4. Kirby (2000) gives a computer simulation of how fractionation allows compositionality to emerge in a population of learners. More on this later.

5. Tallerman (2005) cites Jackendoff's (1999) discussion of ordering patterns such as "Agent First," "Focus Last," and Grouping, which are, he suggests, "fossil principles" from protolanguage. They correlate linear order with semantic roles but do not require syntactic structure. However, I remain uncomfortable with the idea that we can find a hard-and-fast dividing line between "ordering principles" and "syntax." Tallerman asserts that Bickerton (e.g., 1990) has cogently argued that the criterial properties of full syntax are all interdependent. We need instead to adopt a Construction Grammar approach to protolanguages of increasing complexity such as that limned earlier in which diverse constructions can emerge in relative independence of one another, even though subject to later aggregation through generalization.

6. The example of King James and the awful St. Paul's was recently revived at http://stancarey.wordpress.com/tag/etymology/, which is "Sentence first: An Irishman's blog about the English language. Mostly." He observes that the change in meaning is an example of *catachresis. Catachresis* (from the Greek κατάχρησις, "abuse") is, according to the *Penguin Dictionary of Literary Terms and Literary Theory*, "misapplication of a word, especially in a mixed metaphor." Another meaning is to use an existing word to denote something that has no name in the current language. Catachresis can have both positive and negative effects on language: It helps a language evolve and overcome poverty of expression, but it can also lead to miscommunications or make the language of one era incompatible with that of another.

Chapter 11

1. In the almost 30 years since Hill's model was developed, there has been a huge body of research that examines the ways in which children acquire language and develops conceptual and computational models of the processes involved. Most of these studies are broadly consistent with the perspective offered here but, of course, probe very much deeper, thus offering further material for our search for the key properties of the language-ready brain. MacWhinney (2010) provides the introduction to a special issue of the *Journal of Child Language* that provides an excellent selection of recent articles on computational models of child language learning.

2. Confusingly, the latest version of Chomsky's syntactic theory, the Minimalist Program, does not provide language universals of a kind that would simplify language acquisition for the child—see the brief comments within "Universal Grammar or Unidentified Gadgets?" of Chapter 2. It seems to me that the most recent Chomskian theory that does offer linguistic universals in a form appropriate (but, I believe, inadequate) for a model of language acquisition is that of Principles and Parameters. Baker (2001) offers an accessible account of the theory that provides many insights into properties shared across languages that are useful even for readers who do not accept that these principles are innate. David Lightfoot is a linguist who sees the Principles and Parameters approach to Universal Grammar as providing the key to language learning in the child and has argued that this supports a child-centered theory of historical patterns of language change (Lightfoot, 2006). I don't want to burden this volume with further critique of the Chomskian approach, but I have argued against both aspects of Lightfoot's theory elsewhere (Arbib, 2007). The key point of the present chapter is to offer, briefly, a theory of language acquisition related to Construction Grammar that is harmonious with our account of the evolution of the language-ready brain.

3. Hill and I in the early 1980s spoke of templates rather than constructions, but I have used the latter word in the present exposition. Our work was completed before the introduction of Construction Grammar (Fillmore, Kay, & O'Connor, 1988). We can now see Hill's templates as anticipating later work applying Construction Grammar to language acquisition. For example, Michael Tomasello's research group has conducted a large body of research very much in the same spirit as our early work. See *Constructing a Language: A Usage-Based Theory of Language Acquisition* (Tomasello, 2003a) for a comprehensive overview.

4. "[A]ny number of impressions, from any number of sensory sources, falling simultaneously on a mind which has not yet experienced them separately, will fuse into a single undivided object for that mind. ... The baby, assailed by eyes, ears, nose, skin, and entrails at once, feels it all as one great blooming, buzzing confusion; and to the very end of life, our location of all things in one space is due to the fact that the original extents or bignesses of all the sensations which came to our notice at once, coalesced together into one and the same space" (James, 1890, p. 488).

5. The relevance of Construction Grammar to language acquisition extends also to historical linguistics (Chapter 13), the study of how languages emerge and change over time (see, e.g., Croft, 2000).

Chapter 12

1. This chapter is based in large part on one of my articles (Arbib, 2009). My thanks to Virginia Volterra, Wendy Sandler, and Derek Bickerton for their thoughtful suggestions for updating the material.

2. There are interesting parallels between the Al-Sayyid Bedouin and Deaf communities that arose in America (e.g., Nantucket) as a consequence of recessive deafness in a closed community (Lane, Pillard, & French, 2000, 2002).

3. These notes on deafness are based in great part on Polich (2005).

4. However, this pattern is by no means unique. The phenomenon of the younger having more linguistic skill than the older is seen in the difference between pidgin and creole speakers in, for example, Hawaii (but see Bickerton, 1984; and Roberts, 2000, for contrasting analyses of the emergence of Hawaiian Creole) and in the different levels of attainment typically found when parents and children simultaneously acquire the same second language.

5. The video clips from which the frames of Figure 12-1 were drawn can be viewed at Science Online at http://www.sciencemag.org/cgi/content/full/305/5691/1779/DC1).

6. This section is based on Polich (2005).

7. The process also occurs in many "advanced" sign languages, as signers seek to find signs for words that they have met in spoken or written form. But the process also occurs in spoken languages as well. For example, the Spanish debated whether to simply "Spanify" *computer* to get *computador* or go for the more distinctive *ordenador*, while the Germans alternate between *Computer* and *Rechner*.

8. Scott et al. (in 1995) estimated that there were about 125 congenitally deaf individuals distributed throughout the community.

9. Note that the analysis of the data employs syntactic categories to describe ABSL at the second-generation stage, even though some of the categories may still remain more semantic than syntactic. From a more general perspective, Slobin (2008) cautions against using the form of grammars established for, for example, the written language in use in the surrounding hearing community as the basis for formalizing the grammar of a sign language. Such grammars presuppose categories of discrete elements that are combined into various sorts of structures, whereas sign languages incorporate gradient elements of signs—such as rate and intensity and expansiveness of movement—that reflect the communicative and

physical settings in which signs are produced. Of course, gradient phenomena—such as intonation patterns, and rate and intensity of vocal production—are also employed by speakers, but because almost all of these prosodic devices are missing from writing systems, they have been excluded from most linguistic descriptions of languages. Slobin suggests that sign language linguists can benefit from using new linguistic terms such as *body-partitioning, surrogates, buoys, ion-morphs, iconic mapping, indicating verbs, interacting and noninteracting handshapes,* and *richly grounded symbols* that are now being discussed in such journals as *Sign Language & Linguistics, Sign Language Studies,* and *Cognitive Linguistics.*

10. See also Laudanna and Volterra (1991) for an early comparison of the order of words, signs, and gestures, and Schembri, Jones, and Burnham (2005) for comparison of action gestures and classifier verbs of motion in Australian Sign Language, Taiwan Sign Language, and nonsigners gesturing without speech.

11. Cormier, Schembri, and Tyrone (2008), building on the earlier work of Brentari and Padden (2001), discuss ways in which gestures or foreign signs may become nativized as signs within a sign language They note, for example, that some color signs in ASL all share a common movement and location. For example, the ASL signs BLUE, YELLOW, GREEN, and PURPLE are all nativized from the finger spelling of the initial letter of the English word by having repeated rotation of the radio-ulnar and radio-humeral joints (i.e., components of the elbow) in neutral space.

12. An early version of the discussion of children raised in isolation was prepared in response to a question that Christine Kenneally asked several researchers to answer for the epilogue of her book on language evolution (Kenneally, 2007): "If we shipwrecked a boatload of babies on the Galapagos Islands, and they had all the food, water and shelter they needed to thrive, would they produce language in any form when they grew up? And if they do, what form might it take, how many individuals would you need for it to take off, and how would it change over the generations?" Different experts had very different opinions!

Chapter 13

1. The following subsections are based on sections of Arbib (2011a), which were heavily influenced by the research on stone tools conducted and reviewed by Dieter Stout (2011).

2. This formulation is somewhat updated from that of Arbib (2011a).

3. My thinking on historical linguistics owes a great deal to the books of Dixon (1997) and Lass (1997).

4. This forms part of a broader movement of what has been called Revival Linguistics. Working within the Australian context, Zuckermann and Walsh (2011) offer lessons from the revival of Hebrew in Israel, which they see as applicable to the reclamation of aboriginal languages.

5. Modern work in grammaticalization starts in the 1970s (see Givón, 1971). Examples of further work can be found in Heine, Claudi, and Hünnemeyer (1991); Heine and Kuteva (2002); Hopper and Traugott (2003); Traugott and Hopper (1993). The present section is based in part, and with permission, on Bernd Heine's presentation "On the Origin of Grammar" to the Summer Institute on *The Origins*

of Language, Université du Québec à Montréal, June 21–30, 2010, as well as papers with his colleagues (Heine & Kuteva, 2011; Heine & Stolz, 2008).

6. The section on Pidgins, Creoles, and Protolanguage is based in part, with permission, on Claire Lefebvre's presentation "On the relevance of pidgins and creoles in the debate on the origins of language" to the Summer Institute on The Origins of Language, Université du Québec à Montréal, June 21–30, 2010, and it has benefited from the comments of Derek Bickerton.

References

Aboitiz, F., & García, R. (2009). Merging of phonological and gestural circuits in early language evolution. *Reviews in the Neurosciences, 20*(1), 71–84.

Aboitiz, F., García, R., Brunetti, E., & Bosman, C. (2006). The origin of Broca's area and its connections from an ancestral working memory network. In Y. Grodzinsky & K. Amunts (Eds.), *Broca's region* (pp. 3–16). Oxford, England: Oxford University Press.

Aboitiz, F., & Garcia, V. R. (1997). The evolutionary origin of the language areas in the human brain. A neuroanatomical perspective. *Brain Research and Brain Research Review, 25*(3), 381–396.

Adolphs, R. (2009). The social brain: Neural basis of social knowledge. *Annual Review of Psychology, 60*, 693–716.

Anderson, J. R., Bothell, D., Byrne, M. D., Douglass, S., Lebiere, C., & Qin, Y. (2004). An integrated theory of the mind. *Psychological Review, 111*, 1036–1060.

Anisfeld, M. (2005). No compelling evidence to dispute Piaget's timetable of the development of representational imitation infancy. In S. Hurley & N. Chater (Eds.), *Imitation, human development, and culture* (pp. 107–132). Cambridge, MA: MIT Press.

Arbib, M. A. (1964). *Brains, machines and mathematics.* New York: McGraw-Hill.

Arbib, M. A. (1972). *The metaphorical brain: An introduction to cybernetics as artificial intelligence and brain theory.* New York: Wiley-Interscience.

Arbib, M. A. (1981). Perceptual structures and distributed motor control. In V. B. Brooks (Ed.), *Handbook of physiology—The nervous system II. Motor control* (pp. 1449–1480). Bethesda, MD: American Physiological Society.

Arbib, M. A. (1989a). *The metaphorical brain 2: Neural networks and beyond.* New York: Wiley-Interscience.

Arbib, M. A. (1989b). Visuomotor coordination: Neural models and perceptual robotics. In J.-P. Ewert & M. A. Arbib (Eds.), *Visuomotor coordination: Amphibians, comparisons, models, and robots* (pp. 121–171). New York: Plenum Press.

Arbib, M. A. (1990). Cooperative computation in brains and computers. In M. A. Arbib & J. A. Robinson (Eds.), *Natural and artificial parallel computation* (pp. 123–154). Cambridge, MA: MIT Press.

Arbib, M. A. (2001). Co-evolution of human consciousness and language. in Cajal and consciousness: Scientific approaches to consciousness on the centennial of Ramon y Cajal's Textura [Special issue, P. C. Marijuan, Ed.], *Annals of the New York Academy of Sciences, 929*, 195–220.

Arbib, M. A. (2002). The mirror system, imitation, and the evolution of language. In K. Dautenhahn & C. L. Nehaniv (Eds.), *Imitation in animals and artifacts. Complex adaptive systems* (pp. 229–280). Cambridge, MA: The MIT Press.

Arbib, M. A. (2005a). From monkey-like action recognition to human language: An evolutionary framework for neurolinguistics. *Behavioral and Brain Sciences, 28*(2), 105–124; discussion 125–167.

Arbib, M. A. (2005b). Interweaving protosign and protospeech: Further developments beyond the mirror. *Interaction Studies: Social Behavior and Communication in Biological and Artificial Systems, 6,* 145–171.

Arbib, M. A. (2006a). A sentence is to speech as what is to action? *Cortex, 42*(4), 507–514.

Arbib, M. A. (2006b). Aphasia, apraxia and the evolution of the language-ready brain. *Aphasiology, 20,* 1–30.

Arbib, M. A. (2007, Feb. 08). How new languages emerge (Review of D. Lightfoot, 2006, How new languages emerge, Cambridge University Press). *Linguist List,* 18–432. Retrieved November 2001, from http://linguistlist.org/issues/17/17-1250.html

Arbib, M. A. (2008). Holophrasis and the protolanguage spectrum. *Interaction Studies: Social Behavior and Communication in Biological and Artificial Systems, 9*(1), 151–165.

Arbib, M. A. (2009). Invention and community in the emergence of language: A perspective from new sign languages. In S. M. Platek & T. K. Shackelford (Eds.), *Foundations in evolutionary cognitive neuroscience: Introduction to the discipline* (pp. 117–152). Cambridge, England: Cambridge University Press.

Arbib, M. A. (2011a). From mirror neurons to complex imitation in the evolution of language and tool use. *Annual Review of Anthropology, 40,* 257–273.

Arbib, M. A. (2011b). Niche construction and the evolution of language: Was territory scavenging the one key factor? *Interaction Studies, 12*(1), 162–193.

Arbib, M. A. (Ed.). (2012). *Language, music and the brain, a mysterious relationship.* Cambridge, MA: The MIT Press.

Arbib, M. A., & Bickerton, D. (Eds.). (2010). *The emergence of protolanguage: Holophrasis vs compositionality.* Philadelphia: John Benjamins Publishing Company.

Arbib, M. A., Bischoff, A., Fagg, A. H., & Grafton, S. T. (1994). Synthetic PET: Analyzing large-scale properties of neural networks. *Human Brain Mapping, 2,* 225–233.

Arbib, M. A., & Bonaiuto, J. (2008). From grasping to complex imitation: Modeling mirror systems on the evolutionary path to language. *Mind and Society, 7,* 43–64.

Arbib, M. A., Bonaiuto, J., Jacobs, S., & Frey, S. H. (2009). Tool use and the distalization of the end-effector. *Psychological Research, 73*(4), 441–462.

Arbib, M. A., & Caplan, D. (1979). Neurolinguistics must be computational. *Behavioral and Brain Sciences, 2,* 449–483.

Arbib, M. A., Caplan, D., & Marshall, J. C. (Eds.). (1982). *Neural models of language processes.* New York: Academic Press.

Arbib, M. A., Conklin, E. J., & Hill, J. C. (1987). *From schema theory to language.* New York: Oxford University Press.

Arbib, M. A., Fagg, A. H., & Grafton, S. T. (2002). Synthetic PET imaging for grasping: From primate neurophysiology to human behavior. In F. T. Soomer & A. Wichert (Eds.), *Exploratory analysis and data modeling in functional neuroimaging* (pp. 231–250). Cambridge, MA: MIT Press.

Arbib, M. A., & Hesse, M. B. (1986). *The construction of reality*. Cambridge, England: Cambridge University Press.

Arbib, M. A., & Hill, J. C. (1988). Language acquisition: Schemas replace universal grammar. In J. A. Hawkins (Ed.), *Explaining language universals* (pp. 56–72). Oxford, England: Basil Blackwell.

Arbib, M. A., & Iriki, A. (2012). Evolving the language- and music-ready brain. In M. A. Arbib (Ed.), *Language, music and the brain, a mysterious relationship*. Cambridge, MA: The MIT Press.

Arbib, M. A., & Lee, J. (2007). Vision and action in the language-ready brain: From mirror neurons to SemRep. In F. Mele (Ed.), *BVAI 2007 (Brain Vision and Artificial Intelligence, 2007), LNCS 4729* (pp. 104–123). Berlin, Germany: Springer-Verlag.

Arbib, M. A., & Lee, J. (2008). Describing visual scenes: Towards a neurolinguistics based on construction grammar. *Brain Research, 1225*, 146–162.

Arbib, M. A., Liebal, K., & Pika, S. (2008). Primate vocalization, gesture, and the evolution of human language. *Current Anthropology, 49*(6), 1053–1076.

Arbib, M. A., & Mundhenk, T. N. (2005). Schizophrenia and the mirror system: An essay. *Neuropsychologia, 43*(2), 268–280.

Arbib, M. A., & Rizzolatti, G. (1997). Neural expectations: A possible evolutionary path from manual skills to language. *Communication and Cognition, 29*, 393–424.

Arikuni, T., Watanabe, K., & Kubota, K. (1988). Connections of area 8 with area 6 in the brain of the macaque monkey. *Journal of Comparative Neurology, 277*(1), 21–40.

Arkin, R. C. (1998). *Behavior-based robotics*. Cambridge, MA: The MIT Press.

Armstrong, D. F., Stokoe, W. C., & Wilcox, S. E. (1995). *Gesture and the nature of language*. Cambridge, England: Cambridge University Press.

Armstrong, D. F., & Wilcox, S. E. (2007). *The gestural origin of language*. Oxford, England: Oxford University Press.

Arnold, K., & Zuberbühler, K. (2006a). The alarm-calling system of adult male putty-nosed monkeys, *Cercopithecus nictitans martini. Animal Behaviour, 72*, 643–653.

Arnold, K., & Zuberbühler, K. (2006b). Language evolution: Semantic combinations in primate calls. *Nature, 441*, 303.

Aronoff, M., Meir, I., Padden, C., & Sandler, W. (2008). The roots of linguistic organization in a new language. *Interaction Studies, 9*(1), 133–153.

Baker, M. (2001). *The atoms of language: The mind's hidden rules of grammar*. New York: Basic Books.

Baldwin, J. M. (1896). A new factor in evolution. *American Naturalist, 30*, 441–451, 536–533.

Bard, K. A. (1990). Social tool use by free-ranging orangutans: A Piagetian and developmental perspective on the manipulation of an animate object. In S. T. Parker & K. R. Gibson (Eds.), *Language and intelligence in monkeys and apes. Comparative developmental perspectives* (pp. 356–378). New York: Cambridge University Press.

Bartlett, F. C. (1932). *Remembering*. Cambridge, England: Cambridge University Press.

Bates, E., Benigni, L., Bretherton, I., Camaioni, L., & Volterra, V. (1979). *The emergence of symbols: Cognition and communication in infancy*. New York: Academic Press.

Bates, E., Camaioni, L., & Volterra, V. (1975). The acquisition of performatives prior to speech. *Merrill-Palmer Quarterly, 21*(3), 205–226.

Bates, E., & Volterra, V. (1984). On the invention of language: An alternative view. *Monographs of the Society for Research in Child Development, 49*(3–4), 130–142.

Bellugi, U. (1980). The structuring of language: Clues from the similarities between signed and spoken language. In U. Bellugi & M. Studdert-Kennedy (Eds.), *Signed and spoken language: Biological constraints on linguistic form (Dahlem Konferenzen)* (pp. 115–140). Deerfield Beach, FL: Verlag Chemie.

Benga, O. (2005). Intentional communication and the anterior cingulate cortex. *Interaction Studies, 6*, 201–221.

Bickerton, D. (1984). The language bioprogram hypothesis. *Behavioral and Brain Sciences, 7*, 173–221.

Bickerton, D. (1990). *Language and species*. Chicago: University of Chicago Press.

Bickerton, D. (1995). *Language and human behavior*. Seattle: University of Washington Press.

Bickerton, D. (2009). *Adam's tongue. How humans made language, how language made humans*. New York: Hill & Wang.

Bigelow, H. J. (1850). Dr. Harlow's case of recovery from the passage of an iron bar through the head. *American Journal of the Medical Sciences, 19*, 13–22.

Bischoff-Grethe, A., Crowley, M. G., & Arbib, M. A. (2003). Movement inhibition and next sensory state predictions in the basal ganglia. In A. M. Graybiel, M. R. Delong, & S. T. Kitai (Eds.), *The basal ganglia VI* (pp. 267–277). New York: Kluwer Academic/Plenum Publishers.

Bloom, P. (2000). *How children learn the meanings of words*. Cambridge, MA: MIT Press.

Bloom, P. (2004). Can a dog learn a word? *Science, 304*(5677), 1605–1606.

Boesch, C., & Boesch, H. (1982). Optimisation of nut-cracking with natural hammers by wild chimpanzees. *Behavioural Brain Research, 83*(3/4), 265–286.

Boesch, C., & Boesch, H. (1990). Tool use and tool making in wild chimpanzees. *Folia Primatologica, 54*, 86–99.

Bonaiuto, J. B., & Arbib, M. A. (2010). Extending the mirror neuron system model, II: What did I just do? A new role for mirror neurons. *Biological Cybernetics, 102*, 341–359.

Bonaiuto, J. B., Rosta, E., & Arbib, M. A. (2007). Extending the mirror neuron system model, I: Audible actions and invisible grasps. *Biological Cybernetics, 96*, 9–38.

Boyd, R., & Richerson, P. J. (1985). *Culture and the evolutionary process*. Chicago, IL: University of Chicago Press.

Boyd, R., Richerson, P. J., & Henrich, J. (2011). Rapid cultural adaptation can facilitate the evolution of large-scale cooperation. *Behavioral Ecology and Sociobiology, 65*(3), 431–444.

Boyd, R., & Silk, J. B. (2000). *How humans evolved* (2nd ed.). New York: W. W. Norton.

Brentari, D., & Padden, C. (2001). Native and foreign vocabulary in American Sign Language: A lexicon with multiple origins. In D. Brentari (Ed.), *Foreign vocabulary:*

A cross-linguistic investigation of word formation (pp. 87–119). Mahwah, NJ: Erlbaum.

Bridgeman, B. (2005). Action planning supplements mirror systems in language evolution. *Behavioral and Brain Sciences, 28,* 129–130.

Bril, B., Rein, R., Nonaka, T., Wenban-Smith, F., & Dietrich, G. (2010). The role of expertise in tool use: Skill differences in functional action adaptations to task constraints. *Journal of Experimental Psychology: Human Perception and Performance, 36,* 825–839.

Broca, P. P. (1861). Perte de la parole. *Bulletins de la Societé Anthropologique de Paris, 2,* 235–238.

Brodmann, K. (1905). Beitrage zur histologische Localisation der Grosshirnrinde. Dritte Mitteilung. Die Rindenfelder der niederen Affen. *Journal of Psychology and Neurology (Leipzig), 4,* 177–226.

Brothers, L. (1997). *Friday's footprint: How society shapes the human mind.* Oxford, England: Oxford University Press.

Buccino, G., Lui, F., Canessa, N., Patteri, I., Lagravinese, G., Benuzzi, F., ... Rizzolatti, G. (2004). Neural circuits involved in the recognition of actions performed by nonconspecifics: An FMRI study. *Journal of Cognitive Neuroscience, 16*(1), 114–126.

Butterworth, G. (2003). Pointing is the royal road to language for babies. In S. Kita (Ed.), *Pointing: Where language, culture, and cognition meet* (pp. 9–33). Mahwah, NJ: Erlbaum.

Buxbaum, L. J., Kyle, K. M., Tang, K., & Detre, J. A. (2006). Neural substrates of knowledge of hand postures for object grasping and functional object use: Evidence from fMRI. *Brain Research, 1117*(1), 175–185.

Byrne, R. W. (2003). Imitation as behavior parsing. *Philosophical Transactions of the Royal Society of London B, 358,* 529–536.

Byrne, R. W., & Byrne, J. M. E. (1993). Complex leaf-gathering skills of mountain gorillas (*Gorilla g. beringei*): Variability and standardization. *American Journal of Primatology, 31,* 241–261.

Byrne, R. W., & Russon, A. E. (1998). Learning by imitation: A hierarchical approach. *Behavioral and Brain Sciences, 21*(5), 667–684; discussion 684–721.

Byrne, R. W., & Whiten, A. (Eds.). (1988). *Machiavellian intelligence: Social expertise and the evolution of intellect in monkeys, apes and humans.* Oxford, England: Clarendon Press.

Calvo-Merino, B., Glaser, D. E., Grezes, J., Passingham, R. E., & Haggard, P. (2005). Action observation and acquired motor skills: An FMRI study with expert dancers. *Cerebral Cortex, 15*(8), 1243–1249.

Capirci, O., Iverson, J. M., Pizzuto, E., & Volterra, V. (1996). Gestures and words during the transition to two-word speech. *Journal of Child Language, 23,* 645–673.

Capirci, O., & Volterra, V. (2008). Gesture and speech. The emergence and development of a strong and changing partnership. *Gesture, 8*(1), 22–44.

Carey, D. P., Perrett, D. I., & Oram, M. W. (1997). Recognizing, understanding, and producing action. In M. Jeannerod & J. Grafman (Eds.), *Handbook of neuropsychology. Vol. 11: Action and cognition* (pp. 111–130). Amsterdam, Netherlands: Elsevier.

Caro, T. M., & Hauser, M. D. (1992). Is there teaching in nonhuman animals? *The Quarterly Review of Biology, 67,* 151–174.

Carpenter, M., Akhtar, N., & Tomasello, M. (1998). 14-through 18-month-old infants differentially imitate intentional and accidental actions. *Infant Behavior and Development, 21*, 315–330.

Carruthers, P. (2002). The cognitive functions of language. *Behavioral and Brain Science, 25*(6), 657–674; discussion 674–725.

Cheney, D. L., & Seyfarth, R. M. (1990). *How monkeys see the world: Inside the mind of another species*. Chicago, IL: University of Chicago Press.

Cheney, D. L., & Seyfarth, R. M. (2005). Constraints and preadaptations in the earliest stages of language evolution. *The Linguistic Review, 22*, 135–159.

Cheney, D. L., & Seyfarth, R. M. (2007). Baboon metaphysics: The evolution of a social mind. Chicago, IL: University Of Chicago Press.

Chomsky, N. (1956). *Syntactic structures*. The Hague, Netherlands: Mouton.

Chomsky, N. (1965). *Aspects of the theory of syntax*. Cambridge, MA: MIT Press.

Chomsky, C. (1969). *The acquisition of syntax in children from 5 to 10*. Cambridge, MA: The MIT Press.

Chomsky, N. (1972). *Language and mind*. New York: Harcourt Brace.

Chomsky, N. (1981). *Lectures on government and binding*. Dordrecht, Netherlands: Foris.

Chomsky, N. (1992). A minimalist program for linguistic theory. In K. H. a. S. J. Keyser (Ed.), *The view from building 20: Essays in linguistics in honor of Sylvan Bromberger* (pp. 1–52). Cambridge, MA: MIT Press.

Chomsky, N. (1995). *The minimalist program*. Cambridge, MA: MIT Press.

Clark, J. D. (2001). Variability in primary and secondary technologies of the Later Acheulian in Africa. In S. Miliken & J. Cook (Eds.), *A very remote period indeed: Papers on the Palaeolithic presented to Derek Roe* (pp. 1–18). Oakville, CT: Oxbow Books.

Clayton, N. S., & Dickinson, A. (1998). Episodic-like memory during cache recovery by scrub jays. *Nature, 395*, 272–274.

Coppola, M. (2002). *The emergence of grammatical categories in home sign: Evidence from family-based gesture systems in Nicaragua*. Unpublished Ph.D. dissertation, University of Rochester, NY.

Corballis, M. C. (2002). *From hand to mouth, the origins of language*. Princeton, NJ: Princeton University Press.

Corina, D. P., Poizner, H., Bellugi, U., Feinberg, T., Dowd, D., & O'Grady-Batch, L. (1992). Dissociation between linguistic and nonlinguistic gestural systems: A case for compositionality. *Brain and Language, 43*(3), 414–447.

Corkin, S., Amaral, D. G., Gonzalez, R. G., Johnson, K. A., & Hyman, B. T. (1997). H. M.'s medial temporal lobe lesion: Findings from magnetic resonance imaging. *Journal of Neuroscience, 17*(10), 3964–3979.

Cormier, K., Schembri, A., & Tyrone, M. E. (2008). One hand or two? Nativisation of fingerspelling in ASL and BANZSL. *Sign Language and Linguistics, 11*(1), 3–44.

Corp, N., & Byrne, R. W. (2002). Ontogeny of manual skill in wild chimpanzees: Evidence from feeding on the fruit of Saba Florida. *Behavior, 139*, 137–168.

Coudé, G., Ferrari, P. F., Rodà, F., Maranesi, M., Borelli, E., Veroni, V., ...Fogassi, L. (2011). Neurons controlling voluntary vocalization in the macaque ventral premotor cortex. *PLoS ONE, 6*(11), e26822. doi: 10.1371/journal.pone.0026822

Coulmas, F. (2003). *Writing systems: An introduction to their linguistic analysis*. Cambridge, England: Cambridge University Press.

Critchley, M., & Critchley, E. A. (1998). *John Hughlings Jackson. Father of English neurology.* Oxford, England: Oxford University Press.

Croft, W. (2000). *Explaining language change: An evolutionary approach.* Harlow, England: Longman.

Croft, W. (2001). *Radical construction grammar: Syntactic theory in typological perspective.* Oxford, England: Oxford University Press.

Croft, W., & Cruse, D. A. (2005). *Cognitive linguistics.* Cambridge, England: Cambridge University Press.

Cross, I. (2003). Music, cognition, culture and evolution. In I. Peretz & R. J. Zatorre (Eds.), *The cognitive neuroscience of music* (pp. 42–56). Oxford, England: Oxford University Press.

Crosson, B., Benefield, H., Cato, M. A., Sadek, J. R., Moore, A. B., Wierenga, C. E., ... Brigs, R. W. (2003). Left and right basal ganglia activity during language generation: Contributions to lexical, semantic and phonological processes. *Journal of the International Neuropsychological Society, 9*, 1061–1077.

D'Errico, F., Henshilwood, C., & Nilssen, P. (2001). An engraved bone fragment from c. 70,000-year-old Middle Stone Age levels at Blombos Cave, South Africa: Implications for the origin of symbolism and language. *Antiquity, 75*, 309–318.

Dąbrowska, E. (2011). Individual differences in native language attainment: A review article. *University of Sheffield.* Retrieved November 2011, from http://www.cogling.group.shef.ac.uk/publications/Ind_diffs_review.pdf

Damasio, A. (1994). *Descartes' error: Emotion, reason, and the human brain.* New York: Putnam Publishing.

Damasio, H., Grabowski, T., Frank, R., Galaburda, A. M., & Damasio, A. R. (1994). The return of Phineas Gage: Clues about the brain from the skull of a famous patient. *Science, 264*(5162), 1102–1105.

Dapretto, M., Davies, M. S., Pfeifer, J. H., Scott, A. A., Sigman, M., Bookheimer, S. Y., & Iacoboni, M. (2006). Understanding emotions in others: Mirror neuron dysfunction in children with autism spectrum disorders. *Nature Neuroscience, 9*(1), 28–30.

Darwin, C. (1871). *The descent of man and selection in relation to sex.* London: John Murray.

Darwin, C. (1872/1965). *The expression of the emotions in man and animals.* Chicago, IL: University of Chicago Press.

Dawkins, C. R. (1976). *The selfish gene.* Oxford, England: Oxford University Press.

De Renzi, E. (1989). Apraxia. In F. Boller & J. Grafman (Eds.), *Handbook of neuropsychology, Vol. 2* (pp. 245–263). Amsterdam: Elsevier.

de Waal, F. B. M. (2001). *The ape and the sushi master: Cultural reflections of a primatologist.* New York: Basic Books.

de Waal, F. B. M. (2006). *Primates and philosophers: How morality evolved.* Princeton, NJ: Princeton University Press.

Deacon, T. W. (1992). Cortical connections of the inferior arcuate sulcus cortex in the macaque brain. *Brain Research, 573*(1), 8–26.

Deacon, T. W. (1997). *The symbolic species: The co-evolution of language and the brain.* New York: W. W. Norton.

DeCasper, A. J., & Fifer, W. P. (1980). Of human bonding: Newborns prefer their mothers' voices. *Science, 208*(4448), 1174–1176.

DeCasper, A. J., & Spence, M. J. (1991). Auditorily mediated behavior during the perinatal period: A cognitive view. In M. J. S. W. a. P. R. Zelazo (Ed.), *Newborn attention: Biological constraints and the influence of experience*. Norwood, NJ: Ablex.

Decety, J., & Ickes, W. J. (Eds.). (2009). *The social neuroscience of empathy*. Cambridge, MA: MIT Press.

di Pellegrino, G., Fadiga, L., Fogassi, L., Gallese, V., & Rizzolatti, G. (1992). Understanding motor events: A neurophysiological study. *Experimental Brain Research, 91*(1), 176–180.

Didday, R. L. (1970). *The simulation and modelling of distributed information processing in the frog visual system*. Unpublished Ph.D. dissertation, Stanford University, Palo Alto, CA.

Dinstein, I., Thomas, C., Behrmann, M., & Heeger, D. J. (2008). A mirror up to nature. *Current Biology, 18*(1), R13–18.

Dissanayake, E. (2000). Antecedents of the temporal arts in early mother-infant interaction. In N. L. Wallin, B. Merker, & S. Brown (Eds.), *The origins of music* (pp. 389–410). Cambridge, MA: MIT Press.

Dixon, R. M. W. (1997). *The rise and fall of languages*. Cambridge, England: Cambridge University Press.

Dominey, P. F., Arbib, M. A., & Joseph, J.-P. (1995). A model of corticostriatal plasticity for learning oculomotor associations and sequences. *Journal of Cognitive Neuroscience, 7*(3), 311–336.

Dominey, P. F., & Inui, T. (2009). Cortico-striatal function in sentence comprehension: Insights from neurophysiology and modeling. *Cortex, 45*, 1012–1018.

Donald, M. (1991). *Origins of the modern mind: Three stages in the evolution of culture and cognition*. Cambridge, MA: Harvard University Press.

Donald, M. (1993). Precis of origins of the modern mind: Three stages in the evolution of culture and cognition. *Behavioral and Brain Sciences, 16*, 737–791.

Donald, M. (1998). Mimesis and the executive suite: Missing links in language evolution. In J. R. Hurford, M. Studdert-Kennedy, & C. Knight (Eds.), *Approaches to the evolution of language: Social and cognitive bases* (pp. 44–67). Cambridge, England: Cambridge University Press.

Donald, M. (1999). Preconditions for the evolution of protolanguages. In M. C. Corballis & E. G. Stephen (Eds.), *The descent of mind: Psychological perspectives on hominid evolution* (pp. 138–154). Oxford, England: Oxford University Press.

Doupe, A. J., & Kuhl, P. K. (1999). Birdsong and human speech: Common themes and mechanisms. *Annual Review of Neuroscience, 22*, 567–631.

Doupe, A. J., Perkel, D. J., Reiner, A., & Stern, E. A. (2005). Birdbrains could teach basal ganglia research a new song. *Trends in Neuroscience, 28*(7), 353–363.

Draper, B. A., Collins, R. T., Brolio, J., Hanson, A. R., & Riseman, E. M. (1989). The schema system. *International Journal of Computer Vision, 2*, 209–250.

Dryer, M. S. (1996). Word order typology. In J. Jacobs (Ed.), *Handbook on syntax* (Vol. 2, pp. 1050–1065). Berlin: Walter de Gruyter Publishing.

Dunbar, R. (1993). Co-evolution of neocortex size, group size and language in humans. *Behavioral and Brain Sciences, 16*, 681–735.

Dunbar, R. (1996). *Grooming, gossip and the evolution of language*. London: Faber and Faber Ltd.

Durkheim, E. (1915). *Elementary forms of the religious life: A study in religious sociology (translated from the French original of 1912 by Joseph Ward Swain)*. London: Macmillan.

Edwards, S. W. (2001). A modern knapper's assessment of the technical skills of the Late Acheulean biface workers at Kalambo Falls. In J. D. Clark (Ed.), *Kalambo Falls prehistoric site. Vol. 3: The earlier cultures: Middle and Earlier Stone Age* (pp. 605–611). Cambridge, England: Cambridge University Press.

Emmorey, K. (2002). *Language, cognition, and the brain: Insights from sign language research*. Mahwah, NJ: Erlbaum.

Emmorey, K. (2005). Sign languages are problematic for a gestural origins theory of language evolution. *Behavioral and Brain Sciences, 28*(2), 130–131.

Emmorey, K., Damasio, H., McCullough, S., Grabowski, T., Ponto, L. L. B., Hichwa, R. D., & Bellugi, U. (2002). Neural systems underlying spatial language in American Sign Language. *NeuroImage, 17*(2), 812–824.

Emmorey, K., McCullough, S., Mehta, S., Ponto, L. L. B., & Grabowski, T. J. (2011). Sign language and pantomime production differentially engage frontal and parietal cortices. *Language and Cognitive Processes, 26*(7), 878–901.

Evans, N. (2003). Culture and structuration in the languages of Australia. *Annual Review of Anthropology, 32,* 13–40.

Ewert, J-P., & von Seelen, W. (1974). Neurobiologie and System-Theorie eines visuellen Muster-Erkennungsmechanismus bei Kroten. *Kybernetik, 14,* 167–183.

Fadiga, L., Fogassi, L., Pavesi, G., & Rizzolatti, G. (1995). Motor facilitation during action observation: a magnetic stimulation study. *J Neurophysiol, 73*(6), 2608-2611.

Fagg, A. H., & Arbib, M. A. (1998). Modeling parietal-premotor interactions in primate control of grasping. *Neural Networks, 11*(7–8), 1277–1303.

Farnell, B. (1995). *Do you see what I mean? Plains Indian sign talk and the embodiment of action*. Austin: University of Texas Press.

Fellous, J-M., & Arbib, M. A. (Eds.). (2005). *Who needs emotions: The brain meets the robot*. Oxford, England: Oxford University Press.

Fellous, J-M., & Ledoux, J. E. (2005). Toward basic principles for emotional processing: What the fearful brain tells the robot. In J-M. Fellous & M. A. Arbib (Eds.), *Who needs emotions: The brain meets the robot* (pp. 79–115). Oxford, England: Oxford University Press.

Ferrari, P. F., Gallese, V., Rizzolatti, G., & Fogassi, L. (2003). Mirror neurons responding to the observation of ingestive and communicative mouth actions in the monkey ventral premotor cortex. *European Journal of Neuroscience, 17*(8), 1703–1714.

Ferrari, P. F., Visalberghi, E., Paukner, A., Fogassi, L., Ruggiero, A., & Suomi, S. J. (2006). Neonatal imitation in rhesus macaques. *PLoS Biology, 4*(9), e302.

Ferreira, F., Ferraro, V., & Bailey, K. G. D. (2002). Good-enough representations in language comprehension. *Current Directions in Psychological Science, 11,* 11–15.

Ferreira, F., & Patson, N. D. (2007). The 'good enough' approach to language Comprehension. *Language and Linguistics Compass, 1*(1–2), 71–83.

Fillmore, C. J., Kay, P., & O'Connor, M. K. (1988). Regularity and idiomaticity in grammatical constructions: The case of let alone. *Language and Cognitive Processes, 64,* 501–538.

Fitch, W. T. (2010). *The evolution of language*. Cambridge, England: Cambridge University Press.

Fitch, W. T., & Reby, D. (2001). The descended larynx is not uniquely human. *Proceedings of the Royal Society for Biological Sciences, 268,* 1669–1675.

Fogassi, L., & Ferrari, P-F. (2004). Mirror neurons, gestures and language evolution. *Interaction Studies: Social Behavior and Communication in Biological and Artificial Systems, 5,* 345–363.

Fogassi, L., & Ferrari, P-F. (2007). Mirror neurons and the evolution of embodied language. *Current Directions in Psychological Science, 16*(3), 136–141.

Fogassi, L., Gallese, V., Buccino, G., Craighero, L., Fadiga, L., & Rizzolatti, G. (2001). Cortical mechanism for the visual guidance of hand grasping movements in the monkey: A reversible inactivation study. *Brain, 124*(Pt 3), 571–586.

Fogassi, L., Gallese, V., Fadiga, L., & Rizzolatti, G. (1998). Neurons responding to the sight of goal directed hand/arm actions in the parietal area PF (7b) of the macaque monkey. *Society of Neuroscience Abstracts, 24,* 257.

Fusellier-Souza, I. (2001). La création gestuelle des individus sourds isolés: de l'édification conceptuelle et linguistique à la sémiogenèse des langues des signes. *Acquisition et Interaction en Langue Étrangère (AILE), 15,* 61–95.

Fusellier-Souza, I. (2006). Emergence and development of signed languages: From a semiogenetic point of view. *Sign Language Studies, 7*(1), 30–56.

Fuster, J. M. (2004). Upper processing stages of the perception-action cycle. *Trends in Cognitive Science, 8*(4), 143–145.

Gallese, V., Fadiga, L., Fogassi, L., & Rizzolatti, G. (1996). Action recognition in the premotor cortex. *Brain, 119,* 593–609.

Gallese, V., Fogassi, L., Fadiga, L., & Rizzolatti, G. (2002). Action representation and the inferior parietal lobule. In W. Prinz & B. Hommel (Eds.), *Attention and performance XIX. Common mechanisms in perception and action.* Oxford, England: Oxford University Press.

Gallese, V., & Goldman, A. (1998). Mirror neurons and the simulation theory of mind-reading. *Trends in Cognitive Science, 2,* 493–501.

Gamble, C. (1994). *Timewalkers: The prehistory of global colonization.* Cambridge, MA: Harvard University Press.

Gardner, R. A., & Gardner, B. (1969). Teaching sign language to a chimpanzee. *Science, 165,* 664–672.

Gazzola, V., Aziz-Zadeh, L., & Keysers, C. (2006). Empathy and the somatotopic auditory mirror system in humans. *Current Biology, 16*(18), 1824–1829.

Gentilucci, M., & Corballis, M. C. (2006). From manual gesture to speech: A gradual transition. *Neuroscience Biobehavioral Review, 30*(7), 949–960.

Gentilucci, M., Santunione, P., Roy, A. C., & Stefanini, S. (2004). Execution and observation of bringing a fruit to the mouth affect syllable pronunciation. *European Journal of Neuroscience, 19,* 190–202.

Gentilucci, M., Stefanini, S., Roy, A. C., & Santunione, P. (2004). Action observation and speech production: study on children and adults. *Neuropsychologia, 42*(11), 1554–1567.

Gibson, J. J. (1979). *The ecological approach to visual perception.* Boston, MA: Houghton Mifflin.

Givón, T. (1971). Historical syntax and synchronic morphology: An archaeologist's field trip. *Chicago Linguistic Society, 7,* 394–415.

Givón, T. (1998). Toward a neurology of grammar. *Behavioral and Brain Sciences, 21,* 154–155.

Goldin-Meadow, S. (1982). The resilience of recursion: A study of a communication system developed without a conventional language model. In E. Wanner & L. R.

Gleitman (Eds.), *Language acquisition: The state of the art* (pp. 51–77). Cambridge, England: Cambridge University Press.

Goldin-Meadow, S. (2003). *The resilience of language: What gesture creation in deaf children can tell us about how all children learn language.* New York: Psychology Press.

Goldin-Meadow, S. (2005). Watching language grow. *Proceedings of the National Academy of Sciences USA, 102,* 2271–2272.

Goldin-Meadow, S., & Mylander, C. (1984). Gestural communication in deaf children: The effects and noneffects of parental input on early language development. *Monographs of the Society for Research in Child Development, 49*(3-4), 1–151.

Goldin-Meadow, S., & Mylander, C. (1998). Spontaneous sign systems created by deaf children in two cultures. *Nature, 391*(15), 279–281.

Goldin-Meadow, S., Yalabik, E., & Gershkoff-Stowe, L. (2000). *The resilience of ergative structure in language created by children and by adults.* Paper presented at the Proceedings of the 24th Annual Boston University Conference on Language Development, Vol. 1, Somerville, MA.

Goldstein, L., Byrd, D., & Saltzman, E. (2006). The role of vocal tract gestural action units in understanding the evolution of phonology In M. A. Arbib (Ed.), *From action to language via the mirror system* (pp. 215–249). Cambridge, England: Cambridge University Press.

Goodale, M. A., Milner, A. D., Jakobson, L. S., & Carey, D. P. (1991). A neurological dissociation between perceiving objects and grasping them. *Nature, 349*(6305), 154–156.

Goodall, J. (1986). *The chimpanzees of Gombe: Patterns of behaviour.* Cambridge, England: The Belknap Press of Harvard University Press.

Gould, S. J., & Vrba, E. (1982). Exaptation—a missing term in the science of form. *Paleobiology, 8,* 4–15.

Grafton, S. T., Arbib, M. A., Fadiga, L., & Rizzolatti, G. (1996). Localization of grasp representations in humans by positron emission tomography. 2. Observation compared with imagination. *Experimental Brain Research, 112*(1), 103–111.

Graybiel, A. M. (1997). The basal ganglia and cognitive pattern generators. *Schizophrenia Bulletin, 23*(3), 459–469.

Grodzinsky, Y., & Amunts, K. (2006). *Broca's region: Mysteries, facts, ideas, and history.* New York: Oxford University Press.

Gross, C. G. (1992). Representation of visual stimuli in inferior temporal cortex. In V. Bruce, A. Cowey, & A. W. Ellis (Eds.), *Processing the facial image* (pp. 3–10). New York: Oxford University Press.

Groves, C. P. (1989). *A theory of human and primate evolution.* Oxford, England: Clarendon Press/Oxford University Press.

Hagoort, P. (2005). On Broca, brain, and binding: A new framework. *Trends in Cognitive Science, 9*(9), 416–423.

Hanson, A. R., & Riseman, E. M. (1978). VISIONS: A computer system for interpreting scenes. In A. R. Hanson & E. M. Riseman (Eds.), *Computer vision systems* (pp. 129–163). New York: Academic Press.

Hare, B., Brown, M., Williamson, C., & Tomasello, M. (2002). The domestication of social cognition in dogs. *Science, 298,* 1634–1636.

Harlow, J. M. (1848). Passage of an iron rod through the head. *Boston Medical and Surgical Journal, 39,* 389–393.

Harlow, J. M. (1868). Recovery from the passage of an iron bar through the head. *Publications of the Massachusetts Medical Society, 2,* 327–347.

Hast, M. H., Fischer, J. M., Wetzel, A. B., & Thompson, V. E. (1974). Cortical motor representation of the laryngeal muscles in Macaca mulatta. *Brain Research, 73*(2), 229–240.

Hauk, O., Johnsrude, I., & Pulvermüller, F. (2004). Somatotopic representation of action words in human motor and premotor cortex. *Neuron, 41*(2), 301–307.

Hauser, M. D. (1996). *The evolution of communication.* Cambridge, MA: Bradford Books/The MIT Press.

Hauser, M. D., Chomsky, N., & Fitch, W. T. (2002). The language faculty: What is it, who has it, and how did it evolve? *Science, 298,* 1568–1579.

Heine, B., Claudi, U., & Hünnemeyer, F. (1991). *Grammaticalization: A conceptual framework.* Chicago, IL: University of Chicago Press.

Hayes, K. J., & Hayes, C. (1951). The intellectual development of a home-raised chimpanzee. *Proceedings of the American Philosophical Society, 95,* 105–109.

Head, H., & Holmes, G. (1911). Sensory disturbances from cerebral lesions. *Brain, 34,* 102–254.

Heine, B., & Kuteva, T. (2002). *World lexicon of grammaticalization.* Cambridge, England: Cambridge University Press.

Heine, B., & Kuteva, T. (2007). *The genesis of grammar: A reconstruction.* Oxford, England: Oxford University Press.

Heine, B., & Kuteva, T. (2011). Grammaticalization theory as a tool for reconstructing language evolution. In M. Tallerman & K. Gibson (Eds.), *The Oxford handbook of language evolution* (pp. in press). Oxford, England: Oxford University Press.

Heine, B., & Stolz, T. (2008). Grammaticalization as a creative process. *STUF (Sprachtypologie und Universalienforschung), 61*(4), 326–357.

Hewes, G. W. (1973). Primate communication and the gestural origin of language. *Current Anthropology, 12*(1–2), 5–24.

Hickok, G., & Poeppel, D. (2004). Dorsal and ventral streams: A framework for understanding aspects of the functional anatomy of language. *Cognition, 92*(1-2), 67–99.

Hihara, S., Yamada, H., Iriki, A., & Okanoya, K. (2003). Spontaneous vocal differentiation of coo-calls for tools and food in Japanese monkeys. *Neuroscience Research, 45,* 383–389.

Hill, J. C. (1983). A computational model of language acquisition in the two-year-old. *Cognition and Brain Theory, 6,* 287–317.

Hillix, W. A., & Rumbaugh, D. M. (2003). *Animal bodies, human minds: Ape, dolphin, and parrot language skills.* : Springer.

Hilts, P. J. (1995). *Memory's ghost: The strange tale of Mr. M and the nature of memory.* New York: Simon and Schuster.

Hockett, C. F. (1960). The origin of speech. *Scientific American, 203,* 88–96.

Hoff, B., & Arbib, M. A. (1993). Models of trajectory formation and temporal interaction of reach and grasp. *Journal of Motor Behavior, 25*(3), 175-192.

Hopper, P. J., & Traugott, E. C. (2003). *Grammaticalization.* Cambridge, England: Cambridge University Press.

Horner, V., & Whiten, A. (2005). Causal knowledge and imitation/emulation switching in chimpanzees (*Pan troglodytes*) and children (*Homo sapiens*). *Animal Cognition, 8*(3), 164–181.

Hurford, J. R. (2004). Language beyond our grasp: What mirror neurons can, and cannot, do for language evolution. In D. K. Oller & U. Griebel (Eds.), *Evolution of communication systems: A comparative approach* (pp. 297–313). Cambridge, MA: MIT Press.

Hurford, J. R. (2011). *The origins of grammar II: Language in the light of evolution.* New York: Oxford University Press.

Indurkhya, B. (1992). *Metaphor and cognition.* Dordrecht, Netherlands: Kluwer Academic Publishers.

Ingle, D. J. (1968). Visual releasers of prey catching behaviour in frogs and toads. *Brain, Behavior, and Evolution, 1,* 500–518.

Iriki, A., Tanaka, M., & Iwamura, Y. (1996). Coding of modified body schema during tool use by macaque postcentral neurones. *Neuroreport, 7,* 2325–2330.

Iriki, A., & Taoka, M. (2012). Triadic (ecological, neural, cognitive) niche construction: A scenario of human brain evolution extrapolating tool use and language from the control of reaching actions. *Philosophical Transactions of the Royal Society B: Biological Sciences, 367,* 10–23.

Iverson, J. M., Capirci, O., & Caselli, M. C. (1994). From communication to language in two modalities. *Cognitive Development, 9,* 23–43.

Iverson, J. M., & Goldin-Meadow, S. (1998). Why people gesture when they speak. *Nature, 396,* 228.

Jablonka, E., & Lamb, M. J. (2005). *Evolution in four dimensions. Genetic, epigenetic, behavioral, and symbolic variation in the history of life.* Cambridge, MA: Bradford Books/MIT Press.

Jackendoff, R. (1987). The status of thematic relations in linguistic theory. *Linguistic Inquiry, 18,* 369–411.

Jackendoff, R. (1999). Possible stages in the evolution of the language capacity. *Trends in Cognitive Science, 3*(7), 272–279.

Jackendoff, R. (2002). *Foundations of language: Brain, meaning, grammar, evolution.* New York: Oxford University Press.

Jackendoff, R. (2010). The ecology of English noun-noun compounds. In *Meaning and the lexicon: The parallel architecture 1975–2010.* New York: Oxford University Press.

Jakobson, R. (1956). Two aspects of language and two types of linguistic disturbance. In R. Jakobson & M. Halle (Eds.), *Fundamentals of language* (pp. 58). The Hague, Netherlands: Mouton.

James, W. (1890). *Principles of psychology.* New York: Holt.

Jarvis, E. D. (2004). Learned birdsong and the neurobiology of human language. *Annals of the New York Academy of Sciences, 1016,* 749–777.

Jarvis, E. D. (2007). Neural systems for vocal learning in birds and humans: A synopsis. *Journal of Ornithology, 148,* 35–44.

Jarvis, E. D. (2007). The evolution of vocal learning systems in birds and humans. In J. H. Kaas (Ed.), *Evolution of nervous systems* (pp. 213–227). Oxford, England: Academic Press.

Jeannerod, M. (1994). The representing brain. Neural correlates of motor intention and imagery. *Behavioral and Brain Sciences, 17,* 187–245.

Jeannerod, M. (1997). *The cognitive neuroscience of action.* Oxford, England: Blackwell.

Jeannerod, M., Arbib, M. A., Rizzolatti, G., & Sakata, H. (1995). Grasping objects: The cortical mechanisms of visuomotor transformation. *Trends in Neuroscience, 18*(7), 314–320.

Jeannerod, M., & Biguer, B. (1982). Visuomotor mechanisms in reaching within extra-personal space. In D. J. Ingle, R. J. W. Mansfield, & M. A. Goodale (Eds.), *Advances in the analysis of visual behavior* (pp. 387–409). Cambridge, MA: MIT Press.

Jeannerod, M., Decety, J., & Michel, F. (1994). Impairment of grasping movements following a bilateral posterior parietal lesion. *Neuropsychologia, 32*(4), 369–380.

Jespersen, O. (1921/1964). *Language: Its nature, development and origin*. New York: Norton.

Jones, S. S. (1996). Imitation or exploration. *Child Development, 67*, 1952–1969.

Jourdan, C., & Keesing, R. M. (1997). From Pisin to Pidgin: Creolization in process in the Solomon Islands. *Language and Society, 26*(3), 401–420.

Jürgens, U. (2002). Neural pathways underlying vocal control. *Neuroscience and Biobehavioral Reviews, 26*(2), 235–258.

Jusczyk, P. W., Goodman, M. B., & Baumann, A. (1999). Nine-month-olds' attention to sound similarities in syllables. *Journal of Memory and Language, 40*(1), 62–82.

Kaminski, J., Call, J., & Fischer, J. (2004). Word learning in a domestic dog: Evidence for "fast mapping." *Science, 304*(5677), 1682–1683.

Karchmer, M. A., & Mitchell, R. E. (2003). Demographic and achievement characteristics of deaf and hard of hearing students. In M. M. a. P. E. Spencer (Ed.), *Oxford handbook of deaf studies, language, and education* (pp. 21–37). New York: Oxford University Press.

Kegl, J. (2002). Language emergence in a language-ready brain: Acquisition. In G. Morgan & B. Woll (Eds.), *Directions in sign language acquisition* (pp. 207–254). Amsterdam, Netherlands: John Benjamins.

Kegl, J., Senghas, A., & Coppola, M. (1999). Creation through contact: Sign language emergence and sign language change in Nicaragua. In M. DeGraff (Ed.), *Comparative Grammatical Change: The Intersection of Language Acquisition, Creole Genesis, and Diachronic Syntax* (pp. 179–237). Cambridge, MA: MIT Press.

Keller, H. (1903/1954). *Story of my life*. New York: Doubleday.

Kellogg, W. N., & Kellogg, L. A. (1933). *The ape and the child: A comparative study of the environmental influence upon early behavior*. New York and London: Hafner.

Kemmerer, D. (2000a). Grammatically relevant and grammatically irrelevant features of verb meaning can be independently impaired. *Aphasiology, 14*, 997–1020.

Kemmerer, D. (2000b). Selective impairment of knowledge underlying prenominal adjective order: Evidence for the autonomy of grammatical semantics. *Journal of Neurolinguistics, 13*, 57–82.

Kemmerer, D. (2006). Action verbs, argument structure constructions, and the mirror neuron system. In M. A. Arbib (Ed.), *Action to language via the mirror neuron system* (pp. 347–373). Cambridge, England: Cambridge University Press.

Kendon, A. (1988). *Sign languages of Aboriginal Australians*. Cambridge, England: Cambridge University Press.

Kenneally, C. (2007). *From screech to sonnet: Cracking the completely impossible problem of language evolution*. New York: Viking.

Kettlewell, J. (2004). Children create new sign language. *BBC News*. Retrieved November 2011, from http://news.bbc.co.uk/2/hi/science/nature/3662928.stm

Kimura, D. (1993). *Neuromotor mechanisms in human communication*. New York : Oxford University Press.

Kirby, S. (2000). Syntax without natural selection: How compositionality emerges from vocabulary in a population of learners. In C. Knight, M. Studdert-Kennedy, & J. R. Hurford (Eds.), *The evolutionary emergence of language* (pp. 99–119). Cambridge, England: Cambridge University Press.

Kisch, S. (2004). Negotiating (genetic) deafness in a Bedouin community. In J. V. V. Cleve (Ed.), *Genetics, disability and deafness* (pp. 148–173). Washington, DC: Gallaudet University Press.

Klima, E., & Bellugi, U. (1979). *The signs of language*. Cambridge, MA: Harvard University Press.

Kohler, E., Keysers, C., Umilta, M. A., Fogassi, L., Gallese, V., & Rizzolatti, G. (2002). Hearing sounds, understanding actions: Action representation in mirror neurons. *Science, 297*(5582), 846–848.

Kotz, S. A., Schwartze, M., & Schmidt-Kassow, M. (2009). Non-motor basal ganglia functions: A review and proposal for a model of sensory predictability in auditory language perception. *Cortex, 45*(8), 982–990.

Laidre, M. E. (2011). Meaningful gesture in monkeys? Investigating whether Mandrills create social culture. *PLoS ONE, 6*(2), e14610.

Lakoff, G., & Johnson, M. (1980). *Metaphors we live by*. Chicago, IL: University Of Chicago Press.

Lane, H., Pillard, R. C., & French, M. (2000). Origins of the American deaf-world: Assimilating and differentiating societies and their relation to genetic patterning. *Sign Language Studies, 1*, 17–44.

Lane, H., Pillard, R., & French, M. (2002). Origins of the American deaf-world: Assimilating and differentiating societies and their relation to genetic patterning. In K. a. L. Emmorey, H. (Ed.), *The signs of language revisited: An anthology to honor Ursula Bellugi and Edward Klima* (pp. 77–100). Mahwah, NJ: Erlbaum.

Langacker, R. W. (1986). *Foundations of cognitive grammar* (Vol. 1). Palo Alto, CA: Stanford University Press.

Langacker, R. W. (1991). *Foundations of cognitive grammar* (Vol. 2). Palo Alto, CA: Stanford University Press.

Lashley, K. S. (1951). The problem of serial order in behavior. In L. Jeffress (Ed.), *Cerebral mechanisms in behavior: The Hixon Symposium* (pp. 112–136). New York: Wiley.

Lass, R. (1997). *Historical linguistics and language change*. Cambridge, England: Cambridge University Press.

Laudanna, A., & Volterra, V. (1991). Order of words, signs and gestures: A first comparison. *Applied Psycholinguistics, 12*, 135–150.

Leavens, D. A., Hopkins, W. D., & Bard, K. A. (1996). Indexical and referential pointing in chimpanzees (*Pan troglodytes*). *Journal of Comparative Psychology, 110*(4), 346–353.

Leavens, D. A., Hopkins, W. D., & Bard, K. A. (2005). Understanding the point of pointing. Epigenesis and ecological validity. *Current Directions in Psychological Science, 14*(4), 185–189.

Leavens, D. A., Hopkins, W. D., & Thomas, R. K. (2004). Referential communication by chimpanzees (*Pan troglodytes*). *Journal of Comparative Psychology, 118*(1), 48–57.

Ledoux, J. E. (2000). Emotion circuits in the brain. *Annual Review of Neuroscience, 23*, 155–184.

Lee, L., Friston, K., & Horwitz, B. (2006). Large-scale neural models and dynamic causal modelling. *Neuroimage, 30*(4), 1243–1254.

Lefebvre, C. (1998). *Creole genesis and the acquisition of grammar: The case of Haitian creole.* Cambridge, England: Cambridge University Press.

Lefebvre, C. (2004). *Issues in the study of Pidgin and Creole languages.* Amsterdam, Netherlands: John Benjamins.

Lefebvre, C. (2010). *On the relevance of Pidgins and Creoles in the debate on the origins of language.* Presentation at the Summer Institute on The Origins of Language, Université du Québec à Montréal, Canada, June 21–30.

Lesser, V. R., Fennel, R. D., Erman, L. D., & Reddy, D. R. (1975). Organization of the HEARSAY-II speech understanding system. *IEEE Transactions on Acoustics, Speech, and Signal Processing, 23*, 11–23.

Lettvin, J. Y., Maturana, H., McCulloch, W. S., & Pitts, W. H. (1959). What the frog's eye tells the frog brain. *Proceedings of the IRE, 47*, 1940–1951.

Leyton, A. S. F., & Sherrington, C. S. (1917). Observations on the excitable cortex of the chimpanzee, orang-utan, and gorilla. *Quarterly Journal of Experimental Physiology, 11*, 135–222.

Liberman, A. M., & Mattingly, I. G. (1989). A specialization for speech perception. *Science, 243*, 489–494.

Liebal, K., & Call, J. (2011). The origins of nonhuman primates' manual gestures. *Philosophical Transactions of the Royal Society B.*

Liebal, K., Pika, S., & Tomasello, M. (2004). Social communication in siamangs (*Symphalangus Syndactulus*): Use of gestures and facial expression. *Primates, 45*(2), 41–57.

Liebal, K., Pika, S., & Tomasello, M. (2006). Gestural communication of orangutans (*Pongo pygmaeus*). *Gesture, 6*(1), 1–38.

Lieberman, M. D. (2007). Social cognitive neuroscience: A review of core processes. *Annual Review of Psychology, 58*(1), 259–289.

Lieberman, P. (1991). *Uniquely human: The evolution of speech, thought, and selfless behavior.* Cambridge, MA: Harvard University Press.

Lieberman, P. (2000). *Human language and our reptilian brain: The Subcortical bases of speech syntax and thought.* Cambridge, MA: Harvard University Press.

Lightfoot, D. W. (1999). *The development of language acquisition.* Oxford, England: Blackwell.

Lightfoot, D. W. (2006). *How new languages emerge.* Cambridge, England: Cambridge University Press.

Lillo-Martin, D. (1999). Modality effects and modularity in language acquisition: The acquisition of American Sign Language. In T. Bhatia & W. Ritchie (Eds.), *Handbook of language acquisition* (pp. 531–567). New York: Academic Press.

Liszkowski, U., Carpenter, M., Henning, A., Striano, T., & Tomasello, M. (2004). Twelve-months-olds point to share attention and interest. *Developmental Science, 7*(3), 297–307.

Locke, J. (1690). An essay concerning humane understanding, in four books. London: Printed for Tho. Bassett, and sold by Edw. Mory at the Sign of the Three Bibles in St. Paul's Church-Yard.

Lyons, D. E., Young, A. G., & Keil, F. C. (2007). The hidden structure of overimitation. *Proceedings of the National Academy of Sciences USA, 104*(50), 19751–19756.

MacLean, P. D. (1993). Introduction: Perspectives on cingulate cortex in the limbic system. In B. A. Vogt & M. Gabriel (Eds.), *Neurobiology of cingulate cortex and limbic thalamus: A comprehensive handbook.* Boston, MA: Birkhauser.

Macmillan, M. (2000). *An odd kind of fame: Stories of Phineas Gage.* Cambridge, MA: MIT Press.

Macnamara, J. (1982). *Names for things.* Cambridge, MA: MIT Press.

MacNeilage, P. F. (1998). The frame/content theory of evolution of speech production. *Behavioral and Brain Sciences, 21,* 499–546.

MacNeilage, P. F. (2008). The origin of speech. Oxford, England: Oxford University Press.

MacNeilage, P. F., & Davis, B. L. (2001). Motor mechanisms in speech ontogeny: Phylogenetic, neurobiological and linguistic implications. *Current Opinion in Neurobiology, 11,* 696–700.

MacNeilage, P. F., & Davis, B. L. (2005). The frame/content theory of evolution of speech: Comparison with a gestural origins theory. *Interaction Studies: Social Behavior and Communication in Biological and Artificial Systems, 6,* 173–199.

MacWhinney, B. (2010). Computational models of child language learning: An introduction. *Journal of Child Language, 37,* 477–485.

Maddieson, I. (l999). In search of universals. In *Proceedings of the 14th International Congress of Phonetic Sciences* (Vol. 3, pp. 2521–2528). San Francisco, CA.

Maestripieri, D. (1999). Primate social organization, gestural repertoire size, and communication dynamics. In B. J. King (Ed.), *The origins of language: What nonhuman primates can tell* (pp. 55–77). Santa Fe, NM: School of American Research Press.

Marshall, J., Atkinson, J., Smulovitch, E., Thacker, A., & Woll, B. (2004). Aphasia in a user of British Sign Language: Dissociation between sign and gesture. *Cognitive Neuropsychology, 21,* 537–554.

Matthei, E. (1979). The acquisition of prenominal modifier sequences: Stalking the second green ball. Ph.D. dissertation, Department of Linguistics, University of Massachusetts at Amherst.

McBrearty, S., & Brooks, A. S. (2000). The revolution that wasn't: A new interpretation of the origin of modern human behavior. *Journal of Human Evolution, 39*(5), 453–563.

McGrew, W. C., & Tutin, C. E. G. (1978). Evidence for a social custom in wild chimpanzees? *Man, 13,* 234–251.

McNeill, D. (1992). *Hand and mind.* Chicago, IL: The University of Chicago Press.

McNeill, D. (2005). *Gesture and thought.* Chicago, IL: University of Chicago Press.

Meier, R. P. (1987). Elicited imitation of verb agreement in American Sign Language: Iconically or morphologically determined? *Journal of Memory and Language, 26,* 362–376.

Meier, R. P. (1991). Language acquisition by deaf children. *American Scientist, 79,* 60–70.

Meir, I., Padden, C., Aronoff, M., & Sandler, W. (2007). Body as subject. *Journal of Linguistics, 43,* 531–563.

Meir, I., & Sandler, W. (2008). *A language in space: The story of Israeli Sign Language.* New York: Erlbaum/Taylor & Francis.

Meir, I., Sandler, W., Padden, C., & Aronoff, M. (2010). Emerging sign languages. In M. Marschark & P. E. Spencer (Eds.), *Oxford handbook of deaf studies, language, and education* (Vol. 2). Oxford, England: Oxford University Press.

Meltzoff, A. N., & Moore, M. K. (1977). Imitation of facial and manual gestures by human neonates. *Science, 198*, 75–78.

Michelman, P., & Allen, P. (1994). Forming complex dexterous manipulations from task primitives. In *Proceedings of the 1994 IEEE International Conference on Robotics and Automation*, San Diego, California (pp. 3383–3388).

Miles, H. L., & Harper, S. E. (1994). "Ape language" studies and the study of human language origins. In D. Quiatt & J. Itani (Eds.), *Hominid culture in primate perspective* (pp. 253–278). Denver: University Press of Colorado.

Miller, G. A., Galanter, E., & Pribram, K. H. (1960). *Plans and the structure of behavior*. New York: Holt, Rinehart & Winston.

Mithen, S. (2005). *The singing Neanderthals: The origins of music, language, mind & body*. London: Weidenfeld & Nicholson.

Mithen, S. (2007). The network of brain, body, language, and culture. In W. Henke & I. Tattersall (Eds.), *Handbook of paleoanthropology* (pp. 1965–1999). Berlin and Heidelberg, Germany: Springer

Mühlhäusler, P. (1986). *Pidgin and Creole linguistics [Language in society II]*. Oxford, England: Basil Blackwell.

Mukamel, R., Ekstrom, A. D., Kaplan, J., Iacoboni, M., & Fried, I. (2010). Single-neuron responses in humans during execution and observation of actions. *Current Biology, 20*(8), 750–756.

Myowa-Yamakoshi, M., & Matsuzawa, T. (1999). Factors influencing imitation of manipulatory actions in chimpanzees (*Pan troglodytes*). *Journal of Comparative Psychology, 113*, 128–136.

Myowa-Yamakoshi, M., Tomonaga, M., Tanaka, M., & Matsuzawa, T. (2004). Imitation in neonatal chimpanzees (*Pan troglodytes*). *Developmental Science, 7*(4), 437–442.

Nespor, M., & Sandler, W. (1999). Prosody in Israeli Sign Language *Language and Speech, 42*, 143–176.

Nettl, B. (2000). An ethnomusicologist contemplates universals in musical sound and musical culture. In N. L. Wallin, B. Merker, & S. Brown (Eds.), *The origins of music* (pp. 463–472). Cambridge, MA: MIT Press.

Newmeyer, F. J. (2000). On reconstructing "proto-world" word order. In C. Knight, J. R. Hurford, & M. Studdert-Kennedy (Eds.), *Evolutionary emergence of language: Social functions and the origins of linguistic form* (pp. 372–388). Cambridge, England: Cambridge University Press.

Newport, E. L. (1981). Constraints on structure: Evidence from American Sign Language and language learning. In W. A. Collins (Ed.), *Aspects of the development of competence* (pp. 93–124). Hillsdale, NJ: Erlbaum.

Newport, E. L., & Meier, R. P. (1985). The acquisition of American Sign Language. In D. I. Slobin (Ed.), *The cross-linguistic study of language acquisition. Vol. 1: The data* (pp. 881–938). Mahwah, NJ: Erlbaum.

Nielsen, M., & Tomaselli, K. (2009). Over-imitation in the Kalahari Desert and the origins of human cultural cognition. *Nature Precedings*. Retrieved November 2011, from http://hdl.handle.net/10101/npre.12009.13049.10101

Nishida, T. (1980). The leaf-clipping display: A newly-discovered expressive gesture in wild chimpanzees. *Journal of Human Evolution, 9*, 117–128.

Noble, W., & Davidson, I. (1996). *Human evolution, language and mind: A psychological and archaeological inquiry.* Cambridge, England: Cambridge University Press.

Nowak, M. A., Plotkin, J. B., & Jansen, V. A. (2000). The evolution of syntactic communication. *Nature 404*(6777), 495–498.

Oberzaucher, E., & Grammer, K. (2008). Everything is movement: On the nature of embodied communication. In I. Wachsmuth, M. Lenzen, & G. Knoblich (Eds.), *Embodied communication in humans and machines* (pp. 151–177). Oxford, England: Oxford University Press.

Ochsner, K. N., & Lieberman, M. D. (2001). The emergence of social cognitive neuroscience. *American Psychologist, 56*(9), 717–734.

Odling-Smee, F. J., Laland, K. N., & Feldman, M. W. (2003). *Niche construction: The neglected process in evolution.* Princeton, NJ: Princeton University Press.

Okanoya, K. (2004). The Bengalese Finch, a window on the behavioral neurobiology of birdsong syntax. *Annals of the New York Academy of Sciences, 1016*, 724–735.

O'Keefe, J., & Nadel, L. (1978). *The hippocampus as a cognitive map.* Oxford, England: Oxford University Press.

Olds, J. (1969). The central nervous system and the reinforcement of behavior. *American Psychologist, 24*, 114–132.

Oztop, E., & Arbib, M. A. (2002). Schema design and implementation of the grasp-related mirror neuron system. *Biological Cybernetics, 87*(2), 116–140.

Oztop, E., Arbib, M. A., & Bradley, N. (2006). The development of grasping and the mirror system. In M. A. Arbib (Ed.), *Action to language via the mirror neuron system* (pp. 397–423). Cambridge, England: Cambridge University Press.

Oztop, E., Bradley, N. S., & Arbib, M. A. (2004). Infant grasp learning: A computational model. *Experimental Brain Research, 158*(4), 480–503.

Oztop, E., Imamizu, H., Cheng, G., & Kawato, M. (2006). A computational model of anterior intraparietal (AIP) neurons. *Neurocomputing, 69*(10–12), 1354–1361.

Padden, C., Meir, I., Sandler, W., & Aronoff, M. (2010). Against all expectations: Encoding subjects and objects in a new language. In D. B. Gerdts, J. C. Moore, & M. Polinsky (Eds.), *Hypothesis A/hypothesis B: Linguistic explorations in honor of David M. Perlmutter.* Cambridge, MA: MIT Press.

Papeo, L., Negri, G. A. L., Zadini, A., & Rumiati, R. (2010). Action performance and action-word understanding: Evidence of double dissociations in left-damaged patients. *Cognitive Neuropsychology, 27*, 428–461.

Parr, L. A., Waller, B. M., Burrows, A. M., Gothard, K. M., & Vick, S. J. (2010). Brief communication: MaqFACS: A muscle-based facial movement coding system for the rhesus macaque. *American Journal of Physical Anthropology, 143*(4), 625–630.

Patterson, F. (1978). Conversations with a gorilla. *National Geographic, 134*(4), 438–465.

Patterson, K. E., & Shewell, C. (1987). Speak and spell: Dissociations and word class effects. In M. Coltheart, G. Sartori, & R. Job (Eds.), *The cognitive neuropsychology of language* (pp. 273–294). London: Erlbaum.

Patterson, N., Richter, D. J., Gnerre, S., Lander, E. S., & Reich, D. (2006). Genetic evidence for complex speciation of humans and chimpanzees. *Nature, 441*(7097), 1103–1108.

Paus, T. (2001). Primate anterior cingulate cortex: Where motor control, drive and cognition interface. *Nature Reviews Neuroscience, 2,* 417–424.

Pearson, H. (2004). The birth of a language. *Nature News.* Retrieved November 2011, from http://www.nature.com/news/2004/040913/full/040913-19.html.

Peirce, C. S. (1931–58). *The collected papers of C. S. Peirce* (Volumes 1–6, eds. Charles Hartshorne and Paul Weiss; Volumes 7–8, ed. Arthur W. Burks). Cambridge, MA: Harvard University Press.

Pelegrin, J. (1990). Prehistoric lithic technology: Some aspects of research. *Archaeological Review from Cambridge, 9,* 116–125.

Pepperberg, I. M. (2008). *Alex & Me: How a Scientist and a Parrot Discovered a Hidden World of Animal Intelligence—and Formed a Deep Bond in the Process.* New York: Harper.

Perrett, D. I., Mistlin, A. J., & Chitty, A. J. (1987). Visual neurons responsive to faces. *Trends in Neuroscience, 10,* 358–364.

Perrett, D. I., Mistlin, A. J., Harries, M. H., & Chitty, A. J. (1990). Understanding the visual appearance and consequence of hand actions. In M. A. Goodale (Ed.), *Vision and action: The control of grasping* (pp. 163–180). Norwood, NJ: Ablex.

Peters, M., & Ploog, D. (1973). Communication among primates. *Annual Review of Physiology, 35,* 221–242.

Petersson, K. M., Reis, A., Askelof, S., Castro-Caldas, A., & Ingvar, M. (2000). Language processing modulated by literacy: A network analysis of verbal repetition in literate and illiterate subjects. *Journal of Cognitive Neuroscience, 12*(3), 364–382.

Petrides, M., & Pandya, D. N. (2009). Distinct parietal and temporal pathways to the homologues of Broca's area in the monkey. *PLoS Biology, 7*(8), e1000170.

Piaget, J. (1952). *The origins of intelligence in children.* New York: Norton.

Piaget, J. (1954). *The construction of reality in a child.* New York: Norton.

Pika, S., & Mitani, J. C. (2006). Referential gesturing in wild chimpanzees (*Pan troglodytes*). *Current Biology, 16*(6), 191–192.

Pika, S., & Mitani, J. C. (2009). The directed scratch: Evidence for a referential gesture in chimpanzees? In R. Botha & C. Knight (Eds.), *The prehistory of language* (pp. 166–180). Oxford, England: Oxford University Press.

Pika, S., Liebal, K., Call, J., & Tomasello, M. (2005). The gestural communication of apes. *Gesture, 5*(1/2), 41–56.

Pika, S., Liebal, K., & Tomasello, M. (2003). Gestural communication in young gorillas (*Gorilla gorilla*): Gestural repertoire, learning and use. *American Journal of Primatology, 60*(3), 95–111.

Pika, S., Liebal, K., & Tomasello, M. (2005). Gestural communication in subadult bonobos (*Pan paniscus*): Repertoire and use. *American Journal of Primatology, 65*(1), 39–61.

Pinker, S., & Bloom, P. (1990). Natural language and natural selection. *Behavioral and Brain Sciences, 13,* 707–784.

Pizzuto, E., Capobianco, M., & Devescovi, A. (2005). Gestural-vocal deixis and representational skills in early language development. *Interaction Studies, 6,* 223–252.

Poizner, H., Klima, E., & Bellugi, U. (1987). *What the hands reveal about the brain.* Cambridge, MA: MIT Press.

Polich, L. (2005). *The emergence of the deaf community in Nicaragua: "With sign language you can learn so much."* Washington, DC: Gallaudet University Press.

Popper, K., & Eccles, J. C. (1977). *The self and its brain: An argument for interactionism.* Berlin, Germany: Springer Verlag.

Potter, S. (1950). *Our language.* Harmondsworth, England: Penguin Books.

Prather, J. F., Peters, S., Nowicki, S., & Mooney, R. (2008). Precise auditory-vocal mirroring in neurons for learned vocal communication. *Nature, 451*(7176), 305–310.

Pribram, K. H. (1960). A review of theory in physiological psychology. *Annual Review of Psychology, 11,* 1–40.

Pulvermüller, F. (2005). Brain mechanisms linking language and action. *Nature Reviews Neuroscience, 6*(7), 576–582.

Ratiu, P., Talos, I. F., Haker, S., Lieberman, D., & Everett, P. (2004). The tale of Phineas Gage, digitally remastered. *Journal of Neurotrauma, 21*(5), 637–643.

Rauschecker, J. P. (1998). Cortical processing of complex sounds. *Current Opinion in Neurobiology, 8*(4), 516–521.

Redshaw, M., & Locke, K. (1976). The development of play and social behaviour in two lowland gorilla infants. *Jersey Wildland Preservation Trust, 13th Annual Report,* 71–86.

Rendell, L., Boyd, R., Enquist, M., Feldman, M. W., Fogarty, L., & Laland, K. N. (2011). How copying affects the amount, evenness and persistence of cultural knowledge: Insights from the social learning strategies tournament. *Philosophical Transactions of the Royal Society B: Biological Sciences, 366*(1567), 1118–1128.

Rhesus Macaque Genome Sequencing and Analysis Consortium, Gibbs, R. A., Rogers, J., Katze, M. G., Bumgarner, R., Weinstock, G. M., ... Zwieg, A. (2007). Evolutionary and biomedical insights from the rhesus macaque genome. *Science, 316*(5822), 222–234.

Richerson, P. J., & Boyd, R. (2010). Why possibly language evolved. *Biolinguistics, 4,* 289–306.

Rizzolatti, G., & Arbib, M. (1998). Language within our grasp. *Trends in Neurosciences, 21,* 188–194.

Rizzolatti, G., Camarda, R., Fogassi, L., Gentilucci, M., Luppino, G., & Matelli, M. (1988). Functional organization of inferior area 6 in the macaque monkey. II. Area F5 and the control of distal movements. *Experimental Brain Research, 71,* 491–507.

Rizzolatti, G., & Craighero, L. (2004). The mirror-neuron system. *Annual Review of Neuroscience, 27,* 169–192.

Rizzolatti, G., Fadiga, L., Gallese, V., & Fogassi, L. (1996). Premotor cortex and the recognition of motor actions. *Cognitive Brain Research, 3,* 131–141.

Rizzolatti, G., Fadiga, L., Matelli, M., Bettinardi, V., Paulesu, E., Perani, D., & Fazio, F. (1996). Localization of grasp representations in humans by PET: 1. Observation versus execution. *Experimental Brain Research, 111*(2), 246–252.

Rizzolatti, G., Fogassi, L., & Gallese, V. (2001). Neurophysiological mechanisms underlying the understanding and imitation of action. *Nature Reviews Neuroscience, 2*(9), 661–670.

Rizzolatti, G., & Luppino, G. (2001). The cortical motor system. *Neuron, 31*(6), 889–901.

Rizzolatti, G., & Luppino, G. (2003). Grasping movements: Visuomotor transformations. In M. A. Arbib (Ed.), *The handbook of brain theory and neural networks* (2nd ed., pp. 501–504). Cambridge, MA: MIT Press.

Rizzolatti, G., Luppino, G., & Matelli, M. (1998). The organization of the cortical motor system: New concepts. *Electroencephalography and Clinical Neurophysiology, 106*(4), 283–296.

Rizzolatti, G., & Sinigaglia, C. (2008). *Mirrors in the brain: How our minds share actions, emotions, and experience* (Frances Anderson, Trans.). Oxford, England: Oxford University Press.

Rizzolatti, G., & Sinigaglia, C. (2010). The functional role of the parieto-frontal mirror circuit: Interpretations and misinterpretations. *Nature Reviews Neuroscience, 11*(4), 264–274.

Roberts, J. M. (1989). Echolalia and comprehension in autistic children. *Journal of Autism Development Disorder, 19*(2), 271–281.

Roberts, S. J. (2000). Nativisation and the genesis of Hawaiian Creole. In J. McWorther (Ed.), *Language change and language contact in Pidgins and Creoles* (pp. 257–300). Amsterdam, Netherlands: John Benjamins.

Roberts, S. J., & Bresnan, J. (2008). Retained inflectional morphology in pidgins: A typological study. *Linguistic Typology, 12,* 269–302.

Roche, H. (2005). From simple flaking to shaping: Stone knapping evolution among early hominins. In V. Roux & B. Bril (Eds.), *Stone knapping: The necessary conditions for a uniquely hominin behaviour* (pp. 35–48). Cambridge, England: McDonald Institute for Archaeological Research.

Rolls, E. T. (2005). What are emotions, why do we have emotions, and what is their computational role in the brain? In J-M. Fellous & M. A. Arbib (Eds.), *Who needs emotions: The brain meets the robot* (pp. 117–146). Oxford, England: Oxford University Press.

Romaine, S. (1992). *Language, education, and development: Urban and rural Tok Pisin in Papua New Guinea.* Oxford, England: Oxford University Press.

Romanski, L. M. (2007). Representation and integration of auditory and visual stimuli in the primate ventral lateral prefrontal cortex. *Cerebral Cortex, 17*(Suppl 1), i61–i69.

Romanski, L. M., Tian, B., Fritz, J., Mishkin, M., Goldman-Rakic, P. S., & Rauschecker, J. P. (1999). Dual streams of auditory afferents target multiple domains in the primate prefrontal cortex. *Nature Neuroscience, 2*(12), 1131–1136.

Rosenbloom, P. S., Laird, J. E., Newell, A., & McCarl, R. (1991). A preliminary analysis of the Soar architecture as a basis for general intelligence. *Artificial Intelligence, 47*(1–3), 289–325.

Rothi, L. J., Ochipa, C., & Heilman, K. M. (1991). A cognitive neuropsychological model of limb praxis. *Cognitive Neuropsychology, 8,* 443–458.

Russo, T., & Volterra, V. (2005). Comment on "Children creating core properties of language: Evidence from an emerging sign language in Nicaragua." *Science, 309,* 56.

Sakaki, Y., Watanabe, H., Fujiyama, A., Hattori, M., Toyoda, A., & Taylor, T. D. (2002). Chimpanzee genome project for understanding ourselves. *International Congress Series, 1246,* 183–187.

Sallandre, M. A., & Cuxac, C. (2002). Iconicity in sign language: A theoretical and methodological point of view. In *Gesture and sign language in human-computer interaction, lecture notes in computer science 2298* (pp. 13–35). Berlin/Heidelberg, Germany: Springer-Verlag.

Sandler, W., Aronoff, M., Meir, I., & Padden, C. (2011). The gradual emergence of phonological form in a new language. *Natural Language and Linguistic Theory*, DOI: 10.1007/s11049-11011-19128-11042.

Sandler, W., & Lillo-Martin, D. (2006). *Sign language and linguistic universals.* Cambridge, England: Cambridge University Press.

Sandler, W., Meir, I., Dachkovsky, S., Padden, C., & Aronoff, M. (2011). The emergence of complexity in prosody and syntax. *Lingua*, in press.

Sandler, W., Meir, I., Padden, C., & Aronoff, M. (2005). The emergence of grammar: Systematic structure in a new language. *Proceedings of National Academy of Sciences USA, 102*(7), 2661–2665.

Saussure, F. (1916). *Cours de linguistique générale* (C. Bally, A. Sechehaye, A. Riedlinger, Eds.). Lausanne and Paris: Payot.

Savage-Rumbaugh, E. S., Shanker, S. C., & Taylor, T. J. (1998). *Apes, language and the human mind.* Oxford, England: Oxford University Press.

Schaal, S., Sternad, D., Osu, R., & Kawato, M. (2004). Rhythmic arm movement is not discrete. *Nature Neuroscience, 7,* 1136–1143.

Schembri, A., Jones, C., & Burnham, D. (2005). Comparing action gestures and classifier verbs of motion: Evidence from Australian Sign Language, Taiwan Sign Language, and non-signers gestures without speech. *The Journal of Deaf Studies and Deaf Education, 10*(3), 272–290.

Schmid, W. P. (1987). "Indo-European"–"Old European." (On the reexamination of two linguistic terms). In S. N. Skomal & E. C. Polomé (Eds.), *Proto-Indo-European: The archaeology of a linguistic problem. Essays in honor of Marija Gimbutas* (pp. 322–338). Washington, DC: Institute for the Study of Man.

Schultz, W. (2006). Behavioral theories and the neurophysiology of reward. *Annual Review of Psychology, 57,* 87–115.

Scott, D., Carmi, R., Eldebour, K., Duyk, G., Stone, E., & Sheffield, V. (1995). Nonsyndromic autosomal recessive deafness is linked to the DFNB1 locus in a large inbred Bedouin family from Israel. *American Journal of Human Genetics, 57,* 965–968.

Scoville, W. B., & Milner, B. (1957). Loss of recent memory after bilateral hippocampal lesions (Reprinted in *Journal of Neuropsychiatry and Clinical Neuroscience* 2000, 12, pp. 103–113). *Journal Neurology, Neurosurgery and Psychiatry, 20,* 11–21.

Searle, J. R. (1979). *Expression and meaning: Studies in the theory of speech acts.* Cambridge, England: Cambridge University Press.

Seidenberg, M. S., & Petitto, L. A. (1987). Communication, symbolic communication, and language: Comment on Savage-Rumbaugh, McDonald, Sevcik, Hopkins, and Rupert. *Journal of Experimental Psychology: General, 116*(3), 279–287.

Semaw, S. (2000). The world's oldest stone artefacts from Gona, Ethiopia: Their implications for understanding stone technology and patterns of human evolution between 2.6-1.5 million years ago. *Journal of Archaeological Science, 27*(12), 1197–1214.

Semaw, S., Rogers, M., & Stout, D. (2009). The Oldowan-Acheulian transition: Is there a "developed Oldowan" artifact tradition? In M. Camps & P. Chauhan

(Eds.), *Sourcebook of paleolithic transitions: Methods, theories, and interpretations* (pp. 173–193). New York: Springer.

Senghas, A. (2003). Intergenerational influence and ontogenetic development in the emergence of spatial grammar in Nicaraguan Sign Language. *Cognitive Development, 18*, 511–531.

Senghas, A., & Coppola, M. (2001). Children creating language: How Nicaraguan Sign Language acquired a spatial grammar. *Psychological Science, 12*(4), 323–328.

Senghas, A., Kita, S., & Özyürek, A. (2004). Children creating core properties of language: Evidence from an emerging sign language in Nicaragua. *Science, 305*, 1779–1782.

Senghas, R. J. (1997). *An "unspeakable, unwriteable" language: Deaf identity, language and personhood among the first cohorts of Nicaraguan signers.* Unpublished Ph.D. dissertation, University of Rochester, NY.

Seyfarth, R. M., & Cheney, D. L. (1997). Some general features of vocal development in nonhuman primates. In C. Snowdon & M. Hausberger (Eds.), *Social influences on vocal development* (pp. 249–273). Cambridge, England: Cambridge University Press.

Seyfarth, R. M., & Cheney, D. L. (2002). The structure of social knowledge in monkeys. In M. Bekoff, C. Allen, & G. M. Burghardt (Eds.), *The cognitive animal: Empirical and theoretical perspectives in animal cognition* (pp. 379–384). Cambridge, MA: MIT Press.

Seyfarth, R. M., Cheney, D. L., & Bergman, T. J. (2005). Primate social cognition and the origins of language. *Trends in Cognitive Sciences, 9*(6), 264–266.

Simonyan, K., & Jürgens, U. (2002). Cortico-cortical projections of the motorcortical larynx area in the rhesus monkey. *Brain Research, 949*(1–2), 23–31.

Slobin, D. I. (2005). From ontogenesis to phylogenesis: What can child language tell us about language evolution? In J. Langer, S. T. Parker, & C. Milbrath (Eds.), *Biology and knowledge revisited: From neurogenesis to psychogenesis.* Mahwah, NJ: Erlbaum.

Slobin, D. I. (2008). Breaking the molds: Signed languages and the nature of human language. *Sign Language Studies, 8*(2), 114–130.

Slocombe, K. E., Waller, B. M., & Liebal, K. (2011). The language void: The need for multimodality in primate communication research. *Animal Behaviour, 81*(5), 919–924.

Smith, A. D. M. (2008). Protolanguage reconstructed. *Interaction Studies: Social Behavior and Communication in Biological and Artificial Systems, 9*(1), 100–116.

Spivey, M. J., Richardson, D. C., & Fitneva, S. A. (2005). Thinking outside the brain: Spatial indices to visual and linguistic information. In J. M. Henderson & F. Ferreira (Eds.), *The interface of language, vision, and action: Eye movements and the visual world* (pp. 161–190). New York: Psychology Press.

Squire, L. R., & Zola-Morgan, S. (1991). The medial temporal lobe memory system. *Science, 253*(5026), 1380–1386.

Steiper, M. E., Young, N. M., & Sukarna, T. Y. (2004). Genomic data support the hominoid slowdown and an Early Oligocene estimate for the hominoid-cercopithecoid divergence. *Proceedings of the National Academy of Sciences USA, 101*(49), 17021–17026.

Stokoe, W. C. (1960). *Sign language structure: An outline of the visual communication systems of the American deaf.* Buffalo, NY: University of Buffalo.

Stokoe, W. C. (2001). *Language in hand: Why sign came before speech*. Washington, DC: Gallaudet University Press.

Stout, D. (2010). Possible relations between language and technology in human evolution. In A. Nowell & I. Davidson (Eds.), *Stone tools and the evolution of human cognition* (pp. 159–184). Boulder: University Press of Colorado.

Stout, D. (2011). Stone toolmaking and the evolution of human culture and cognition. *Philosophical Transactions of the Royal Society B: Biological Sciences, 366*, 1050–1059.

Stout, D., Semaw, S., Rogers, M. J., & Cauche, D. (2010). Technological variation in the earliest Oldowan from Gona, Afar, Ethiopia. *Journal of Human Evolution, 58*(6), 474–491.

Stringer, C. (2003). Human evolution: Out of Ethiopia. *Nature, 423*(6941), 692–695.

Studdert-Kennedy, M. (2002). Mirror neurons, vocal imitation and the evolution of particulate speech. In M. Stamenov & V. Gallese (Eds.), *Mirror neurons and the evolution of brain and language* (pp. 207–227). Amsterdam, Netherlands: John Benjamins.

Suddendorf, T., & Corballis, M. C. (1997). Mental time travel and the evolution of the human mind. *Genetic, Social, and General Psychology Monographs, 123*(2), 133–167.

Suddendorf, T., & Corballis, M. C. (2007). The evolution of foresight: What is mental time travel, and is it unique to humans? *Behavioral and Brain Sciences, 30*, 299–351.

Supalla, T., & Newport, E. L. (1978). How many seats in a chair? The derivation of nouns and verbs in American Sign Language. In P. Siple (Ed.), *Understanding language through sign language research* (pp. 91–159). New York: Academic Press.

Sutton, D., Larson, C., & Lindeman, R. C. (1974). Neocortical and limbic lesion effects on primate phonation. *Brain Research, 17*, 61–75.

Sutton, R. S. (1988). Learning to predict by the methods of temporal differences. *Machine Learning, 3*, 9–44.

Tagamets, M. A., & Horwitz, B. (2000). A model of working memory: Bridging the gap between electrophysiology and human brain imaging. *Neural Networks, 13*(8–9), 941–952.

Taira, M., Mine, S., Georgopoulos, A. P., Murata, A., & Sakata, H. (1990). Parietal cortex neurons of the monkey related to the visual guidance of hand movement. *Experimental Brain Research, 83*, 29–36.

Tallerman, M. (2006). A holistic protolanguage cannot be stored, cannot be retrieved. In A. Cangelosi, A. D. M. Smith, & K. Smith (Eds.), *The evolution of language: Proceedings of the 6th International Conference (EVOLANG6)* (pp. 447–448). Singapore: World Scientific.

Tallerman, M. (2007). Did our ancestors speak a holistic protolanguage? *Lingua, 117* 579–604.

Talmy, L. (2000). *Towards a cognitive semantics*. Cambridge, MA: The MIT Press.

Tanner, J. E., & Byrne, R. W. (1993). Concealing facial evidence of mood. Perspective taking in a captive gorilla. *Primates, 34*(4), 451–457.

Tennie, C., Call, J., & Tomasello, M. (2009). Ratcheting up the ratchet: On the evolution of cumulative culture. *Philosophical Transactions of the Royal Society of London B: Biological Sciences, 364*(1528), 2405–2415.

Tessari, A., & Rumiati, R. I. (2004). The strategic control of multiple routes in imitation of actions. *Journal of Experimental Psychology: Human Perception and Performance, 30*(6), 1107–1116.

Tomasello, M. (1999). The human adaptation for culture. *Annual Review of Anthropology, 28,* 509–529.

Tomasello, M. (2003a). *Constructing a language: A usage-based theory of language acquisition.* Cambridge, MA: Harvard University Press.

Tomasello, M. (2003b). On the different origins of symbols and grammar. In M. H. Christiansen & S. Kirby (Eds.), *Language evolution* (pp. 94–110). Oxford, England: Oxford University Press.

Tomasello, M. (2008). *Origins of human communication.* Cambridge, MA: Bradford Books/MIT Press.

Tomasello, M. (2009). *Why we cooperate (with responses by Carol Dweck, Joan Silk, Brian Skyrms, and Elizabeth Spelke).* Cambridge, MA: MIT Press.

Tomasello, M., & Call, J. (1997). *Primate cognition.* New York: Oxford University Press.

Tomasello, M., Carpenter, M., Call, J., Behne, T., & Moll, H. (2005). Understanding and sharing intentions: The origins of cultural cognition. *Behavioral and Brain Sciences, 28,* 1–17.

Tomasello, M., Kruger, A. C., & Ratner, H. H. (1993). Cultural learning. *Behavioral and Brain Sciences, 16,* 495–552.

Toth, N. (2001). Experiments in quarrying large flake blanks at Kalambo Falls. In J. D. Clark (Ed.), *Kalambo Falls prehistoric site. Vol. 3: The earlier cultures: Middle and Earlier Stone Age* (pp. 600–604). Cambridge, England: Cambridge University Press.

Traugott, E. C., & Hopper, P. J. (1993). *Grammaticalization.* Cambridge, England: Cambridge University Press.

Turella, L., Pierno, A. C., Tubaldi, F., & Castiello, U. (2009). Mirror neurons in humans: Consisting or confounding evidence? *Brain and Language, 108*(1), 10–21.

Umiltà, M. A., Escola, L., Intskirveli, I., Grammont, F., Rochat, M., Caruana, F., ... Rizzolatti, G. (2008). When pliers become fingers in the monkey motor system. *Proceedings of the National Academy of Sciences USA, 105*(6), 2209–2213.

Umiltà, M. A., Kohler, E., Gallese, V., Fogassi, L., Fadiga, L., Keysers, C., & Rizzolatti, G. (2001). I know what you are doing: A neurophysiological study. *Neuron, 31,* 155–165.

Ungerleider, L. G., & Mishkin, M. (1982). Two cortical visual systems. In D. J. Ingle, M. A. Goodale, & R. J. W. Mansfield (Eds.), *Analysis of visual behavior* (pp. 549–586). Cambridge, MA: MIT Press.

Vaccari, O., & Vaccari, E. E. (1961). *Pictorial Chinese-Japanese characters* (4th ed.). Tokyo: Charles E. Tuttle.

Van Essen, D. C. (2005). Surface-based comparisons of macaque and human cortical organization. In S. Dehaene, J-R. Duhamel, M. D. Hauser & G. Rizzolatti (Eds.), *From monkey brain to human brain* (pp. 3–19). Cambridge, MA: MIT Press.

Vea, J. J., & Sabater-Pi, J. (1998). Spontaneous pointing behaviour in the wild pygmy chimpanzee (Pan paniscus). *Folia Primatologica, 69,* 289–290.

Vick, S-J., Waller, B. M., Parr, L. A., Smith Pasqualini, M., & Bard, K. A. (2007). A cross-species comparison of facial morphology and movement in humans and chimpanzees using the facial action coding system (FACS). *Journal of Nonverbal Behavior, 31*(1), 1–20.

Visalberghi, E., & Fragaszy, D. (2001). Do monkeys ape? Ten years after. In K. Dautenhahn & C. Nehaniv (Eds.), *Imitation in animals and artifacts* (pp. 471–500). Cambridge, MA: The MIT Press.

Voelkl, B., & Huber, L. (2000). True imitation in marmosets. *Animal Behaviour, 60*, 195–202.

Volterra, V., & Erting, C. J. (Eds.). (1994). *From gesture to language in hearing and deaf children*. Washington, DC: Gallaudet University Press.

Walker, W., & Sarbaugh, J. (1993). The early history of the Cherokee syllabary. *Ethnohistory, 40*(1), 70–94.

Webelhuth, G. (1995). X-Bar theory and case theory. In G. Webelhuth (Ed.), *Government and binding theory and the minimalist program* (pp. 15–95). Oxford, England and Cambridge, MA: Blackwell.

Wernicke, C. (1874). Der aphasische symptomencomplex. Breslau, Germany: Cohn and Weigert.

Whiten, A., Goodall, A. G., McGrew, W. C., Nishida, T., Reynolds, V., Sugiyama, Y., ... Boesch, C. (2001). Charting cultural variation in chimpanzees. *Behaviour, 138*, 1489–1525.

Whiten, A., Hinde, R. A., Laland, K. N., & Stringer, C. B. (2011). Culture evolves. *Philosophical Transactions of the Royal Society B: Biological Sciences, 366*(1567), 938–948.

Whiten, A., Horner, V., & Marshall-Pescini, S. (2003). Cultural panthropology. *Evolutionary Anthropology: Issues, News, and Reviews, 12*(2), 92–105.

Wicker, B., Keysers, C., Plailly, J., Royet, J. P., Gallese, V., & Rizzolatti, G. (2003). Both of us disgusted in my insula: The common neural basis of seeing and feeling disgust. *Neuron, 40*(3), 655–664.

Wiener, N. (1948). *Cybernetics: or control and communication in the animal and the machine*. New York: Technology Press and John Wiley & Sons.

Wilkins, W., & Wakefield, J. (1995). Brain evolution and neurolinguistic preconditions. *Brain and Behavioral Science, 18*, 161–226.

Wilkinson, K. M., Dube, W. V., & McIlvane, W. J. (1998). Fast mapping and exclusion (emergent matching) in developmental language, behavior analysis, and animal cognition research. *Psychological Record, 48*(3), 407–422.

Williams, S. M., White, L. E., & Mace, A. C. (2007). *Sylvius 4: An Interactive Atlas and Visual Glossary of Human Neuroanatomy*. Sunderland, MA: Sinauer Associates, in association with Pyramis Studios.

Winder, R., Cortes, C. R., Reggia, J. A., & Tagamets, M. A. (2007). Functional connectivity in fMRI: A modeling approach for estimation and for relating to local circuits. *NeuroImage, 34*(3), 1093–1107.

Wittgenstein, L. (1953). *Philosophical investigations*. Oxford, England: Blackwell.

Wohlschläger, A., Gattis, M., & Bekkering, H. (2003). Action generation and action perception in imitation: An instance of the ideomotor principle. *Philosophical Transactions of the Royal Society of London, 358*, 501–515.

Woodruff, G., & Premack, D. (1979). Intentional communication in the chimpanzee: The development of deception. *Cognition, 7*, 333–352.

Wray, A. (1998). Protolanguage as a holistic system for social interaction. *Language and Communication, 18*, 47–67.

Wray, A. (2000). Holistic utterances in protolanguage: The link from primates to humans. In C. Knight, M. Studdert-Kennedy, & J. Hurford (Eds.), *The evolutionary emergence of language: Social function and the origins of linguistic form* (pp. 285–202). Cambridge, England: Cambridge University Press.

Wray, A. (2002). *The transition to language.* Oxford, England: Oxford University Press.

Wynn, T. (2009). Hafted spears and the archaeology of mind. *Proceedings of the National Academy of Sciences USA, 106*(24), 9544–9545.

Wynn, T., & Coolidge, F. L. (2004). The expert Neandertal mind. *Journal of Human Evolution, 46*(4), 467–487.

Yaguello, M. (1998). *Language through the looking glass: Exploring language and linguistics.* New York: Oxford University Press.

Zuberbühler, K. (2002). A syntactic rule in forest monkey communication. *Animal Behaviour, 63,* 293–299.

Zuberbühler, K., Cheney, D. L., & Seyfarth, R. M. (1999). Conceptual semantics in a nonhuman primate. *Journal of Comparative Psychology, 113*(1), 33–42.

Zuckermann, G., & Walsh, M. (2011). Stop, revive, survive: Lessons from the Hebrew revival applicable to the reclamation, maintenance and empowerment of aboriginal languages and cultures. *Australian Journal of Linguistics, 31,* 111–127.

Zukow-Goldring, P. (1996). Sensitive caregivers foster the comprehension of speech: When gestures speak louder than words. *Early Development and Parentint, 5,* 195–211.

Zukow-Goldring, P. (2001). Perceiving referring actions: Latino and Euro-American infants and caregivers comprehending speech. In K. L. Nelson, A. Aksu-Koc, & C. Johnson (Eds.), *Children's language* (Vol. 11, pp. 139–165). Hillsdale, NJ: Erlbaum.

Zukow-Goldring, P. (2006). Assisted imitation: affordances, effectivities, and the mirror system in early language development. In M. A. Arbib (Ed.), *Action to language via the mirror neuron system* (pp. 469–500). Cambridge, England: Cambridge University Press.

Zukow-Goldring, P., & Arbib, M. A. (2007). Affordances, effectivities, and assisted imitation: Caregivers and the directing of attention. *Neurocomputing, 70,* 2181–2193.

Name Index

Subject Index

ABSL. *See* Al-Sayyid Bedouin Sign
     Language
abstract language
     compositional semantics and, 273
     episodic memory and, 272
     mental time travel and, 271–72, 274
     roots in embodiment, 271–75
accommodation, in schema theory,
     17–18
Acheulian tool making, 325–28
     Homo sapiens and, 328–29
action-level imitation
     in apes and monkeys, 187
     behavior parsing compared to, 209
     complex imitation and, 188–89
action-oriented framework, for language,
     54–59
     action-perception cycle of, 9–10, 55
     communicative actions in, 56
     cultural evolution in, 58
     language production in, 56
     perception grammar in, 57
     production grammar in, 56–57
     semantic structure in, 57
     sentence-planning strategy for, 57–58
action-oriented perception, 6, 9
action-perception cycle, 9–10, 55
action recognition neurons, 132
action-word processing, semantic
     somatotopy model of, 222–23
active form, 62–63
affordances
     in human infant imitation, 199–200
     in rhesus macaque monkey brain, 110

aggression, language changes as result
     of, 334
American Notes (Dickins), 227–28
American Sign Language (ASL)
     British Sign Language and, 42
     French Sign Language and, 42
     in Nicaraguan Deaf community, 306
     space exploitation in, 40
amnesia. *See* anterograde amnesia
amygdala, 100–01
     cerebral cortex and, 101
analytic languages, 353
animal calls. *See also* call systems, among
     monkeys
     auditory systems and, 118
     protolanguage from, 255–56
animals. *See specific animals*
anterograde amnesia, 102–03
apes. *See also* imitation, in apes and
     monkeys; Kanzi; vocalization, by
     monkeys and apes
     action-level imitation in, 187
     deictic gestures among, 81–82
     facial expressions among, 77–78
     gestures among, 78–83
     human-supported ritualization by,
     82, 218
     language learning by, 83–85
     lexigrams and, communication
     with, 84
     observational priming for, 185
     ontogenetic ritualization in, for manual
     gestures, 79–82, 215
     play hitting among, 80

395